Assessment and Treatment Methods for Manual Therapists

Of related interest

**Advanced Osteopathic and Chiropractic
Techniques for Manual Therapists**
**Adaptive Clinical Skills for Peripheral
and Extremity Manipulation**
Giles Gyer and Jimmy Michael
ISBN 978 0 85701 394 1
eISBN 978 0 85701 395 8

**Osteopathic and Chiropractic
Techniques for Manual Therapists**
**A Comprehensive Guide to Spinal and
Peripheral Manipulations**
Jimmy Michael, Giles Gyer, and Ricky Davis
ISBN 978 1 84819 326 0
eISBN 978 0 85701 281 4

Palpation and Assessment in Manual Therapy
Learning the Art and Refining Your Skills
Leon Chaitow
Foreword by Jerrilyn Cambron
ISBN 978 1 90914 134 6
eISBN 978 1 91208 515 6

Spine and Joint Articulation for Manual Therapists
Giles Gyer, Jimmy Michael, and Ben Calvert-Painter
ISBN 978 1 90914 131 5
eISBN 978 1 91208 518 7

ASSESSMENT AND TREATMENT METHODS FOR MANUAL THERAPISTS

The Most Effective and Efficient Treatment Every Time

Jeffrey Burch

Illustrated by Peter Anthony

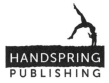
HANDSPRING
PUBLISHING

First published in Great Britain in 2024 by Handspring Publishing,
an imprint of Jessica Kingsley Publishers
Part of John Murray Press

I

The information contained in this book is not intended to replace the services of trained medical
professionals or to be a substitute for medical advice. You are advised to consult a doctor on any matters
relating to your health, and in particular on any matters that may require diagnosis or medical attention.

A CIP catalogue record for this title is available from the British Library and the Library of Congress

ISBN 978 1 83997 874 6
eISBN 978 1 83997 875 3

Printed and bound in Great Britain by CPI Group

Jessica Kingsley Publishers' policy is to use papers that are natural, renewable and recyclable
products and made from wood grown in sustainable forests. The logging and manufacturing
processes are expected to conform to the environmental regulations of the country of origin.

Handspring Publishing
Carmelite House
50 Victoria Embankment
London EC4Y 0DZ

www.handspringpublishing.com

John Murray Press
Part of Hodder & Stoughton Limited
An Hachette UK Company

For my daughters
Meaghan and Belle

Acknowledgements

Jean-Pierre Barral DO for his excellent teaching and his many innovations, some of which are described in this book.

Alain Gehin DE for his excellent teaching and modeling of good writing.

Mark Thomas DC and Maggie Cooper PT for many years of collegial discussions through which all our manual therapy skills grew.

Mary Frost and Jack Nelson PhD who each edited earlier drafts of portions of this text.

My parents Paul and Velma Burch for gifts of many kinds, including my first anatomical models at age nine.

My wife Janhavi McKenzie for her loving support.

Contents

Acknowledgements 7

Invitation 11

How to Use This Book. 13

1. Foundations. 15
   Concepts and history   15

2. Assessment Methods 29
   Introduction   29
   Assessment algorithm   30
   General assessment methods   31
      Assessment method 1: general listening   33
      Assessment method 2: general lift   39
      Assessment method 3: general tap   42

   Local assessment methods   45
      Assessment method 4: local listening   45
      Assessment method 5: local lift   51
      Assessment method 6: local tap   53
      Assessment method 7: layer awareness   55
      Assessment method 8: layer palpation   56
      Assessment method 9: layer listening   58
      Assessment method 10: manual thermal
      evaluation   60
      Assessment method 11: ultraslow mobility
      testing   63
      Assessment method 12: ruling out false
      positives on orthopedic tests   67

   Assessment methods useful for both
   general and local assessment   71
      Assessment method 13: mobility testing   71

   Assessment method 14: yes–no questions
   (applied kinesiology and a variant)   75
   Assessment method 15: developing intuition 77
   Assessment method 16: introduction
   to use of the craniosacral rhythm as an
   assessment tool   79

   Extended assessment methods   84
      Assessment method 17: extended listening   85
      Assessment method 18: listening from a
      symptomatic area   88
      Assessment method 19: assessment algorithm 90

3. Treatment Methods 93
   Introduction to treatment techniques   93

   Treatment methods in which therapeutic
   engagement is made by the client's
   system and unwinding is used   97
      Treatment method 1: classic unwinding   97
      Treatment method 2: augmented unwinding   107
      Treatment method 3: alternate interrupt
      unwinding   113

   Treatment techniques in which tissue
   engagement is made by the therapist and
   unwinding is used   119
      Treatment method 4: near first barrier stack 119
      Treatment method 5: far first barrier stack   126
      Treatment method 6: mixed directions of
      near and far first barrier stack   131
      Treatment method 7: stack-restack: a
      sequence of single release stacks   138
      Treatment method 8: walking through
      the spectrum of barriers   145
      Treatment method 9: stack and borrow   151

Treatment method 10: standing adaptation of the sacro-occipital technique (SOT) type 4 correction: an application of the stack and borrow technique 159

Treatment method 11: scrubbing the walls 161

Treatment method 12: pendulum wall scrubbing 170

Techniques in which therapeutic engagement is made by the therapist and unwinding is not used 178

Treatment method 13: recoil 178

Treatment method 14: accordion technique, also known as alternating decompression 185

Treatment method 15: centralizing (Hoover) technique 192

Treatment method 16: induction of a bodily rhythm 200

Treatment method 17: reconstructed A. T. Still technique 206

Treatment method 18: listen and follow 214

Treatment method 19: load and tap 218

Techniques in which therapeutic engagement is made by the therapist and unwinding may or may not occur 224

Treatment method 20: first barrier stretch 224

Treatment method 21: first barrier shear 231

Treatment method 22: middle barrier technique 238

Treatment method 23: flossing 245

Treatment method 24: circle flossing 253

Leverage principles that may be used with many techniques 261

4. Five In-Depth Treatment Protocols. . . 265

5. Appendices 277

Appendix 1: Recommended reading 277

Appendix 2: How this book came to be: a biographical appendix 280

Appendix 3: Mechanical force types 283

Appendix 4: Space between the stars 286

About the Author 287

Invitation

How to deliver the most effective and efficient treatment, aye, that is the question. How to accomplish the most for your client in a reasonable time and, oh, by the way, comfortably for both client and therapist, that is the question burning in the heart of manual therapists through the ages.

Many great minds have contributed partial answers, supplying better and better assessment methods and more effective treatment methods, and then a funny thing happened. Actually, a couple of funny things. A) Methods were not always well shared. B) Some therapists came to believe their methods were not only the best but the only right way.

The truth is there are many assessment and treatment methods because each is useful for some purposes, some of the time. No one assessment method can show everything. Each assessment method has an error rate. Assessing in more than one way is essential.

The book you have in your hands clearly describes 19 assessment methods and 24 treatment methods and how to choose the best ones for the situation at hand. Ah! So, this is a cookbook, right? Nope, it is a chef's manual. Rather than a linear set of instructions like "In situation B use treatment method #4," this book shows you how to find the best method for the uniqueness of each client at each moment.

If you have insatiable curiosity,

if you have the dedication to do the best for each client,

if you prefer uniqueness to uniformity,

if you would rather observe and think than push harder and longer,

if you know you are a reincarnation of Sherlock Holmes,

this is the book for you.

How to Use This Book

Start by reading the foundations section. The history and concepts presented in it set the stage for understanding the assessment methods and treatment methods presented in this book. Then as you read the descriptions of the methods described in the book, refer to the foundations section to continue to deepen your understanding.

Next, read the introductions at the beginning of the assessment section and the treatment section.

You may want to skim through the assessment and treatment methods to get a sense of the scope of methods presented. If so, let this preview wash over you, to get a general sense of the subject matter. The details will come later.

Now begin studying the individual methods. Read an assessment method and begin to practice it. Soon, read and begin to practice a treatment method. Skill with each method can increase for the rest of your career. Perfection means only continual growth. Practice is the path to increasing skill.

As you develop some skill with the first methods, read about and begin to practice another method. Give each method practice time. Let each method develop in you before adding another.

Each person will find some methods more compatible than others. You can treat the collection of methods in this book as a buffet from which you choose your favorite foods. By practicing the familiar and compatible methods your clinical skill will grow. Alternatively, you can take on learning all the methods in this book. If you choose this path, do two things. 1) Go to strength, practice, and use the methods which seem easiest, more familiar, and more compatible. In this way your clinical skill will increase rapidly. 2) Also practice methods that are less familiar, less easy, even alien. By learning all the methods in this book, your larger toolbox will contribute to greater treatment efficiency and effectiveness. Whichever path you choose, be patient with yourself. Celebrate each small step.

PART 1

Foundations

CONCEPTS AND HISTORY

Alignment and mobility concepts

Alignment and mobility are two sides of a coin, or better, two facets of the same gem. In our minds as therapists these two facets must always be considered together with goals and methods balanced between them. We do not thrive with lack of movement. For health we must walk, lift, and stretch.

Life is movement. Thus spoke A. T. Still, echoing Aristotle. Even when we are at rest each breath can be felt and seen in all parts of the body. The rhythms of cardiac pulse, craniosacral rhythms, and organ motility are all continuous during life. Together these rhythms form a jazz symphony with multiple rhythms.

Any two points of our body move with respect to each other in complex rhythmic ways. In addition, as we move through life, each two points move with respect to each other in non-rhythmic paths; these movements are often larger than the rhythmic ones. Each pair of neighboring bodily parts are related in ranges of motion.

Since no two points on the body stay in fixed relationship to one another, what do we mean by alignment or position? Position or alignment refers to the portion of the range of motion between two bodily structures which requires no effort or least effort to maintain. This may or may not be in the geographic center of the range of motion. It is the place of minimum effort. Other parts of the range of motion require more effort to occupy. My arm hangs comfortably at my side. No effort on my part is required to keep it here. I use energy to move my arm out of this easy place to accomplish many things.

Mobility in soft tissue has two facets: how far we can move the part, and how much effort is required to move through each portion of the range of motion. Any movement from center requires work. As we move farther from the easy resting place, the effort required to move, and in some cases to maintain a position, increases incrementally.

As a feature of therapeutic assessment, we explore both how far parts can move related to each other, and the effort required to move through each part of the range of motion. We compare our findings with related structures in the same person including neighboring areas and similar areas on the other side of the body. We also compare these findings to our store of memories of other bodies we have worked with. From this exploration and additional data, including what the client can tell us of their internal experience, and what we have learned of the history of the situation, we formulate a plan to improve the total range of motion and the ease of movement within the range. If the zone of central ease is changed, the alignment between the two parts is also changed.

We are never fully symmetrical. Each of us is like all other people in some ways and we each have substantial unique features. Working to achieve standardized range of motion and alignment is procrustean. While we must keep an eye to these standards, the best solution is what is functional and comfortable for each person.

The impossibility of symmetry in our bodies underscores the importance of balanced mobility as a therapeutic goal. Solutions must be found which keep an eye to an approximation of symmetry alongside constant observation of what fluid movement there is throughout a person's body and how comfortable the person is in their body, the later considerations taking precedence when there is a perceived conflict among goals.

History of alignment and mobility in manual therapy

Mechanical engineer and physicist Wilhelm Conrad Roentgen accidentally discovered X-rays in 1895, leading to a Nobel Prize in Physics in 1901. The early decades of the 20th century saw the rapid adoption of diagnostic X-rays in health care practice. The first use in chiropractic was in 1910. At about the same time, osteopaths started to use X-rays.

Although X-ray visualization of motion through the use of fluoroscopy began soon after the use of static X-rays, static films remained more common. Recognition of the dangers of X-ray exposure during fluoroscopy has severely limited its use. The static nature of the X-rays may have contributed to the development of therapy models attending more to static alignment than to movement.

In the late 1940s, osteopath Harold V. Hoover recognized that he and many of his colleagues had become too focused on static alignment, routinely forgetting to consider mobility. In his practice he explored methods to assess and remediate mobility alongside alignment. Hoover brought his colleagues' attention back to movement as an equal partner in therapy in a 1954 landmark address at the annual meeting of the American Osteopathic Association (AOA), subsequently published in the 1954 *Yearbook of the AOA*. In his address and article, Hoover offered a new low force treatment method to improve functional movement in the body.

Since Hoover, many workers in the field have developed a considerable spectrum of functional methods. Some methods used before Hoover's time have been recognized as belonging to this newer category.

Andrew Taylor Still MD, the discoverer of osteopathy, used a wide range of techniques, most of which were not recorded, to improve mobility in the body. One of Still's methods has been painstakingly reconstructed by Richard Van Buskirk DO. An introduction to this method is included in this book.

Many methods to learn and enjoy

Mobility is more complex than static alignment. Therefore, addressing mobility in our bodies requires the larger set of assessment methods. Concurrent with the development of the many functional treatment methods, many new and elegant methods of assessment have been developed.

This book describes many of the functional treatment and assessment methods. Learning any of these methods can improve your therapeutic effectiveness and efficiency. This book can be treated as a buffet from which you can select appealing methods. For full benefit, take the time to learn all of them. You will find some easier to learn than others. Give more time to learning the challenging ones.

In our practices we encounter many different situations. For each situation several treatment methods are usually effective, but some methods will be more effective and/or more efficient than others.

Each assessment method provides some information. No single assessment method provides all information. Each assessment method has an error rate. Using several assessment methods leads to a more complete and accurate understanding of the situation.

If you have previously learned some of the methods in this book, you may find a method presented here differently than the way you learned. You may wonder which way is correct. If we understand "correct" to mean effective, the answer is both the variation you learned earlier and the variation in this book are correct. Additional variations not described here are also beneficial. Many variations have been created and they are all effective. Enjoy them all.

Assessment concepts

In therapeutic assessment, two questions must be answered:

1. Where in the body should I work?
2. What should I do in that location?

This therapeutic localization does not mean that the effect of treatment is only local. On the contrary, changing anything will change many things. Some of this change will be immediate, and change will continue for weeks.

Another way to say this is, as therapists, we must perpetually have in our minds the question: To make the most positive change for the whole person, where can I work on this person and what can I do from that location?

We use several assessment methods to answer these questions. No single assessment method can show us everything. Two or more assessment methods may confirm each other's findings. One assessment method may show features another assessment will miss.

This book describes several assessment methods that provide useful answers to our perpetual questions. Typically, there is not a single answer, but rather a cluster of solutions that could be useful. Among this cluster of useful solutions, one may be a more effective and/or more efficient intervention than others. We always seek efficiency: the way to provide the greatest positive change in the least time, with the least effort, and the greatest comfort for our client.

Certain attitudes or mindsets are useful as we apply any assessment methods.

- Openness to experience—I am open to new and surprising things.
- Vibrant curiosity—Every aspect of the universe intrigues me.
- Complete suspension of expectations—I approach my client without expectations. I observe accurately what is.
- Genuine compassion—I have an authentic interest in my client's viewpoint, suffering, and joys. I seek the highest good for all.
- Excellent boundaries in every sense—There is a precise and knowable set of boundaries between my client and me. It is beneficial to all concerned to discover and live on the right side of those boundaries.

Mechanisms of action

How do the treatment methods work? The short and true answer is, we don't know. More can be said about the state of our understanding of this question.

There are currently three dominant hypotheses for modes of action of manual therapy:

- neurologic mechanisms
- fascial plasticity
- tissue hydration.

Each mechanism of action has its proponents. No one mechanism has been proven to be the sole mechanism of therapeutic change.

It is usual for therapeutic processes to have more than one mode of action. For example, corticosteroids reduce inflammation by at least four mechanisms, two local and two systemic. In addition to biochemistry, we must remember the placebo effect.

Robert Schleip PhD investigated the viscoelasticity of fascia and demonstrated that viscoelasticity cannot be the sole mechanism of action for manual therapy. Continuing to search for answers, Schleip and his colleagues noted the presence of both contractile tissue and rich proprioceptive innervation in fascia.[1] He and others posit that the connection of these sensors and contractile elements through the nervous system provide a mechanism whereby our touch therapies might alter the length and elasticity of tissue by tactile and proprioceptive conversations with the nervous system. All the components of this system exist and are linked in ways that give strong plausibility to this hypothesis. This does not rule out the possibility that other mechanisms also operate.

Working with fresh human and animal cadavers, I have repeatedly demonstrated that many treatment methods change span and elasticity of tissue where there are no functional neurons. Change in tissue span and elasticity in this situation is greater than half as much as in living, innervated tissue. This demonstrates that the neurologic hypothesis does not provide the whole explanation for therapeutic change from manual therapy.

I am confident that more than one mechanism of action is in play during manual therapy. Research in this arena is more fruitful when it studies the contribution of each mechanism, rather than attempting to prove the exclusive role of one mechanism.

This book says little about the mode of action of each treatment method for the simple reason that sufficient research has not been done. I hope readers will pick up the challenge to do this research. Usually when mechanisms of action are understood, existing therapeutic methods can be refined, and new therapeutic methods developed.

While waiting for the research, we will continue to use these treatment methods because they produce therapeutic results. After aspirin was created by Felix Hoffman in 1897, our first understanding of its mode of action came in 1971. Additional modes of action continue to be investigated. Countless people benefited from aspirin before we knew anything about how it worked.

Introduction to functional methods

Functional treatment methods restore appropriate mobility in a sensitive dialogue between the practitioner and the client's tissue. Function in this context refers to mobility. This contrasts with other therapeutic methods which focus more on alignment and less on mobility. As living creatures, the spatial relationships in our bodies are constantly in motion, never static.

Additional features of functional treatment methods include:

- Forces used range from no force to moderate force. High force is never used. Somewhat stronger forces are used in two situations. A moderately stronger force may be exerted at the surface of the body to deliver a light force deeper into the body. A few methods briefly use forces near end-feel during some phases of treatment.
- Speed of treatment ranges from stillness to moderate speed. An exception is when contact is broken as quickly as possible in the release phase of the recoil treatment technique. High velocity thrusts are not used.
- Precise, detailed assessment is used to discern the best intervention to make at each moment, utilizing a similarly diverse collection of assessment methods

---

1   Schleip, R., Gabbriani, G., Wilke, J., Naylor, I., Hinz, B., Zorn, A., Jäger, H., Breul, R., Schreiner, S., and Klingler, W. (2019) "Fascia is able to actively contract and may thereby influence musculoskeletal dynamics: a histochemical and mechanographic investigation." *Frontiers in Physiology 10*, 336.

developed to guide treatment with functional methods.

Additional features of functional methods

Therapeutic engagement

In ballroom dance, one partner is the lead and the other partner is the follow. After one partner makes the first move, the two dancers collaborate to create beauty. The lead continues to offer more overt control while the follow shapes nuance. How these roles are shared differs with both the type of dance, and with the temperament of the dancers. So it is for manual therapy.

At the beginning of each therapeutic episode, the therapist reaches out to contact the client. This is a neutral contact with respect to control. Then the music starts, and one partner makes the first move, gracefully directing the other. In some functional treatment methods, the client's tissue makes the first move, and the therapist follows. In other functional methods, the therapist makes the first move and the client's tissue responds. Both ways can work well. In some instances, each of these paths will produce better results than the other. No one choreography is always right.

In some treatment methods, the client's body makes the first move and may continue to lead throughout the process. In this situation, the therapist, like a good parent or teacher, is watchful for a couple of different patterns that signal a stalled therapeutic process. If the therapist detects one of these patterns, the therapist offers direction to put the dance back on track. As soon as grace and beauty are restored to the dance, the therapist steps back into a pure follow role.

When the therapist is the lead, some treatment methods allow the client's system more latitude for action than others. Sometimes the direction for the dance is shared more equally, sometimes the therapist is a firmly benevolent guide. In some treatment methods, which partner controls the process changes at different phases of the treatment. The following descriptions of each treatment method specify who makes the first move, and how control of therapeutic process is shared after that.

EFFORT BARRIERS

Tissue may be mobility tested in any direction. If the tissue is stretched or compressed very slowly, at first a certain effort to move the tissue will be perceived. As movement proceeds through the range, increased effort will be required to produce movement. This increase of effort to produce more movement does not follow a smooth curve; it has steps. We call the first step up or increase in this effort the first barrier. This is often but not always a highly beneficial force level at which to treat. Some methods use any other effort barrier up to end-feel.

A benefit of treating at the first barrier, or early barriers, is that pain receptors are usually not engaged, and stretch receptors are engaged in a way that does not provoke even subtle fight or flight responses. Clients will often say they feel nothing. It will then be necessary to demonstrate to them change in range of motion or alignment before and after treatment.

Very important: In equilibrium with the tension of other tissues, any given tissue may rest beyond its first barrier. To identify the first barrier, it is always wise to slack a tissue and then let it slowly spring back toward its resting length.

Force vs deformation curves and the concept of first barrier

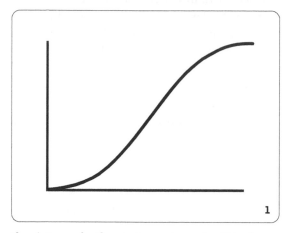

If a substance of uniform texture such as natural latex is stretched or compressed there is a nearly linear relationship between force applied and deformation.

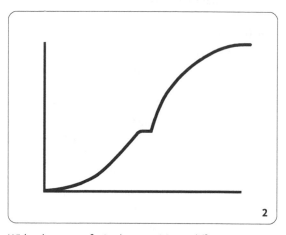

With substances of mixed composition, a different pattern is seen. There will be an initial linear relationship between force and deformation, then there will be a step up in force before further deformation occurs. For example, if liquid latex were mixed with synthetic spandex fibers and allowed to congeal, the resulting force deformation graph would look something like the above.

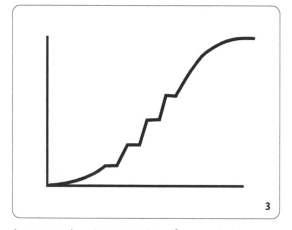

A more complex mixture containing, for example, latex, spandex, Styrofoam pellets, and a few cotton fibers would show several steps in the deformation graph. Human tissues are always mixed in composition so show this stepped deformation curve behavior.

Often, but not always, the most effective force level at which to treat human tissues is at the first barrier. However, in the equilibrium of tensional and compressive forces in the human body, some tissues spend most of their time beyond the first barrier. What this means in terms of treatment strategy is if the therapist wishes to exert a first barrier stretch, it will first be necessary to compress the tissue so the tensional forces on the tissue are less than the first barrier. The tissue is then slowly allowed to spring back towards equilibrium. During this controlled return, the therapist will perceive a sudden decrease in spring within the tissue pushing on his hands. This is the first barrier stretch for the target tissue even though the therapist is still exerting compression on the sum of tissue forces in the region.

END-FEEL AND END RANGE

In mobility testing, the force required to produce movement will increase incrementally. Eventually a state of force and cumulative movement will be achieved at which no further movement is readily available. At this state, the next increment of force required to produce movement may well produce tissue damage, possibly including tearing or dislocation.

Engaging fight and flight responses during treatment will cause the body to engage contractile elements resulting in a wrestling match and may traumatize or re-traumatize the client.

End-feel mobility testing is useful to observe the full range of motion. While many functional methods are performed at a first barrier, some use later barriers including a few that briefly use end-feel.

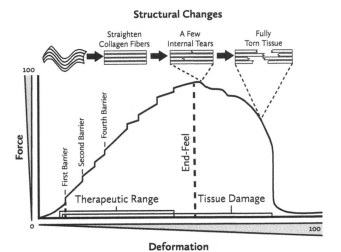

In this chart, Force is the amount of force applied; Deformation is how much the tissue changes shape, which may be lengthening, shortening, bending, or twisting.

PACE

In mobility testing and in treatment pace is important. Stretch receptors (Pacinian corpuscles) respond to both speed of stretch and distance stretched. Through most of the range, speed of stretch produces more neuron firing than distance. At end range, distance plays a larger role. Pace is therefore very important in not engaging fight or flight responses. Feel the responses of the tissue under your hand. Watch your client for the slightest signs of distress.

TISSUE TYPES

For each functional method, we will see how to apply the method to a range of tissue types. Most methods can be used on many different tissue types. Certain methods are contraindicated for some specific tissues for safety reasons. Tissue types treated include but are not limited to:

- skin
- muscle
- fascia
- ligament
- bone
- blood vessel
- nerve
- peritoneum
- pleura
- meninges
- organ parenchyma.

RELEASE SIGNS

Any given bit of tissue may release in any succession or combination of several ways including:

- Unwinding—A progressive unraveling sense with frequent shifts in direction.
- Softening—This will occur in usually

small directional increments, which is different than the generalized softening at the end of a treatment.

Note: If the tissue was slack prior to treatment then the change will be firming rather than softening.

- Temperature change, usually warming.
- Therapeutic pulse—At first this may resemble a cardiac pulse; however, it crescendos and decrescendos in both rate and intensity over a period usually lasting tens of seconds.
- Sense of fluid filling—Subtle edema signals both release and end of treatment in a particular area for that day.

RECOGNIZING WHEN A TREATMENT IS DONE

It is very important to recognize when to stop treating a given structure. Over treating inflames tissue leading to more fibrosis in the weeks and months to follow.

If tissue is very tight it is important to make the right amount of change on a given day, and then return on another day to continue. *It is better to undertreat than to over treat.*

Usually, the tissue treated will change further in the days or weeks between treatments. It is sometimes necessary to treat again in future treatment sessions once or several times.

When to stop may be recognized by any one of several signs:

- A generalized softening of the tissue followed by cessation of unwinding.
- Mobility is restored to normal range.
- A subtle feeling of swelling in the tissue. This is the beginning of edema.

On the way to the point at which one should stop treatment there are usually several increments of release which can be recognized by the release signs listed above, on this and the preceding page.

Six factors describing each functional method

Some of the features described above and additional features are useful to describe, distinguish, and classify each of the functional treatment methods. The following six factor model summarizes these features and is used in the treatment method section of this book to describe and distinguish each of the treatment methods.

1. **Tissue engagement**

   Engagement between the client's tissue and the therapist's hand may be initiated by either party. Often when tissue is contacted with a relaxed hand, inherent movement in the client's tissue will engage the therapist's hand and pull it in a particular direction or sequence of directions. Alternatively, the therapist may initiate the engagement.

2. **Force**

   Amount of force used varies between functional methods. Many methods use low force. A few use moderate force, even fewer briefly use end-feel. For some functional methods, the amount of force used changes from one phase of a treatment to the next phase. For example, recoil uses moderate force in the setup phase and no force in the release.

3. **Speed**

   The speed with which the hands are moved varies between functional methods. Usually, the speed is slow to moderate. In recoil, however, the release is accomplished with a quick movement.

4. **Constraint**

   In some but not all functional methods, tissue is prevented from moving in certain ways. The nature and extent of constraint varies from method to method: ranging from no constraint to complete prevention of movement. For example, in pure unwinding, the therapist offers no constraint to movement, unless one of two special conditions arise. In contrast, Hoover's centralizing technique allows no movement.

5. **Directiveness**

In some functional methods, the therapist requires tissue to move in particular ways; in other methods, no specific movement is required. The nature and extent of this directiveness varies from method to method ranging from non-directive through moderately directive to highly directive. In some methods, directiveness varies between phases of the same treatment.

It is important to clarify the differences between constraint and directiveness. Constraint describes what the therapist does not allow the tissue to do. Directiveness describes what the therapist requires the tissue to do. In both instances, the therapist makes a requirement of the tissue; one forbids action while the other is a call to action. Both may be present in the same treatment method with some things being forbidden while others are required.

6. **Relationship to effort barriers**

In passive range of motion testing, tissue is moved to a comfortable end-feel. If the therapist's hands are kept relaxed and tissue is moved very slowly, the increase in resistance to movement will be felt to be stepwise, rather than a smooth curve. A certain amount of effort is required to displace tissue the first linear or angular distance; then a distinct rise in effort is felt to achieve the next increments of change. This is called the first barrier. With a little further displacement, a second distinct rise of force required to produce positional change will be felt. This is called the second barrier. A sequence of such barriers will be felt at unequal increments until end range is reached. At end range, tissue failure is a possibility, producing pain and damage; do not push into this range.

Some functional methods treat at a first barrier, others treat at forces less than first barrier. Some methods utilize barriers in mid-range between first barrier and end-feel. A few methods briefly use end-feel.

End range is of various types. In mobility testing any tissue, whether assessing a joint range of motion or stretch in soft tissue, there is a distinct anatomic limit beyond which healthy tissue cannot be displaced without pain and/or damage. For some joints such as extension at the elbow, this end-feel has a distinct bony feel. For other healthy joints and soft tissues, there is a gradual incremental rise of force required to produce movement. At the end, a larger increment of force is required and produces little movement. In tissue that is fibrosed, edematous, or both, the effort required to move through the range will be felt to be greater than normal. In that case, the end-feel will have a less sharp rise to end-feel, but rather a more gradual or boggy increase of effort.

If there is conscious or unconscious guarding of an area, attempts by the therapist to produce movement will provoke active muscular contraction opposed to the therapist's intended movement. This may or may not be accomplished by a perception of pain on the part of the client. When guarding is observed, a slower testing speed may produce movement without muscular guarding or pain; if not, the nature of the end-feel is noted, and it is recognized that anatomic end range has not been found. Exploration of and possible reduction of guarding may now become a treatment goal.

Primacy

Our constant question is "Where can I work on this person to make the greatest beneficial change for the whole person?" We call this best area to work the primary lesion. In this context, primary means only the most beneficial structure or area we can work on at this moment. Primary does not mean it is the strongest restriction; in fact, it usually is not the strongest. Primary does not mean it is the oldest restriction; age of restriction has no relationship to primacy.

Our bodies all have many lesions in them. These lesions are all connected to other lesions by any of several pathways including through the connective tissue matrix and the nervous system. Some lesions are connected to a larger number of other lesions, other lesions to fewer. At any given moment, some of these lesions are in the process of change, others are not. Of those restrictions that are changing, some are changing faster than others. Change in any area affects other areas. If we appropriately treat tissue which is in the process of change, the body will readily accept our

intervention as assistance to what it is already trying to do. Because each lesion is connected to other lesions, all interventions we make will affect areas we have not touched. It is most beneficial to treat areas which are changing relatively rapidly and are connected to many other lesions. The most primary lesion has the best mix of rapidly changing and widely connected.

It is possible to identify and characterize several lesions in the body, and to determine their relative primacy. Below is a fictional example of how this might be arranged in a person's body. The actual pattern is unique in each person and changes constantly. The higher up on the list we can treat the greater the benefit for the whole person. Restrictions below the solid line in the list below are not actively changing and therefore make the poorest candidates to treat.

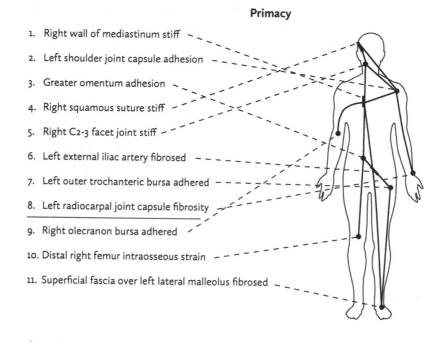

Primacy

1. Right wall of mediastinum stiff
2. Left shoulder joint capsule adhesion
3. Greater omentum adhesion
4. Right squamous suture stiff
5. Right C2-3 facet joint stiff
6. Left external iliac artery fibrosed
7. Left outer trochanteric bursa adhered
8. Left radiocarpal joint capsule fibrosity
9. Right olecranon bursa adhered
10. Distal right femur intraosseous strain
11. Superficial fascia over left lateral malleolus fibrosed

Assessment confirmation

Each test provides some information. No one test can provide all information. All tests can present inaccurate information. Therefore, several tests must be used to provide confirmation. An additional test may also provide information that no other tests will provide. The following Venn diagrams give a visual representation of this.

Test result confirmation

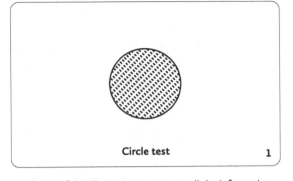

Circle test   **1**

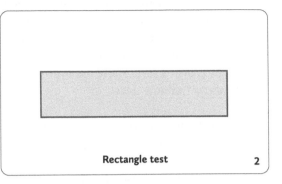

Rectangle test   **2**

The frame of this illustration represents all the information that can be learned about a person's body. The circle represents the information provided by a particular test.

This shaded rectangle represents the information provided by a second test. It overlaps but is not identical with the data set provided by the circle test.

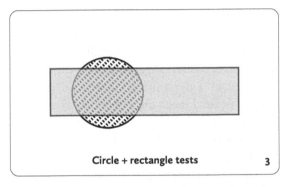

Circle + rectangle tests   **3**

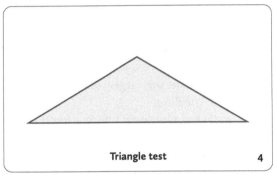

Triangle test   **4**

Here we see the information available from both the circle and rectangle tests. Note the area where the test results can confirm each other. Each test may provide true information which is not confirmable in this way.

A third test looks at a different part of the information about this person which overlaps but is not identical with either of the first two tests.

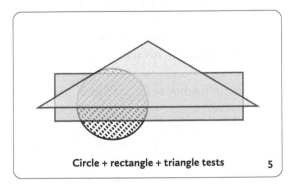

Circle + rectangle + triangle tests   **5**

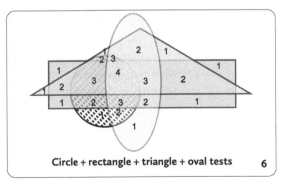

Circle + rectangle + triangle + oval tests   **6**

The potential information provided by each of the first three tests are shown overlapped here.

A fourth test represented by an oval is added. Areas marked 1 are examined by only one test and may be true or not. Areas marked 2 are examined by two tests which is an opportunity for confirmation or disconfirmation. Similarly, areas marked 3 and 4 are examined by more tests providing opportunity for further confirmation or disconfirmation.

Treatment is also a test

Always use at least four tests. Once treatment is initiated, the results of the treatment provide further confirmation or disconfirmation of the findings from the first four or more tests. The treatment is also a test. There are four possible results of treatment as a test.

1. The treatment result is as expected from the assessment, suggesting the assessment was largely correct.
2. The treatment result is somewhat as expected with additional features, suggesting that the assessment was partially correct. Such a treatment result may provide additional clues guiding further treatment.
3. The treatment result is entirely or largely different from expected, suggesting the assessment was largely incorrect. In this case consider:
   a. what additional information the results of treatment provide,
   b. return to earlier steps of assessment to see what may have been missed, and
   c. what additional testing may be useful.
4. Little or no treatment response is observed, suggesting the assessment was incorrect.
   a. Return to earlier steps of assessment to see what may have been missed.
   b. Consider what additional testing may be useful.

Dynamic stabilization

This concept applies to both assessment and treatment.

During passive mobility testing we move one body part relative to a neighboring body part. To accomplish this, we usually stabilize one body part with our hands as a platform on which to move another body part. As an example, to examine the mobility of a finger joint, we stabilize a proximal phalanx and move a middle phalanx on the stabilized proximal phalanx.

There is more than one way to stabilize a body part and exactly how a body part is stabilized strongly influences the results of mobility testing. There is a large contrast between the results of:

- a strong clamping stabilization of a body part preventing any movement, and
- a less forceful dynamic stabilization where any tendency of the stabilized body part to move is met with just enough back force to prevent movement.

Compared to a dynamic stabilization, a strong stabilization which is insensitive to the dynamics of the movement will give a mobility test result of much less both end range, and ease within range.

Because a dynamic stabilization is more like the normal mechanics of the body as we go through life, the larger range of motion demonstrated by testing in this way is more realistic.

Dynamic stabilization requires a constant alertness by the therapist for any tendency of the gently stabilized part to move. The therapist applies an ever-shifting back load just preventing movement of the stabilized part. This back load varies from moment to moment in both direction of load and force of load.

The therapist must maintain constant, moment by moment, detailed awareness of:

- any tendency of the stabilized part to move
- effort required to move the mobile part
- smoothness of movement of the mobile part
- range of motion of the mobile part in a succession of directions
- slightest signs of distress from the client.

One awareness cannot be sacrificed for another, all must be constantly monitored.

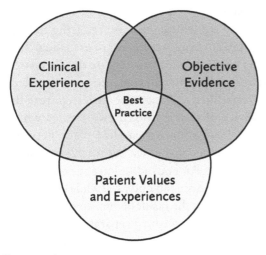

Best practices

Terminology clarification

While a rose by any other name would smell as sweet, we seek names that are both accurately descriptive and succinct. Here is a discussion of terms as they apply to manual therapy: lesions, primacy, and fibrosity, adhesion, and contracture.

Lesions

Problems in the body that we address with manual therapy have sometimes been called "lesions." As one word, this is succinct; however, it is not adequately descriptive, even misleading. The term lesion evokes wounds and infections, neither of which are qualities we treat with manual therapy.

For the purposes of manual therapy, lesion was later defined by Alain Croibier DO as "a localized area of tissue dysfunction." This expression stands better by itself without reference to the term lesion. However, "localized area of tissue dysfunction" is problematic in at least two ways. 1) It is a mouthful to say. We can hope for a more succinct expression. 2) While it is true, we often apply treatment to local areas, the effect of the treatment is always on the whole system. The expression "localized area of tissue dysfunction"

does not adequately relate to the fact that these are entry or leverage points for action on the whole system.

Primacy

The expression "primary restriction" is succinct and somewhat descriptive of what we work on as most of the time we are working on areas of fibrosity that appear "restricted." However, we sometimes work on areas of functional laxity.

An expression, "The point or area on the body which if worked on in this moment will make the most beneficial change for the whole person," is accurate and descriptive but far too long to be practical. The shorthand term primary restriction is used.

"Area of best leverage at this moment" captures enough meaning more succinctly. It is still seven words. Primary lesion is more succinct.

Fibrosity, adhesion, and contracture

The term fibrosity refers to an excessive ingrowth of collagen and elastin fibers during repair of an injured area of connective tissue. It is useful to distinguish two varieties of fibrosity: adhesion and contracture.

ADHESION

In many places in our bodies there are lubricated glide planes between two surfaces, which are not normally mechanically connected to each other. Three examples are: 1) the glide plane between the visceral pleura and the parietal pleura in the thorax; 2) the glide plane within each bursa; 3) the glide plane between an eyeball and the surfaces around it, including the eye socket and the eyelids. Sometime during repair, as the fibroblasts generate new fiber to repair a damaged membrane, some of the fiber grows through the lubricant to attach to the other surface. This is an adhesion.

CONTRACTURE

Sometimes during tissue repair the fibroblasts lay down excessive new fiber so that the tissue being repaired has less elasticity than it originally had. This is referred to as a contracture. The term contracture is somewhat of a misnomer, as it suggests the action of contracting or shortening. A tissue which is fibrosed may become shorter than it was originally, or more commonly that tissue has lost elasticity. It is not as stretchy as before. Thus, the shortness suggested by the name contracture is a loss of ability to elongate, and only less commonly a shortening to less than its original resting length.

FIBROSITY

Fibrosity is the broader term referring to both adhesion and contracture. For us as manual therapists it is important to recognize the distinction between adhesion and contracture. If the fibrosity is within a structure, we wish to restore the elasticity of that tissue. If two tissues which should have a lubricated glide plane between them have become stuck together, we wish to restore glide. For both adhesion and contracture, we seek to restore mobility, and while the process may be similar, the result of our intervention will be different. We wish to separate an adhesion, fully restoring the lubricated glide plane. For a contracture we wish to restore elasticity and we would not want to create a separation between two things.

PART 2

Assessment Methods

INTRODUCTION

For treatment to be effective and efficient we must know several things before we begin. In order these are:

1. What tissue or area is most beneficial to treat at this moment?
2. In detail what is the present condition of this tissue?
3. What is the most effective and efficient method to treat this tissue at this moment?

Each treatment session is usually made up of a succession of several treatments performed on a succession of body parts. The above questions must be answered for each of these body parts.

At the conclusion of each of the treatment moments, the condition of the treated tissue must be reassessed. Assessing the condition of the tissue immediately before and immediately after each treatment moment has three benefits.

1. We get immediate feedback on the results of our work. This is an essential way we grow as therapists.
2. How much the tissue changed in response to the treatment moment compared to how much change we wish to make helps inform whether further treatment can be applied beneficially

to this tissue at this time. Additional factors inform this decision.
3. By making the client aware of the condition of the tissue both before and after:
   a. We demonstrate to the client that change has been made. Many of our treatment methods are so gentle the client may not otherwise immediately recognize change.
   b. The client's overall awareness of their body can increase.

As described in the introduction to this book, each assessment method provides some information; no one assessment method can supply all information. In addition to different tests providing different domains of information, it is also true that each test can provide both true and false information. Tests all provide more truth than falsehood, yet we must be alert to the possibility of false readings. It is essential to use several tests. One test may confirm another. One test may provide information that no other test does.

There is one test that we always use, which is mobility testing. A central goal of functional methods is to normalize range and ease of movement. Thus, we test mobility. Mobility changes promptly with treatment and we can assess this change.

While mobility testing is always performed, poor mobility by itself is never a sufficient reason to treat. Recognition that a body part is stiff or lax is important but is not by itself sufficient reason to treat that area. Another area may be more primary, offering better leverage on the whole system.

Often, change is better made from a distance. Usually, the solution to a problem of mobility and/or pain is not simple; rather, several sometimes surprisingly distant areas must be treated to resolve the local complaint.

The following sections describe several assessment methods, divided into four categories.

- **General assessment methods**

  Some assessment methods are useful to find the vicinity of a primary lesion but give a less detailed understanding of the problem in that area. They are useful as first approximations, to be followed up with other assessment methods that give more detailed information.

- **Local assessment methods**

  Other assessment methods are useful to characterize a lesion in detail. These methods apply to all lesions whether the lesion is primary. Specific assessment methods locate the lesion more precisely, both with respect to landmarks on the surface of the body and depth within the body from the surface. Some methods describe the shape of the lesion. Some of these methods indicate tissue type. Some of them find the nature of the problem in the area.

- **Mixed general and local assessment methods**

  One assessment method is useful both for finding the general area of a primary lesion and for further characterizing it. However, this method has lower reliability than many other methods. All assessment methods are imperfect, which is why we always use several assessment methods for confirmation or disconfirmation findings. While this confirmation process is always important, its use is critical when using any assessment method which has inherently lower reliability.

- **Extended assessment methods**

  Once an area to treat has been located and characterized, a treatment method for that area is chosen. Then, as treatment proceeds, the therapist may become aware of connections to other lesions in the body. These felt connections can be used to amplify the treatment.

The following sections describe in detail the several assessment methods in these groups.

ASSESSMENT ALGORITHM

Rationale and guidelines

In therapeutic assessment, two questions must be answered:

1. Where in the body should I work?
2. What should I do in that location?

This therapeutic localization does not mean that the effect of treatment is only local. On the contrary, changing anything will change many things. Some of this change will be immediate; other elements of change will appear over a period of weeks.

Here is a useful paraphrase of this: as therapists, we must perpetually have in our minds the question: To make the most positive change for the whole person, where can I work on this person and what can I do from that location?

We use several assessment methods to answer these questions. No single assessment method can show everything. One assessment method may show issues another assessment will miss. Two or more assessment methods may confirm each other's findings.

This book describes several assessment methods that provide useful answers to our perpetual questions. Typically, there is not a single answer, but rather a cluster of solutions that could be useful. Among this cluster of useful solutions, however, one may be a more effective and/or more efficient intervention than others. We always seek efficiency: the way to provide the greatest positive change in the least time and for the least effort.

Certain attitudes or mindsets are useful as we apply any assessment methods.

- Openness to experience—I am open to new and surprising things.
- Vibrant curiosity—Every aspect of the universe intrigues me.
- Complete suspension of expectations—I approach my client without expectations. I observe accurately what is.
- Genuine compassion—I treat everyone with equal respect and caring.
- Excellent boundaries in every sense, including this doublethink—There is a precise and knowable set of boundaries between my client and me. It is beneficial to all concerned to recognize and live on the right side of those boundaries.

Inquiry and testing

- Listen on the phone.
- Have the client submit an intake form well before the first appointment.
  - Read the intake.
  - Formulate follow up questions.
- Watch movement and posture as the person walks in.
- Start with open questions.
- Follow up with more closed questions.
- Recognize risk factors.
  - Consider safety of proceeding.
  - Keep in mind things not to do.
- Consider tests to be performed.
- Observe standing alignment—front, side, and back.
- Observe active movement.
- Perform standing passive movement testing.
- As needed, do seated or lying down passive movement testing.
- Do orthopedic testing as indicated.
- Have the client stand again.
- Apply selected tests starting generally and moving to specific. Always include mobility testing as a late step.
- Perform an initial treatment method to the most primary lesion you can find.
- Return to assessment to locate what has now become the next primary restriction.
- Cycle assessment and treatment until the body signals it has had enough treatment for today.

GENERAL ASSESSMENT METHODS

In our search for each primary lesion, we first find a general impression of the restriction's location and then proceed with additional testing to a more detailed understanding of the exact size, shape, depth, and anatomy of the currently primary structure(s).

There are three assessment methods that point specifically to areas of dysfunction which are quite primary. We call these three methods "general" assessments. Each of the three general assessment methods is described in detail in the following pages. Learn and practice all three general assessment methods. Routinely use all three methods to confirm and extend your assessment of the general location of each primary restriction.

In some instances, all three of these general assessment methods provide fairly good information, allowing us to confirm and perhaps begin to refine our understanding of the primary restriction. In other instances, only two of the methods will provide useful information. This still provides a measure of confirmation. Occasionally, only one of the general assessment methods will work well, in which case we can cautiously proceed to more detailed characterization of the primary restriction.

Once you are confident of the general location of a primary restriction, then use local assessment methods to further characterize the restriction. Knowledge of the size, shape, depth from the surface of the body, and tissue type of the restriction allows us to design an effective and efficient treatment.

Each method of assessment whether general or local is imperfect. Any assessment method can give an impression which is largely correct, partially correct, or incorrect. That is why we confirm and extend our understanding by comparing the results of several assessment methods. The fewer the number of assessment methods available the less confidence we have in our results. The effects of treatment are always a further and often final test. Results of treatment may be as expected, partially as expected, or not at all as expected.

Many assessment methods point to an area of dysfunction in the body. Knowing about the presence of a dysfunction does not tell us how primary the dysfunction is. In this context, "primary" means that treating the restriction will have the greatest beneficial effect on the whole person.

Assessment method 1: general listening

Origin

Various listening assessment methods have been in use by osteopaths since at least the 1930s. This method was developed by Jean-Pierre Barral DO.

Concept

One of the most important keys to successful treatment is addressing the lesions in the right order. As therapists, we have the constant question of what to do first and what to do next. Fortunately, if we know how to listen, the body will tell us what structure to work on next at every step of treatment.

Each of our bodies has several areas of fibrosity and sometimes areas of laxity. These areas are all linked by multiple pathways: connective tissue fibers, nervous system, vascular, lymphatic, emotional, and hormonal. We won't always know all the pathways by which lesions are linked, but we can discover the body's priority for which one we should work on first to have the strongest therapeutic effect on the whole person.

The body is constantly revising its system of compensations. New events happen to our bodies, our bodies age, and our bodies constantly try to find the best compromises that will leave it the most available adaptive capacity to meet new challenges. What we therapists want to find is the part of the lesional chain which is most ready to destabilize. The area which is about to change anyway. If we treat this area of imminent destabilization, it will be relatively easy to change, and the therapeutic effect will strongly ripple out to the rest of the body.

We call this focus of strains, which is about to change, the "primary restriction." It is primary *only* in the sense that it is the one we should work on first. It usually did not occur first historically. It is usually not the strongest restriction in the body. In this context "primary" only means it is the one we should work on first.

Method

Lesions are areas with lack of support, or lack of "lift," in the body. To find these, have the client stand and put a little more load on the top of their head with your hand. The area of less support will collapse, usually causing the person to lean. To general listen, stand behind your client and place your dominant hand gently but firmly on the top of the person's head, contacting the sagittal suture. Within 3–5 seconds, the client's body will lean in some direction. This lean points toward the primary restriction. When we put the weight of our hand on their head, the column of their body will begin to collapse around a weak spot. This points to the primary restriction.

As the person's body bends, both watch with your eyes and feel the direction it goes: Left? Right? Forward? Backwards? In addition to direction, see how far down the body the bend is. Is the bend at the neck? At the respiratory diaphragm? Near the top of the pelvis? These two factors, direction and distance, point us to the area of the primary restriction. Additional assessment methods will then be used to refine awareness of that area to the precise structure to be treated.

The next step is a method to check if we have the most primary restriction. Leaving your hand on the top of the head, use your other hand to gently touch the area you suspect of being the primary restriction. As you touch, give subtle support, and have an intention to temporarily remove the effects of this lesion from the body's system of compensations. By your touch you are asking the question, "If I were to treat this area, how would it change the system?" As you make this inhibitory touch, one of two things will happen. Either the leaned body will right itself or not. If the body rights itself, this confirms your assessment of primacy. If the person's body does not right itself, this tells you that you did not find the primary restriction.

Thirteen more points

1. The weight and/or restrictiveness of glasses, watches, pagers, cell phones, other electronics, and heavier jewelry may skew the results of listening. Ask clients to remove these before you begin. Lighter rings and earrings may be left in place.

2. From the client's perspective, it may feel odd to have you step behind them and ask them to close their eyes while you place a hand on their head. One way to handle this is to say you are going to check some postural things. Step behind the client, check the heights of the iliac crests with your hands, then check shoulder levels with your hands. Finally, ask the client to close their eyes for a moment and put your hand on the top of their head.

3. For general listening, stand at a comfortable distance behind the client. If you are too close it will be harder to see how the client leans in response to the load on their head. If you are too far away there will be strain in your arm, which can skew results. Stand as far away as you comfortably can.

4. It is important to be centered behind the person you are listening to; otherwise, you may unintentionally pull them in a particular direction. If your client is much taller than you are, get on a chair or other stable support so you don't have tension in your arm which could also skew the pattern of movement.

5. If a person's eyes are open, they may use their visual reference to stay level, and you will not feel the listening. Having the client shut their eyes may be useful. However, if they have balancing problems, this may be counterproductive.

6. Qualities of your approach to the person's head with your hand are critically important. If you come in too slowly, hovering before you touch, results will not be reliable. Coming in too fast can feel like an impact on the top of the person's head, eliciting guarding. Approach at a moderate and somewhat decelerating rate, so you get there quickly but do not hover. The full weight of your hand can be on the person's head, but not the load of your whole arm. At the same time, you must hold the weight of your arm out of the contact, and you must be as relaxed as possible to allow movement to happen.

7. If a person has practiced chi-gong or some other energetic practices, they may not deflect to your touch. If you suspect this, ask about their practice history; if they use these methods, ask them to turn it off for the time being.

8. General listening happens within the first five seconds of contact, usually less. It often happens immediately when you contact. If you are there longer than five seconds, you may feel the body do many interesting things, but none of those things point you to what you should work on first.

9. The very first direction of lean is the important one. After the first one, the body may go a second, third, or fourth direction. After the first direction, this information is not useful. The first motion may be quite small and latter motions much larger. Do not be distracted by these larger movements. Find the first movement.

10. There is a variation of general listening you will need in a certain situation, such as if the person seems to bend near the hips, or if it is difficult to decide if the bend is in the legs or in the trunk. To check this, have the person sit down and general listen again. If the seated listening is the same as standing, then the lesion is above the sitz bones. If the seated

listening is different than the standing, then the primary lesion is below the sitz bones.

11. Listen from the surface of the body, do not sink your awareness into the body. Entirely, let the information come to you. If you sink into the body for listening, the results may be inaccurate. There is a more advanced technique which utilizes this. See below.

12. In addition to location, the shape of the collapse in the body provides clues to the size of the area to be treated, and sometimes to anatomy. If the lean, fold, or break is sharp or focal, this suggests a small area. A larger area of bending suggests a larger primary restriction. If the deflection is larger, watch for whether the deflection is in a single direction or if it is curvilinear. If it is curved, this shape may give an additional clue to anatomy.

13. The response to general listening will look different than usual for three areas of the body:

   a. If the primary restriction is in the head, it will feel like a twist under your hand, but the head will not be seen or felt to displace on the neck. Be sure to distinguish this from an upper cervical primary restriction where the head, as a whole, may rotate on the top of the neck.

   b. If the primary restriction is in the upper limb, there will be a lateral lean in the upper thorax. If you see a lateral lean in the upper thorax, inhibit at the olecranon process on that side. If this olecranon contact rights the person, the primary restriction is in that upper limb. The upper limb includes the shoulder girdle as well as the arm.

We say the olecranon process "witnesses" the whole upper limb.

   c. If the primary restriction is very close to the centerline of the torso, i.e., near the front of the spine, the person will not deflect; their body will also feel woody, with no sense of spring. To confirm and refine this, make a gliding inhibitory contact along the spine. When you arrive at the level of the primary restriction, the person's head will rise up a little and their body will feel springier under your hand on their head.

General listening in brief

1. Ask your client to remove glasses, watches, electronics, and most jewelry. Small rings or earrings with little weight can be left in place.

2. Center yourself behind your client. If your client is much taller than you, get on a step stool or chair.

3. You may wish to have your client close their eyes. This eliminates visual righting reflexes which may mask results of this assessment method.

4. Quickly and gently lay the palm of your dominant hand on their sagittal suture.

5. Observe the *first* direction in which their body moves. This will happen well within five seconds.

6. If the primary restriction seems to be at or below the pelvis, then have the person sit down and do it again. Is the result the same as standing?

7. Touch the suspected area of primary lesion with your nondominant hand, with an inhibitory intention. Does the lean of the body change or stay the same?

General listening

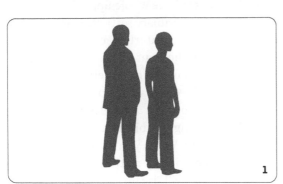

Stand behind the client at a distance at which you will be able to place the palm of your hand on the client's head without straining, but not closer.

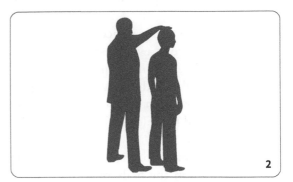

As you place the palm of your hand on the top of the client's head, both see with your eyes and feel which direction the person falls and how far down their body they bend.

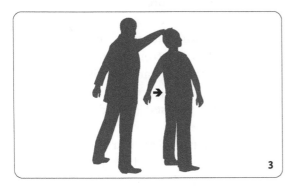

In this example, the client bends left at the waist.

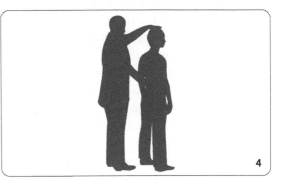

With your other hand, touch the client's body at the area where they appear to bend in response to the pressure on their head. Use this second hand to provide subtle support. If the person straightens up in response to this touch, this confirms that this is the primary area.

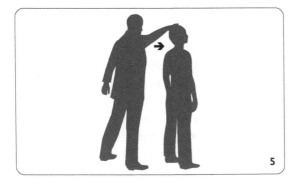

In this example, the client bends in the neck.

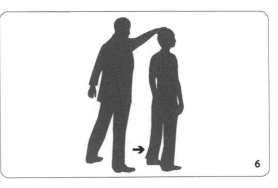

In this example, the client bends at the ankle.

General listening special cases

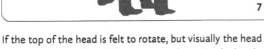

7

If the top of the head is felt to rotate, but visually the head does not move, this indicates a primary lesion in the head.

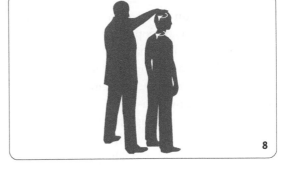

8

In contrast, if the top of the head is felt to move and the head is seen to rotate on the neck, this indicates an upper cervical primary lesion.

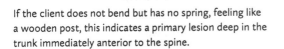

9

If the client does not bend but has no spring, feeling like a wooden post, this indicates a primary lesion deep in the trunk immediately anterior to the spine.

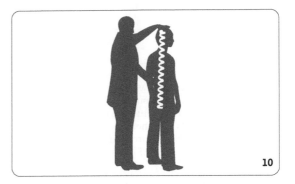

10

In this situation of too stiff steadiness, a gliding inhibitory contact down the spine will identify the level of the primary lesion by restoring the springiness of the spine.

11

A side shift or lean in the upper thorax may indicate either an upper thoracic primary lesion, or a primary lesion in the upper limb. The witness point for the whole upper limb including the shoulder girdle is the olecranon process.

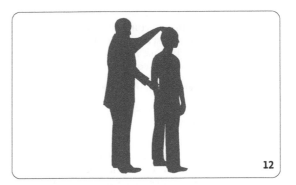

12

If an inhibitory contact on the olecranon process brings the person back upright this indicates the primary restriction is in the upper limb. If the olecranon process inhibitory contact does not right the person this points to an upper thoracic primary restriction.

Witness points for use with general assessment methods
Origin

The original concept and application were developed by early osteopaths; the exact origins have been lost. Additional witness points were discovered by others later. The middle scalene, left triangular ligament, and lateral malleolus were discovered by Jean-Pierre Barral DO. The greater trochanter and digit tips were discovered by Jeffrey Burch. There are likely more witness points yet to be discovered. Happy hunting.

Witness point	Witnesses these structures
Cranial vertex	Cranial vault structures
Occipital squama	Cranial base structures
Maxillae	Facial bones and related structures (Each maxilla witnesses the maxilla, nasal bone, and zygoma on that side. Each maxilla also witnesses the vomer and ethmoid. Neither maxilla witnesses the mandible. Sutures and soft tissues are also witnessed.)
Middle scalene muscle	All parietal pleura and wall of the mediastinum on the same side
Olecranon process	Whole upper limb on the same side, including all features of the shoulder girdle
Left triangular ligament of the liver	All of the structures suspending the liver from the respiratory diaphragm (left and right triangular ligaments and anterior and posterior coronary ligaments)
Greater trochanter	Lower limb on the same side
Lateral malleolus	Foot and ankle
Tips of each finger or toe	The ray associated with that digit from the tip of the finger or toe up to the carpo-metacarpal joint of tarso-metatarsal joint

How to identify new witness points

First, find a primary restriction using the general listening.

Next, touch additional anatomically related points using inhibitory contact. If one of these other points is found to also correct the leaning or tilting shown by general listening, this other point may be a witness point.

From the anatomical relationship of the two points found which both inhibit general listening, form a hypothesis about the anatomic territory which the possible witness point may witness.

In future treatment with many clients, any time a primary restriction is found near this hypothesized witness point, make an inhibitory contact on the possible witness point to see if it also inhibits the general listening lean or tilt. Use this type of testing with many people to try to disconfirm your hypothesis.

If the hypothesized witness point often rights the body, this both supports the hypothesis and starts to define the anatomical area witnessed by the point, which may or may not be identical with the originally hypothesized territory.

If the hypothesized witness point stands up over time, test it with respect to primary restrictions a little farther away to further define the territory witnessed by the new witness point.

Note, it is possible to listen from a witness point. If a primary restriction is found within the realm witnessed by a point, then the next task is to determine where within that realm the primary restriction is. One step toward this is to listen from the witness point. This will point toward the lesion, but not fully define it. This method tends to provide a grainy image, which must be followed up with additional assessment methods. This method was developed by Rihab Yakub.

Assessment method 2: general lift

Origin
Jeffrey Burch.

Concept
In the general listening assessment method, we put pressure down on the top of the head. In response to this pressure, the client's body folds around the primary restriction and leans in that direction.

If the body is lifted up, areas that are flexible lengthen, bound areas do not. This results in the body leaning toward the areas that cannot lengthen. The body will feel tethered down to that area.

The results of the general lift test often match the results of general listening but not always. Areas of laxity are less likely to be found with general lift. Lesions superior to the areas of contact for general lift will not be found. General listening is also imperfect. When the results of general listening and general lift are different, the discrepancy can be resolved using local listening and inhibition.

Method
Ask the client to stand in a relaxed fashion. Gently contact as described below and slowly lift. It may be useful to have the client slump a little or to slightly compress the client down before lifting up.

As you slowly and gently lift, notice the first direction of lean and/or felt sense of tethering down. Note how far down the body the tethering is.

Lifting can be done from several locations. Lifting from each location somewhat shifts the focus of the lift, including more of certain body areas and excluding other areas. Lifting will provide information about tissues below the contact for lifting but not above the areas lifted. Making a succession of lifts at progressively more inferior areas until the lean vanishes is one way to localize the restriction. Similarly, moving upward with a succession of lifts until a lean appears localizes a restriction.

OCCIPUT AND MANDIBLE
This lift contact is often used and provides information about structures below the head.

OCCIPUT AND SPHENOID
If an occiput and mandible lift does not show a lean, but occiput and sphenoid does, then a cranial base strain is indicated.

FRONTAL AND PARIETAL BONES
If a frontal and parietal lift shows a lean but occiput and sphenoid do not, then a cranial vault restriction is indicated.

ANY CERVICAL VERTEBRA
If an occiput and mandible lift produce a lean but no hold superior to that does, and if the lean appears to be in the neck, then a succession of lifts at progressively more inferior cervical vertebrae will localize the restriction in the neck.

FIRST RIBS HELD ANTERIOR AND SUPERIOR
A lift here may provide more detailed information about a restriction in the thorax than a lift from any part superior to this. More superior contacts may point inferiorly to something in the thorax, but this upper thoracic hold will provide a more detailed picture.

Combining assessment methods
General listening, ultraslow mobility testing (page 63), and lift listening can be combined in this way. With both hands, contact broadly on the top of the head, thumbs together along the midline. Compress down a bit more strongly than for usual general listening. Slowly slack the pressure, feeling the person spring back up in an ultraslow mobility fashion. Once neutral has been reached, continue very slowly lifting the parietal bones.

This method may be adapted for more inferior contacts.

General lift

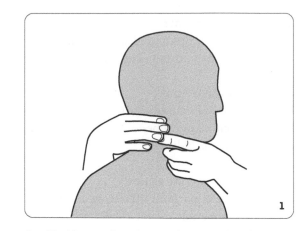

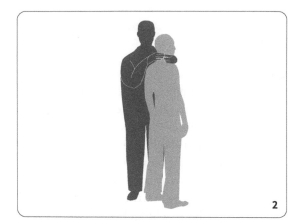

Stand beside your client. Support the occiput broadly with one hand. Support the mandible on the length of the thumb and pointer finger of the other hand with the chin resting on the web of that hand.

With this two hand contact, lift straight up, gently, and at a moderate pace. As you lift, watch and feel for where the body tilts at a point below your lifting hands. Note both the location of the tilt and the direction. These point to a primary lesion.

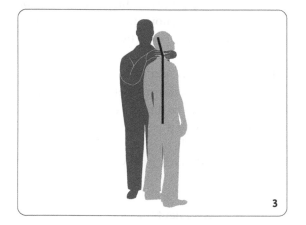

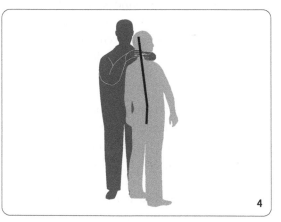

If the primary lesion is in the neck, the head will tilt. Observe both the direction of tilt and exact level in the neck where the tilt occurs. You must catch this "on the fly" as you lift. Once you have lifted the movement is over.

This example shows a tilt at the waist in a left-posterior direction.

With both hands used to lift the occiput and mandible, the lack of a third hand means less opportunity to employ inhibitory contact to confirm and refine the general lift finding. After the location of the apparent primary restriction has been found with a general lift, try a one-handed lift of the occiput, which frees the other hand to use for inhibitory contact. With a single-handed occipital lift, the direction of lift load is somewhat different. Lifting straight up on the occiput without a hand on the mandible would flex the neck. To compensate for this, use the occipital hand to give a slight rotary load posteriorly around a transverse axis through the atlanto-occipital articulation. This is a dynamic rotary load which does not rock the head back but keeps the head going straight up instead of allowing the neck to flex.

General lift (*cont.*)

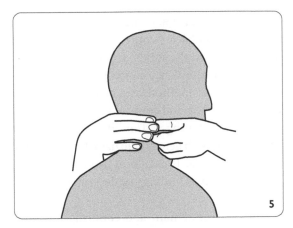

5

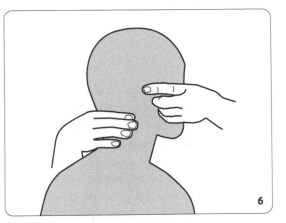

6

Lifting from the occiput and mandible will not find primary restrictions above the lifting hands. Lifting with one hand on the occiput and the other hand under the zygomatic arches provides more information about the lower part of the face, and the relationships between the facial bones and the cranial base.

Lifting from the occiput and sphenoid will provide more information about the cranial base, but not the vault. For the lifts shown in frames 5, 6, and 7, the tissue pulls must be felt. There will be nothing to see.

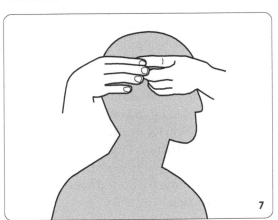

7

Lifting from the parietal bones and frontal bone will provide more information about the cranial vault. Some information about the cranial base will be felt, but in less detail than lifting from the occiput and sphenoid.

Lifting from higher in the head, above the mandible and occiput, provides more information about the head; however, higher lift points may miss some information lower in the body. Therefore, it is best to start with the lift from the occiput and mandible.

Lift listening, general listening, and general tap often point to the same lesion, confirming primacy. In situations where lift listening, general listening, and general tap point to two or more lesions, use local listening and inhibition to learn which of the two or three lesions found with general assessment methods is the most primary.

Once the general location of a primary lesion has been found, other assessment methods are used to refine awareness of the lesion to specific depth in the body and tissue type.

ASSESSMENT
METHOD 2

Assessment method 3: general tap

Origin
Jeffrey Burch.

Concept
Many creatures, including bats and dolphins, learn about their world by emitting sound waves that echo back. The creature interprets the reflected sound to learn about the shape and movement of the world around it. Woodpeckers find grubs in wood by tapping on trees. Humans have learned to use this principle as sonar and ultrasound imaging. Geologists put shock waves through the ground to learn more about the layered structure of rock. Waves used can be audible, supersonic, or subsonic. The general tap assessment method uses a single tap, much as a woodpecker does.

Principle
A single impulse is put into the body perpendicular to the surface. How this ripples out through the body is both seen with the eyes as ripples in the client's body and felt with the hand as reflected impulses.

Method
With a single finger, deliver a tap to the top of the head. Rather than bouncing off the head, leave the now relaxed finger in contact with the head. Both feel with the finger the echo reflected from the body and see with the eyes where tissue moves in response to the tap. With the combined visual and felt sense information locate the primary restriction.

This may be done standing, seated, or supine. Seated will tend to miss information inferior to the sitz bones. Supine will make it harder to see information posterior in the body with the eye; however, posterior information may still be felt with the hand.

Verification and refinement
Sonar taps will lead you to areas of reduced mobility. When the tap is delivered on the top of the head, the disturbance found is usually primary. Other methods can be used to further verify the finding and confirm primacy.

General listening and/or lift listening should be compared with general tap data. Do they point to the same area? If not, local listen and inhibit between the two findings to determine relative primacy.

Further refinement and confirmation then proceed in the usual way which may include any or all of the following, and/or other assessment methods.

- Local listening to an area will show whether an actively changing somatic dysfunction has been found, and if it is actively changing, then local listening will help further localize the issue.
- Manual thermal assessment may provide verification and additional detail.
- Layer listening and/or layer palpation will further help localize the issue.
- If the restriction found by *tap* from the top of the head is a relatively large area of the body, then local *taps* can refine localization.
- Yes/no questions may provide additional information.
- As with all other assessment methods, *always* confirm with mobility testing.

General tap

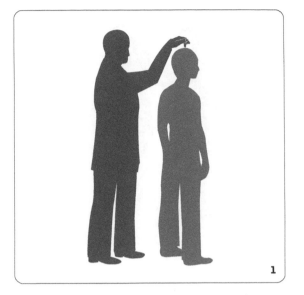

Stand behind the client with the tip of your middle finger poised over the highest point of the client's head.

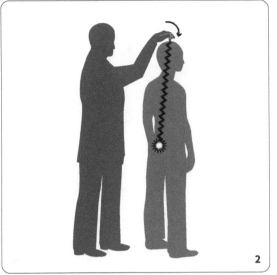

Tap the top of the client's head with the tip (not pad) of your middle finger and stay in contact with the client's head in a relaxed way so you can feel the reflection of your tap impulse back from the person's body. In addition to feeling the echo of the tap, look for a subtle directional ripple in the client's body. In this example, this points to a primary restriction near the left hip.

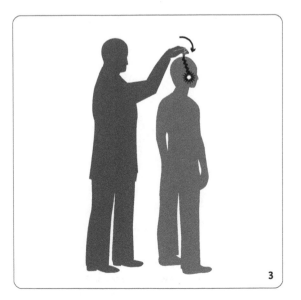

This example points to a primary restriction near the right temporomandibular joint.

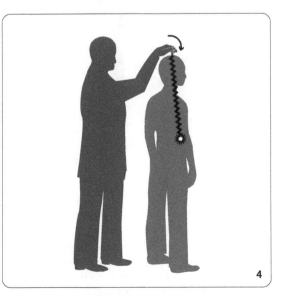

In this example, the reflection and ripple point to the right elbow.

General tap (*cont.*)

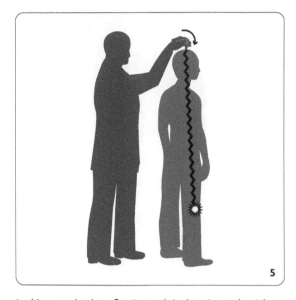

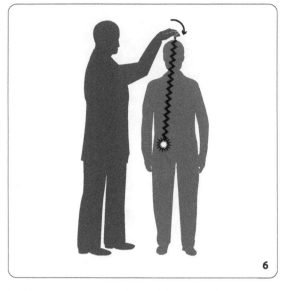

In this example, the reflection and ripple point to the right knee.

In this example, the reflection and ripple point to near the left sacroiliac joint.

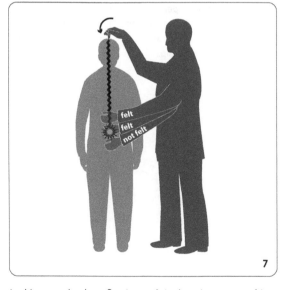

In this example, the reflection and ripple point to something near the upper lumbar spine.

A way to both confirm a general tap finding and to refine your awareness of its location is to place a relaxed hand near the location of the perceived point where the ripple line ends and the reflected impulse seems to come from. With your confirming hand resting comfortably relaxed in this location, tap again. If your confirming hand is on the spot or between your tapping finger and your confirming hand, then your confirming hand will feel the ripple from this new tap. If your confirming hand is beyond the spot, your sensing hand will not feel the ripple.

LOCAL ASSESSMENT METHODS

After using the three general assessment methods to find the location of the primary restriction, we next utilize additional tests to gain a more detailed description of the exact size, shape, depth, and anatomy of the currently primary structure(s).

The more information we have about the primary restriction, the better we can design an effective and efficient treatment.

Several different local assessment methods are always brought to bear on this question. Like general assessment methods, local assessment methods are useful and imperfect.

Each assessment method provides part of the picture. The information provided by each assessment method may be complete—at least as far as that method can go—and may be fully accurate. Usually not. For these reasons we always use several assessment methods, comparing their results.

This section lists and gives detailed instructions for nine local assessment methods. Some of these are very specific tests such as local listening or manual thermal evaluation. Others are broad categories of assessments such as mobility testing or orthopedic testing.

Each of us finds some methods easier to use than others. Often, we have other kinds of preferences for some methods over others. It is essential to learn and be able to use all the assessment methods. Each assessment method has its place, and sometimes no other method will fill the bill.

Assessment method 4: local listening

Origin
Various "listening" assessment methods have been in use by osteopaths since at least the 1930s. This version was developed by Jean-Pierre Barral DO.

Concept
Once the general location of a primary restriction has been found with one or usually more of the three general assessment methods, we next confirm there is actively changing tissue in that area and seek more information about that tissue and its abnormality as a guide to treatment. A much-used early step in this further characterization is local listening.

Method
For treatment with functional methods, we wish to find tissues with a set of three qualities:

1. Tissue texture that is inappropriate; this may be too much fiber or not enough fiber. The problem may be within a tissue or between tissues. No fiber should connect tissues that should glide on each other.

2. Tissues whose tone or elasticity the body is currently changing.

3. Tissues whose distortion is well connected to several other distortions in a chain or web of lesions.

If a tissue with these three characteristics is gently touched, the tissue will respond by pulling the hand in a particular direction. This feels like the first leg of an unwind. An important difference is that the listening pull will go in one direction then stop, while an unwind will continue in a succession of different directions.

For local listening, use a hand surface appropriately sized for the tissue approached. With larger areas, use the heel of the hand. For fine structures, use a fingertip. Avoid using two or more fingertips together as this can lead to confusion.

Qualities of the local listening tissue pull

- The tissue pull may be linear or curved. The smaller the radius of a curve, the deeper in the body the issue is. A spin in place indicates a tissue which is quite deep. A tissue with a straight pull is near the surface. A tissue with a curved pull lies at intermediate depth.
- The pull may be slow or at a moderate pace. Speed has no known meaning.
- The pull may feel weak or moderate in strength. Strength of pull has no known meaning.

Comparing two lesions to decide which to work on first

This process has the not very descriptive name of "inhibition."

If two areas of interest in the body are found with local listening, they can be compared to learn which one is relatively more primary. For most pairs of tissue disturbances, if one is worked on first, it will help release the other one; however, this is usually not a two-way street. Therefore, for efficient work, it is essential to find out which of the two restrictions will have the greater effect on the other when treated. We refer to the disturbance or lesion with the greater effect on the other as "relative primary." In this context, primary means only that we should treat it first. Primary in this context does not mean the lesion is stronger or occurred first in time.

To find out which of two lesions is the more primary, we use a process called "inhibition." In this context "inhibition" means an "as if" treatment, to find out which of the two lesions has

the greater effect on the other. To perform this test, we will arbitrarily label the two lesions as J and K. To perform an inhibition test, touch lesion J with a hand, note the direction of tissue pull, and maintain contact; keep your attention here. As you maintain this contact and attention, use your other hand to touch lesion K. Follow the movement K makes and slightly accentuate this movement at the end. The question is: As you contact, follow, and accentuate the movement of lesion K, does lesion J move again? In effect, we made an "as if" treatment of lesion K; if the faux treatment of K creates a change in J, we know that treating lesion K will cause lesion J to release also, at least partially.

The change in movement of lesion J will most commonly be a reversal of its original movement; however, do not be attached to this. The movement may be any other movement including a resumption of the original movement, or a completely different movement. The direction of the new movement has no known meaning.

If following and exaggerating the movement at K changes J, then K is the more primary of the two. If listening to K does not change J, this does not mean that J is primary to K; finding out if J is primary to K requires a separate test. It is possible there is a nondominance between J and K either way. The testing must be done the other way around: touch K first, following its first movement, then touch, follow, and accentuate J.

To compare three or more lesions, make pairwise comparisons.

Occasionally, neither lesion will cause a change in the other. This means there is something in the body that is substantially more primary than either of these two. Return to general assessment methods to find that area. Look for what you missed in the first round. Sometimes there is a very small first movement followed immediately by a larger second movement which distracts from the first.

It is also possible for each of the two lesions to equally inhibit the other. This may mean the two areas are two parts of the same structure. Think through anatomy to find what may continue between these two points. For example, consider nerve or vascular lesions. Another possibility is the two areas should be treated concurrently.

Important note—Each lesion will exhibit some combination of linear or curved pull with a particular direction. None of these characteristics says anything about the relative primacy of the lesion. Strength or distance of pull is *not* important in determining primacy. Using inhibition, a tissue pull of any strength or direction may be found primary.

Determining the second and subsequent areas to be treated

When two areas are compared, and one is found primary, the more primary should be treated first. Treating this first lesion will alter much of the person's system, well beyond the area treated. We now have no information about what should be treated second. The second lesion tested earlier and found not to be primary is no more likely than anything else in the body to be the new primary. Treating anything in the body shuffles the person's deck. It is essential after each move to go back to the beginning of assessment utilizing general assessment methods.

Local listening

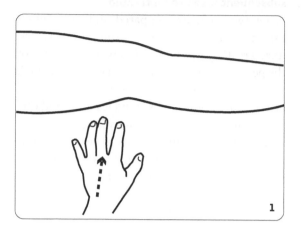

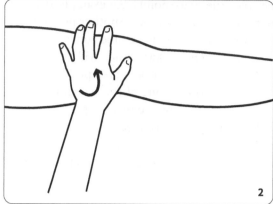

Approach the client's body with a relaxed hand. If there is an actively changing lesion where you touch, the client's tissue will pull your hand in a particular direction. This resembles the first leg of unwinding except it stops at the end of the first movement rather than continuing into further legs of unwind.

If there is a tissue pull, that pull will have a particular direction, speed, and distance and it may be a straight pull or curved. The degree of curve tells us how near the surface of the body the lesion is. Meaning has not been discovered for direction, speed, or distance.

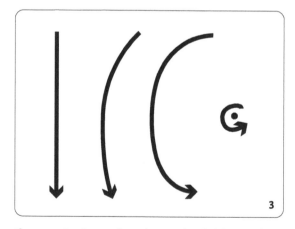

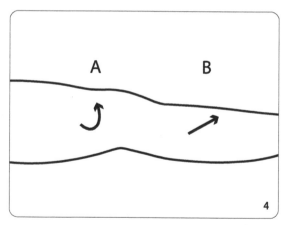

If present, the tissue pull may be straight, slightly curved, more curved, or a rotation in place. A straight pull suggests the lesion is near the surface of the body. The smaller the radius of the curve, the deeper in the body it is. A spin in place suggests the lesion is quite deep in the body.

Two or more tissue pulls may be found at any distance from each other in the body. There is an assessment method to determine which of the two lesions represented by tissue pulls is the relative primary. This method is illustrated in the following frames.

Local listening (*cont.*)

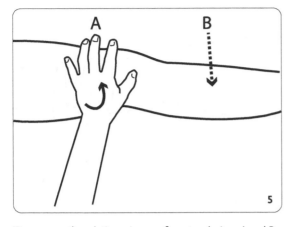

5

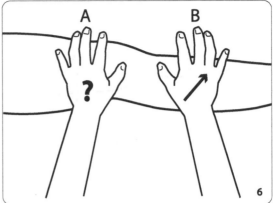

6

To compare the relative primacy of any two lesions A and B we must ask two separate questions: 1) Is lesion B primary to lesion A? and 2) Is lesion A primary to lesion B? The first step is to ask each of these two questions comparing the primacy of two lesions is to touch one of the lesions, in this case A, feel its pull, and once it stops stay in contact with a relaxed hand and aware of this area.

Next, use your other hand to contact the other lesion, in this case B. Watch for immediate movement in lesion A.

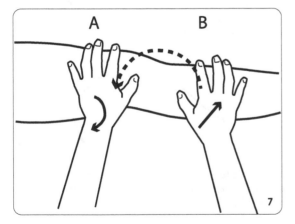

7

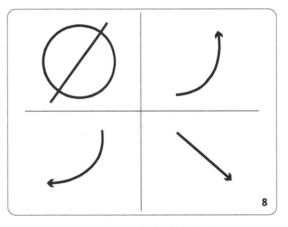

8

If lesion A promptly moves in response to your contact at lesion B, this suggests lesion B is primary to lesion A, which means that if you treat lesion B, lesion A is likely to be changed also. Whether or not lesion A moves in response to your contact at lesion B, remove both hands as soon as this test is complete.

In response to your contact at lesion B, lesion A may or may not move. If lesion A moves in response to your contact at lesion B the movement of lesion A will most often be opposite in direction to its original movement, but it may be further movement in the original direction, or it may be a new different movement. The direction, degree of curve, distance, and speed of the new movement of lesion A is not important for this test. What is important is whether lesion A moves or not.

Local listening (*cont.*)

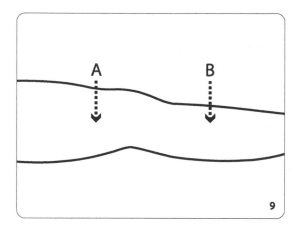

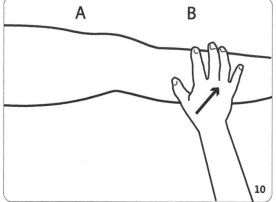

Next, whether lesion B appears to be primary to lesion A or not, perform the test the other way around to ask a new question: Is lesion A primary to lesion B? The process is the same as for the previous question we asked of the body except the order of touching lesions A and B is reversed.

First touch lesion B with a relaxed hand. Note the direction, speed, distance, and degree of curve of the tissue pull. When the tissue pull stops, leave your relaxed hand in place monitoring this area.

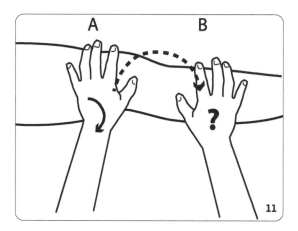

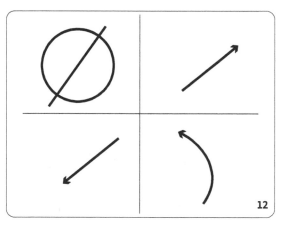

Next, use your other hand to contact lesion A. Note whether the tissue under your hand at lesion B promptly moves or not in response to your contact at lesion A. If lesion B moves that indicates lesion A is primary to lesion B.

In response to your contact at lesion A, lesion B may or may not move. If lesion B moves this indicates that lesion A is primary to lesion B. The direction and other qualities of movement at lesion B in response to your contact at lesion A are unimportant. What is significant is if lesion B moves or not. There may be no movement, movement in a direction opposite to the original movement of lesion B, movement in the same direction as the original movement of lesion B, or movement in a new direction.

The results of asking these two questions about the relative primacy of two lesions may be: A is primary to B, B is primary to A, A and B each affect the other, which can be called co-primacy, or neither A nor B affects the other, which can be called nondominance. Co-primacy may indicate either that the two lesions are very close to each other in degree of relative primacy, or the two areas are part of the same structure, in which case consider anatomy. Nondominance indicates the two lesions are not well connected to each other, in which case there is also usually a third lesion which is primary to both.

Assessment method 5: local lift

Origin
Jeffrey Burch.

Concept
Any portion of a standing person may be lifted to gather more detailed information about primary or relative primary restrictions located inferior to that point of lift.

Method
Ask the client to stand in a relaxed fashion. Gently contact and slowly lift. It may be useful to have the client slump a little or to slightly compress the client down before lifting up.

As you slowly and gently lift, notice the first direction of lean and/or felt sense of tethering down. Note how far down the body the tethering is.

Lifting can be done from diverse locations including, but not limited to:

- Costal margin—If a lift from more superiorly, or information from a different general assessment method, points to something inferior to the costal margin but gives a hazy outline, more detail can be gathered by lifting the costal margin.

- Iliac crests—Similarly, one or both iliac crests can be lifted to provide more detailed information about primary or relative primary restrictions inferior to that level.
- Greater trochanters—In the same way, one or both greater trochanters can be lifted to provide information about structures inferior to that. If a lean appears when lifting an iliac crest but not a greater trochanter, the primary restriction lies between the two.
- Distal femur—Medial and/or lateral malleoli of the ankle.

Combining assessment methods
Ultraslow mobility testing and lift listening can be combined as they were for general lift. With both hands contact the area to be lifted. Compress down to a moderate degree which is comfortable for the client. Slowly slack the compression, feeling the tissue below your hands spring back up in an ultraslow mobility fashion. Once neutral has been reached, continue very slowly lifting the area which had been compressed.

Local lift

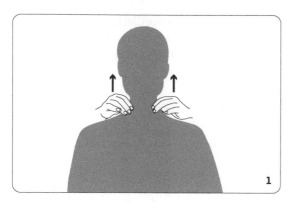

Lift from any cervical vertebra by supporting under the left and right transverse processes.

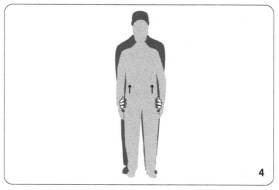

Lift the first ribs, supporting under the medial ends of both the left and right first rib.

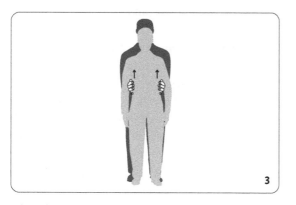

Lift the lower rib cage.

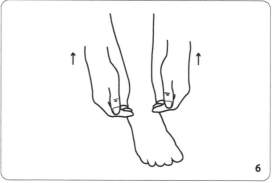

Lift both greater trochanters of the femur.

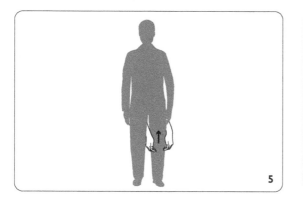

Lift the distal end of the femur supporting under the condyles at the knee joint line.

Lift the lower leg supporting under the medial and lateral malleoli.

The local lift assessment method provides information about portions of the body inferior to the lift point(s). Lifting can be done from many different areas of the body. Six of the many possibilities are shown in these illustrations.

Assessment method 6: local tap

Origin
Jeffrey Burch.

Concept
See the section on general tap for a description of how reflected mechanical waves from sharp impulses are used by many animals and some people to locate things of interest.

Principle
A single impulse is put into the body perpendicular to the surface. How this ripples out through the body is both observed with the eyes and reflections of the impulse are felt with the hand.

Method
After locating a primary restriction with one of the general assessment methods, one way to confirm the existence of the restriction and to further localize it is with local tap. To do this, use a single finger to deliver a tap to an area of the body near but not on the apparent primary. Rather than bouncing off the body, leave the now relaxed finger in contact with the body. Both feel with the finger the echo reflected from the body and see with the eyes where tissue moves in response to the tap.

Next, make a second tap in a new place at a different angle from the apparent primary. Both see and feel the line of ripple from this second impulse, noting where this line crossed the line of ripple from the first local tap. This intersection marks the location of the primary.

Then make a third tap in yet another place at yet a different angle from the apparent primary. Does the ripple from this cross the intersection from the first two? If so, you have a double confirmation. If the new intersection is in a different spot, local listen to both spots. Is there a local listening pull in both spots? If only one has a local listening pull, then it is the primary. If both spots have local listening pulls, inhibit between the two to determine which of the two is more primary.

Variation
The other hand may be placed at another location in the body not on the anticipated primary as an additional receiver.

Verification and refinement
Once the apparent primary is found, other methods are always used to further characterize the finding and determine its size, shape, and depth from the surface of the body.

Local tap

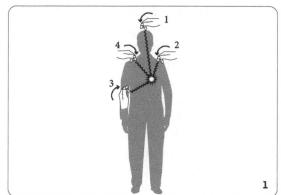

1

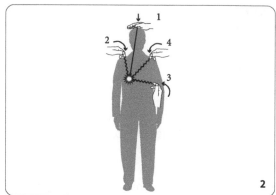

2

General tap points to the vicinity of the left sixth costal cartilage. A succession of single taps at the left acromion process, proximal end of the right clavicle, and the anterolateral portion of the right eighth rib confirm this finding.

General listening points to the lower right anterior rib cage. A succession of single taps at the middle of the right clavicle, the distal end of the left clavicle, and the left costal margin anterolaterally confirm this finding.

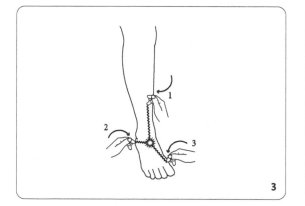

3

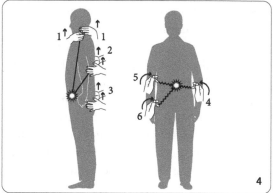

4

General listening points to the right lower limb. Inhibition at the greater trochanter confirms a lesion in the lower limb. Inhibition at the right lateral malleolus points to this primary lesion being in the foot or ankle. A single tap on the distal tibia about 10 cm superior to its distal end points toward the navicular area. Further single taps at the heel and at the distal end of the first metatarsal confirm this finding and refine awareness to the talo-navicular joint.

Lift listening from the mandible and occiput point to the left side of the lower abdomen. Local lift at the inferior margin of the rib cage confirms this. Local lift at the greater trochanters does not show a primary lesion inferior to this lift point, which adds weight to the lower abdomen finding by exclusion. A succession of three single taps at the left anterior superior iliac spine (ASIS), lateral part of the right costal margin, and the right greater trochanter confirm the lower left abdominal finding.

Local tap is used for confirmation and refinement. Any of the three general methods may point toward a primary lesion. A succession of single taps, each from a different point on the body, may both confirm the general finding and further describe its location and size. The examples on this page each start with one of the general assessment methods: listening, tap, or lift. For each example, a succession of several single taps are shown as they are used to both confirm and refine awareness of the lesion. Following the use of local tap, additional assessment methods must be used to determine the depth from the surface at which the lesion lies, its tissue type(s), and its current state of elasticity. The four examples shown are a few of the many thousand possibilities.

Assessment method 7: layer awareness

The general assessment methods show us the general location of the currently primary lesion and may give us a loose idea of the size and shape of the lesion. Next, we use other methods including manual thermal assessment, local tap, and local listening to describe the size and shape of the restriction in more detail.

A further step is to learn how deep in the body the restriction lies. Local listening can give us a loose idea if the restriction is near the surface, very deep, or somewhere in between. We must refine this awareness with additional tests to know exactly what layer the restriction is in.

Learning how to know what layer of tissue the primary restriction is in is a two-step process.

1. Learn and practice distinguishing between layers of tissue in the body by palpating with your hands.
2. Building on this felt sense of layers we next learn to recognize in which layer of tissue the primary restriction resides.

These two skills are described on the following pages.

Assessment method 8: layer palpation

Origin

Classic manual therapy method, origin lost.

Concept

Tissues vary from each other in texture. Some are firmer, others softer. Some are smooth, others more granular. By sinking into the body slowly with the hand, it is easy to distinguish layers of tissue by their texture.

Method

Let your hand and whole upper limb be relaxed. Arrange your hand so the wrist is in the middle half of its range of motion as the client's body is touched. With a very soft hand, touch just the skin and notice its texture. Very slowly and gently, increase the pressure until a texture change is noted. Just under the skin is the superficial fascia, which is also the superficial adipose layer; this feels more liquid than skin. The next layer is the investing fascia, which is a thin, tough layer.

Go slowly; the investing fascia is so thin it is easy to zip past it.

These first three layers are to be found everywhere on the body. Deeper layers vary with location on the body. Sink deeper in with a combination of very gently increasing pressure and with intention. Although pressure must increase a little to reach deeper layers, keep the hand as relaxed as possible.

If you can name the tissue layers as you go, that is very good; if not, note the texture changes and depth. That is enough information to get you to the layer you need.

Practice this component skill on several parts of the body and on several people.

When this skill is developed, build upon it, combining it with local listening to identify the tissue layer containing the primary restriction. This layer listening skill is described in the next section.

Layer palpation

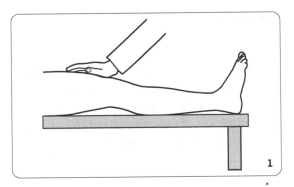

Gently contact the skin and notice its texture.

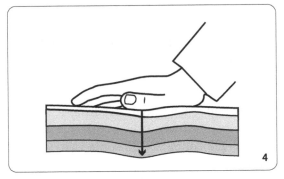

With a mixture of slightly more pressure and intent, sink into the next layer of tissue; notice how its texture differs from the skin.

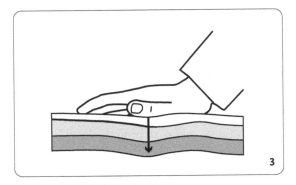

Now slowly sink a little deeper, feeling the texture of the next layer; notice its unique texture. Is it softer or firmer than the one above? Notice the thickness of this layer.

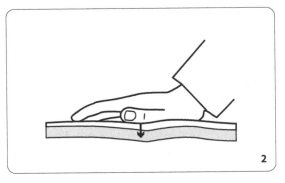

Sink a little deeper, noting the qualities of the next layer of tissue. In what ways is it like earlier layers, and how is it different?

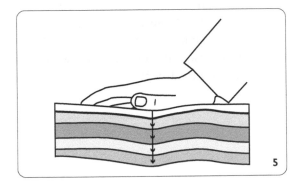

Continue to sink slowly through layers, noting the qualities of each.

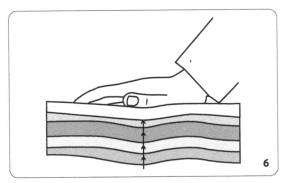

As you back out toward the surface you can again notice the qualities of each layer.

Details will vary depending on where on the body you contact. If you are able to, name the tissues as you feel each one; if not, simply experience the various textures and recognize their depths from the surface. Palpatory recognition of layers of tissue allows treatment to be precisely directed to the relevant layer.

Assessment method 9: layer listening

Origin
Uncertain origin. Taught by Jean-Pierre Barral DO and his associates.

Concept
Once a primary lesion has been located using the general assessment methods, confirmed with inhibition, and further characterized with local assessment methods, it is useful to determine what tissue layer the lesion is in. This may be in any layer from skin down to the deepest layers of bone or internal organs. Knowing depth as well as surface markers allows treatment to be more precisely applied yielding stronger results. Depth localization is accomplished by bringing layer palpation together with local listening and inhibition.

Method
Note the direction, speed, and distance traveled of the first pull when the tissue is contacted. Then break contact. This is the same as local listening.

As you return to the tissue, sink slowly through layers of tissue noting any pull in each layer. Progress slowly deeper until a layer is found which exhibits the same pull initially found. This is the layer to treat.

THE DETAILS

- As you contact the skin, note if the pull in the skin matches the direction, speed, and distance of the local listening pull. If it does, then the primary restriction is in the skin. If the pull in the skin is different in any way, direction, speed, or distance then the skin is not the layer containing the primary restriction. The skin may have no pull, which is certainly different than the local listening pull and a clear message the skin is not primary.

- If the primary restriction is in the skin, choose and apply a treatment technique. If the skin does not demonstrate the local listening pull, sink slightly deeper to the superficial fascia to see if it has the characteristics of the local listening. If not, proceed slowly deeper until the layer with a tissue pull matching the local listening is found.

- Once the layer containing the local listening pull qualities is found, do not proceed to test deeper. This is a waste of time.

- If the layered anatomy is known, think through this as you sink deeper. If the anatomy of the region is not known, simply sink until the layer of the relative primary lesion is found, then engage that layer for treatment.

Layer listening

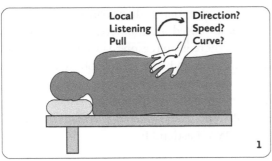

Contact for local listening. Note the qualities of the tissue pull: speed, distance, direction, degree of curve. Then break contact.

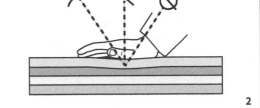

Contact again, being careful to focus on just the skin. Are all the qualities of pull noted in Step 1 present in the skin? If so, the restriction is in the skin. If not, the restriction is in a deeper layer.

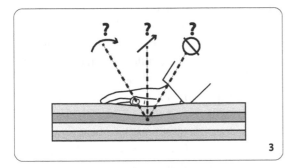

If the skin does not have all the qualities of the local listening pull, sink to the next layer as in layer palpation. If the second layer has all the qualities of the local listening pull, that is the layer to treat.

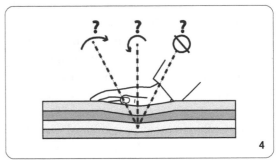

If the second layer of tissue does not have all of the qualities of the local listening pull, then proceed to the third layer to ask the same question. If the local listening pull is not in this layer, continue to the next layer.

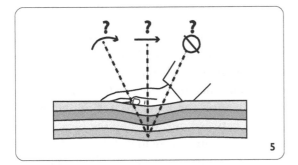

Continue through the layers of tissue one at a time until the layer is found...

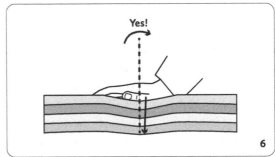

...which has the local listening pull felt at the beginning. This is the layer to treat.

Layer listening brings together the methods of local listening, and layer palpation, to ask the question: In what layer of tissue is the lesion to be treated? In each layer there are three possibilities: 1) All of the tissue pull qualities felt for this area with local listening. 2) A tissue pull partly or completely different from the local listening pull for this area. 3) No tissue pull. The layer that has all of the qualities of the local listening pull is the layer to be treated.

Assessment method 10: manual thermal evaluation

Origin

Manual thermal evaluation was developed by Jean-Pierre Barral DO. One day, Barral was treating a woman in his practice. As he moved his hand toward where he would work next, his hand passed through the air a few inches above her anterior thorax. He noticed a strong focal heat projection. In conversation with the client, Barral learned a mammogram had found a 3 mm tumor at this site.

Concept

Our bodies radiate heat. The temperature of the radiated heat varies from one area of the body to another. Changes in body function and structure change the heat radiated. Our hands are remarkably sensitive to differences in radiated heat between one area of the body and another. The meaning of changes in radiated heat are by themselves nonspecific. Assessment of local radiated heat differences can be combined with other kinds of testing to provide meaning very relevant to treatment design.

Development

After his first experience with palpably greater radiated heat over a small tumor, Barral became curious if other disturbances in the body would alter the heat radiated from the body. Scanning the body with his hand, Barral quickly found heat variations, many of which correlated with disturbances in the body that he found by other means, and which were useful for him to treat.

Using handheld, laser-based thermometers, Barral was able to demonstrate that the human hand scanning about 10 cm off the body can detect differences in temperature from one area to another of less than 1/100 °C. For some years, such a laser thermometer was used by some practitioners to detect disturbances in the body. These laser-based thermometers have fallen out of use as there is no reason to buy an instrument when the human hand can reliably do the job.

Barral developed this into an assessment method which he has published in a book: Barral, J.-P. (1996, 2005) *Manual Thermal Evaluation*. Seattle, WA: Eastland Press.

Additional features

The human hand can detect tiny differences in heat between one area of the body and another; however, when the differences are quite small, the therapist will often not be accurate as to which of two adjacent areas is the warmer and which the cooler. While this is troublesome, the fact that there is a local difference in temperature perceptible to the trained hand is quite useful.

Clothing is insulative and should interfere with perception of radiated heat. In fact, thin clothing does not alter perceived heat projection. Our hands have been demonstrated to also be sensitive to microwaves and adjacent radio frequencies. Apparently, sensitivity to these longer wavelengths accounts for an important part of what we perceive as variations in heat.

Method

Maintain the hand about 10 cm off the body. With the hand open and the palm facing the client's body, move the hand over the body at a rate of about 0.5 meters per second (m/sec).

By moving the hand, heat differences are noticed between one area and the next. Movement of the hand is essential; if the hand stays in one spot over the body, radiated heat will build up between the hand and the client's body and no useful information will be transferred. It is the contrast from one area to the next that informs us.

Always confirm results

Barral has said he never treats based on manual thermal evaluation only. For one thing, manual thermal evaluation tells us there is a disturbance, not its relative primacy. Manual thermal evaluation also does not tell us how deep in the body the lesion is. Always use additional assessment methods to confirm the results of manual thermal evaluation, and to determine their relative primacy.

Manual thermal evaluation

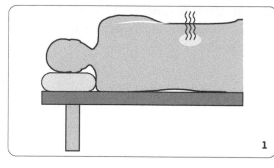

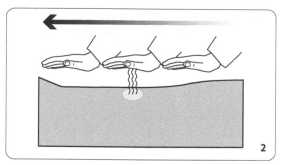

Areas of disturbance in the body are often either warmer or cooler than neighboring areas. The temperature difference may be several degrees or as little as 1/100 degree. Large temperature differences can be felt with hand contact on the skin. For the more common small temperature differences, physical contact will distract from the temperature awareness.

These small temperature differences are best felt as radiated heat about 10 cm off the body. Large temperature differences will also be felt with these sweeps. Sweep your hand over the body at about 0.5 m/sec, feeling for differences in temperature as you sweep. Keep moving; if you hover in one spot you cannot feel the temperature contrast.

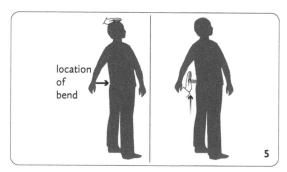

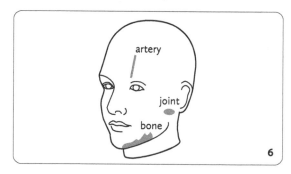

Areas of disturbance may be either warmer or cooler than adjacent areas. For very small temperature differences, our perceptions about whether it is cooler or hotter than adjacent tissue may not be accurate. What is important for us is to recognize the radiated temperature as different from adjacent areas.

The location, size, and shape of the area of radiated heat may suggest anatomy. The radiated heat may have the shape of an organ or may be the size and shape of a joint. Narrow linear heat signatures may represent nerves or vasculature. Manual thermal scanning gives no direct information about depth from the surface of the body.

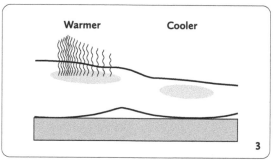

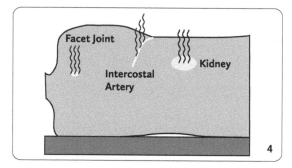

Manual thermal assessment can quickly confirm the presence of a restriction found by a general assessment method and provide additional detail about the shape and size of the restriction.

Usually more than one area of thermal projection can be found. Pairwise comparisons between these several areas can be made using local listening and inhibition to determine relative primacy. See section on local listening and inhibition.

Assessment method 11: ultraslow mobility testing

Origin
Jeffrey Burch.

Concept
For any limitation in joint movement there are usually several limiting factors. Some of these limiting factors will be felt at shorter distances of joint movement than others. Finding and releasing these limitations in order from the one found at the shortest distance of testing to longest often works well. If the therapist moves the joint very slowly, the shortest limiting tissue will be encountered first. If movement is a little faster, the early limitations may not be recognized.

The protocol written below is for joints. The same procedure is adaptable for a wide range of tissues.

Method

1. With the hands as relaxed as practical, contact the tissue on both sides of the joint as close to the joint line as practical. Feel into the joint and maintain awareness in the joint throughout the rest of the procedure; at the same time let your awareness be broad in surrounding tissues.

2. Mobility test the joint to end range. Note the results, both the excursion and the effort required to move through the range. Excursion will be greater in some directions than in others. Some directions may have less than normal range of motions, suggesting fibrosity. Other directions may have greater than normal mobility, suggesting laxity. Note all these differences of normal range, subnormal range, and abnormally large range, as well as the effort required to move through the range.

3. Let the joint settle back to a neutral position.

4. Select a direction of reduced range in which you wish to increase the range of motion. Do *not* choose a direction of laxity for this. Displace the joint to end range in the direction opposite the direction you wish to increase; however, if this is a direction of laxity, exercise caution and restraint displacing the joint to less than full range in the lax direction. Extremely slowly, start to move the joint back toward the direction whose range you wish to increase. Initially, a certain amount of effort will be required to move the joint, but after a short distance a greater amount of effort will be required to further move the joint. Precisely as this increase in effort is noted, feel the direction and location of the tight element that is now resisting movement.

5. With palpation and knowledge of anatomy, discern what this limiting factor is.

6. Return the joint to neutral.

7. Treat to reduce the fibrosity in the limiting area.

8. Retest the overall range of motion. Is it the same as before treatment or has it changed?

9. Again, extremely slowly test the joint mobility as in step 4. Is the first limitation in the same area or in a different area?
   a. If the limitation is in the same area as before, treat it more.
   b. If the limitation is in a new area, return to step 7 for this new area.

10. Cycle through steps 1–9, releasing restrictions found at progressively longer distances.

11. Mobility test to end range. Note how this is different from the original end range mobility tests.

Important elements

- Each joint will have more than one direction of movement. Explore each.
- Each joint will tolerate only so much work on a given day. Too much work will create inflammation. Inflammation will lead to more fibrosity in the long run. At the first tiny hint of swelling or edema, *stop* working on that joint for that day. Either turn your attention to other areas of the body or end the treatment session.
- Avoid pain. Pain is indicative of tissue damage. Ask the client to tell you if there is pain. Some clients will try to be stoic; this is counterproductive. If the client experiences pain, *stop*. Try less force or a different technique. If a way is not found to work on an area comfortably, *stop*. Shift to working on another area.

- An analogy to this process is a weight suspended from the ceiling by not one but by several cords. The cords are not all equal length, so the weight is initially suspended by the shortest one or two. The shortest ones can be seen because of the gravitational load on them. When the shortest cord is lengthened, we then see the next shortest one. One at a time, the cords can be lengthened until the weight is distributed on them all. In this process, any particular cord may be returned to more than once.
- The shortest limiting factor may not be the toughest. How short a tissue is does not correlate with how easy or challenging it is to change. Let yourself be surprised.

Ultraslow mobility testing

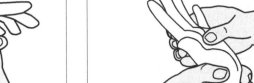

Mobility test the area to be treated. In this case, the goal is to improve wrist flexion. A wide range of diverse tissues may be assessed in this way.

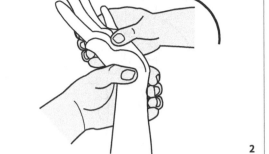

Having noted the end range of flexion and the effort required to move through the range of flexion, then fully extend the wrist.

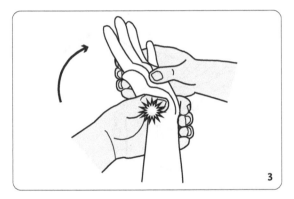

After fully extending the wrist, begin to flex the wrist extremely slowly. Note the location of the first slightest resistance to flexion. This may be at the joint or at some distance.

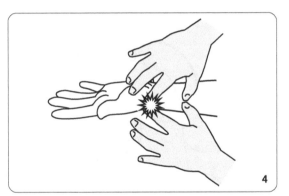

Explore the area of first resistance to flexion discovered in step 3 to further localize and characterize it. Treat that area.

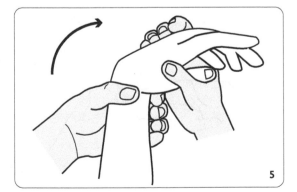

Again, mobility test the full range of wrist flexion noting both end range and effort through the range. At least one and usually both factors will have improved.

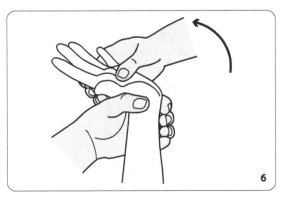

Again, fully extend the wrist as in step 2.

Ultraslow mobility testing (*cont.*)

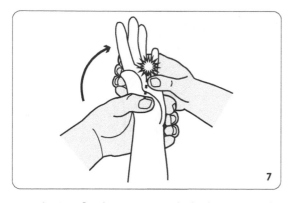

Again, begin to flex the wrist extremely slowly starting at the fully extended position. Note the first hint of resistance. The location of this resistance will likely be at a different location than previously in step 3.

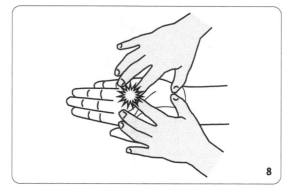

Explore the area where the first resistance was discovered in step 7 to further localize and characterize it. Treat that area. This is the same as step 4 but likely for a different area.

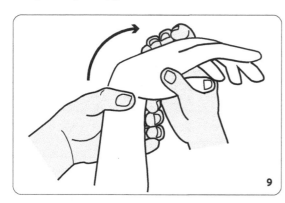

Again, mobility test the full range of flexion, noting both range of motion and effort through the range. At least one and usually both factors will have improved.

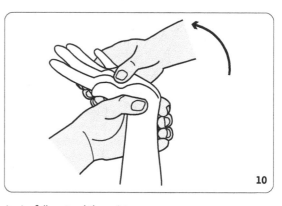

Again, fully extend the wrist.

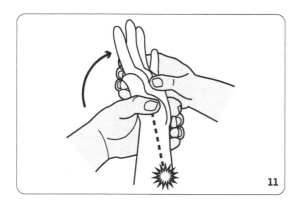

Again, flex the wrist extremely slowly, noting the first slightest resistance to movement. This is the same activity as steps 3 and 7 but will likely lead to a new area.

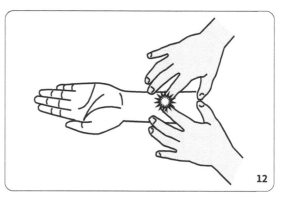

Explore the new area of slight resistance to further localize and characterize it. Treat this area. This is the same activity as in steps 4 and 8 but for a new area.

Assessment method 12: ruling out false positives on orthopedic tests

Origin
Unknown.

Background
Many orthopedic tests have been developed which give suggestive information about the health of certain tissues in the body, often ligaments or cartilages, and sometimes other tissues. The results of orthopedic tests are always suggestive, not definitive. They are good screening tests. Positive results on tests are often followed up with imaging studies to gain more definitive results.

Concept
Orthopedic tests sometimes give either false positive or false negative results. Listening techniques, including inhibition, will sometimes support the result of an orthopedic test. In other instances, inhibition can both suggest that the result of an orthopedic test is false and point toward a way to relieve the complaint.

If a test result appears to be false, then it may be possible to locate a distant tissue, which will relieve a symptomatic area that had exhibited the seemingly false positive on the orthopedic test.

If none of these methods suggest a false positive, this supports the original positive test result. However, while better supported, this is still not definitive.

Method

1. Note a complaint that may have a biomechanical basis.
2. Perform orthopedic tests related to that area. For example, the knee:

Orthopedic test	Test looks for signs of
patellar grind test	chondromalacia patellae

collateral ligament test	laxity in medial and/or lateral collateral ligaments
drawer test	laxity or evulsion of anterior and/or posterior cruciate ligaments
McMurray test	damaged portions of knee menisci

3. When a positive test result is found, try any or all of the following:
   a. Extended listening
   b. Shift from orthopedic testing to first barrier tissue engagement at the area tested. Note any extended listenings. Successively perform inhibition in both directions between the symptomatic area and the area to which the extended listening was felt. If the area of the extended listening inhibits the tissue pull at the symptomatic area, this suggests that the test result was a false positive. If this is found, then redo the orthopedic test while maintaining the inhibition. If the result of the test is now negative, it is likely that treating the area of the extended listening will decrease the symptom.
   c. General listening
   d. Perform general listening. Using inhibition, compare the result of general listening with the symptomatic area. If the area found with general listening inhibits the tissue pull at the symptomatic area, then try redoing the orthopedic test while inhibiting the area found with general listening. If the result of the orthopedic test is now negative, the orthopedic test was likely a false positive and treating the area of the general listening will likely reduce the symptom.
   e. Local listening
   f. Local listen to tissue in several areas

gradually radiating out from the symptomatic area in any direction. Using inhibition, test any tissue pulls found against the symptomatic area with inhibition. If an area is found which inhibits the tissue pull at the symptomatic area, then redo the orthopedic test while inhibiting that area. If the orthopedic test now has a negative result, this both supports the idea that the first test result was a false positive, and it is likely that treating the distant area will reduce the symptom.

Learning to perform orthopedic tests

- Orthopedic tests can be learned in classes. It is wise to get closely supervised instruction to learn to perform tests safely and correctly.
- Some tests are described online, including on YouTube.
- Many books of orthopedic tests are available (included in the recommended reading section at the back of this book).

Example of ruling out false positives on orthopedic tests

THE PATRICK TEST

The Patrick test, also called the FABER test, is understood to indicate dysfunction in iliopsoas muscles, sacroiliac joint, or hip joint. The test method is for the client to lie supine on the table. The tester then passively moves the client's leg which is to be tested, flexing the knee, externally rotating, abducting, and flexing the hip so the ankle of the leg being moved is placed on the client's other thigh just superior to the patella. The tester then allows the knee of the leg being tested to gently rest down toward the table. The name FABER is an acronym for the position of the tested leg: flexion, abduction, and external

rotation. The test is also named Patrick for its developer, neurologist Hugh Talbot Patrick.

Apply this test to each of the two legs in succession, comparing results. Test the asymptomatic leg first to see what a relatively normal test may look like for this person.

A positive test is indicated if the knee of the leg being tested will not rest to, or below, the level of the other knee, and/or the client experiences discomfort at the hip or sacroiliac area on the side being tested.

An adaptation of this test utilizing inhibitory contact can distinguish from where the problem can successfully be treated. This may include distinguishing if the limited movement of the hip can be improved from working on the iliopsoas, sacroiliac, or the hip joint itself. Commonly, more distant areas can also be found which may improve either or both the passive FABER range of the tested hip, and comfort in the hip and/or low back.

FOR THE ADAPTATION OF THIS ORTHOPEDIC TEST:

1. First find the currently primary restriction, using one or more of the general assessment methods. Then, using manual thermal assessment, locate additional areas of interest.
2. Place the client on the table and passively place the leg of interest into the FABER position.
3. One at a time, contact each of the several areas described and/or discovered in step 1, with an inhibitory contact. Start with the hip joint, iliacus, psoas, and sacroiliac joint; next, try the current primary restriction; then move on to other areas discovered with manual thermal assessment. When any of these areas is contacted and the knee being tested settles down any visible degree closer to the table and/or the person's discomfort level

decreases, this indicates that treating that area is likely to improve the result of the FABER test and the comfort and functionality of that hip and/or leg. Prior to treatment, further assessment in the areas indicated by this method will usually be necessary.

4. Other orthopedic tests can be adapted in a similar way. Some creativity will be required to adapt other orthopedic tests which normally require two hands. Some orthopedic tests may be adaptable in this fashion only if an assistant is available.

ASSESSMENT METHOD 12

Patrick test

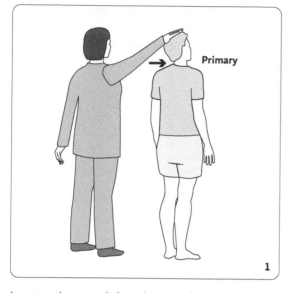

Locate a primary restriction using general assessment methods.

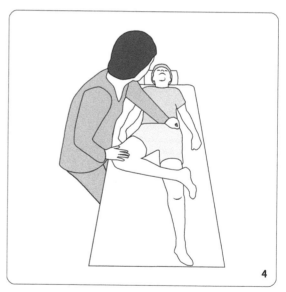

Locate additional actively changing lesions using manual thermal assessment.

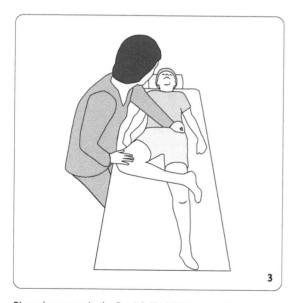

Place the person in the Patrick (FABER) test position. Observe the distance between the knee and the table.

One at a time, successively apply inhibitory contact to the active lesion sites located in steps 1 and 2. If inhibiting any of those sites allows the knee to sink closer to the table without the pelvis rotating, this indicates that treating the lesion at the area inhibited will likely improve the result of the Patrick test, and may reduce hip symptoms.

ASSESSMENT METHODS USEFUL FOR BOTH GENERAL AND LOCAL ASSESSMENT

Some assessment methods have applications both to find the area of primary lesion, and to learn more detail about local lesions. Mobility testing is a core assessment method used in every assessment protocol, sometimes in general assessment and always in local assessment.

Assessment method 13: mobility testing

Before each intervention, it is essential to test range of motion and observe qualities of movement. We must know our starting place. Then, at the conclusion of each intervention, we must mobility test again to know features of the change we made, and to demonstrate those changes to the client. What changes were made? What changes were not yet made?

Recognition of either limited or excessive range of motion is a necessary but *not sufficient* reason to treat. Observations of range of motion and qualities of motion are collectively a core assessment method. Other factors, discernible by other assessment methods, must also be considered to determine when and where to intervene.

Treating parts of the body in a good enough order is critical for effective and efficient treatment. Preconceived protocols are inherently inefficient, and sometimes ineffective. Each person is put together in a unique way, and then each person has individual history. Therefore, we must figure out in detail the condition in which the kittens of life have left this person's skein of yarn, and what is the best path to untangle it. Mobility testing is always a component of this assessment and can never be the whole assessment.

Mobility testing has many facets:

- There are many body areas and parts.
- Tissues are diverse in their qualities.
- Tiny areas can be tested for stretch and for glide of tissues.
- We also make global assessments, examining larger areas of the body at the same time.

- We observe our clients move their own bodies.
- We learn something different when we move parts of our client's bodies.

In addition to how far a structure can move (range of motion), additional factors are important:

- How much effort is required to move through the range?
- Is the movement smooth and uniform, or not?
- What are the qualities of end-feel?

Thorough knowledge of mobility testing can be gained only through good training and extensive practice. The present book includes this introduction to mobility testing, and references to mobility testing elsewhere in the text. Whole large books on mobility testing have been published. See the recommended reading at the end of this book. Further study and practice are necessary. Read the books. Take classes on mobility testing. This book highly values mobility testing, and since that topic has already been well written about, the focus of this book is on other assessment.

Steps to gaining mobility testing expertise are:

- Extensively practice, applying the principles of mobility testing learned in this book and other books and courses to the full range of tissues and areas of the body.

ASSESSMENT METHOD 13

- The recommended reading in this manual has several books with more information about mobility testing.
- Courses in range of motion testing are available from several schools.

Features commonly assessed include joint range of motion and muscle length. Much more can be assessed including:

- skin stretch
- movement of skin over tissue underneath it
- organ glide on other organs, and on the body wall
- stretch of organ support membranes
- stretch and glide of vasculature and nerves
- stretch and glide of the meninges.

Principles of mobility assessment that apply broadly across tissue types and body parts

Strongly avoid pain. If moving a body part is painful for the client, *stop*, and gently release your contact on the body part(s).

- Consider how the test might be modified to be more comfortable; try such a new approach cautiously. Do *not* persist with mobility testing in the presence of pain.
- Shift your investigation to hypothesizing about the origin of the pain. Then seek evidence for and against those hypotheses.
- Consider referrals for further investigation and treatment.

Plan your assessment in detail. Consider what information you hope to gather and how best to collect that information.

- Think through the steps to gather that information. Leave no gaps.

- On the one hand, do not just puddle around in tissue. On the other hand, adapt your assessment plan based on information gathered.

Contact as close to the area being tested as practical. Make your hand contacts as close to the tissue to be tested as practical. This will reduce the confusion of other tissues being tested along with the intended tissues.

Approach slowly.

- Move toward your client's body at a measured pace.
- Sink into or grasp your client's body slowly. Too quick an approach will feel threatening. Even if the client is not consciously disturbed, too fast an approach will result in reflexive tightening which will give a false reading of less range of motion, and/or greater effort to move. Paradoxically, too slow an approach can also elicit apprehension. Find a comfortable middle pace.

Test slowly. Once contact has been made, move the body parts slowly. Too fast movement will feel threatening. Even if the client is not consciously disturbed, too fast movement will result in reflexive tightening which will give a false reading of less range of motion, and/or greater effort to move.

Observe and note qualities of movement. As you move the body part(s) through the range of motion, notice qualities of movement.

- Effort required to move will be different in various parts of the range.
- Some parts of the range may be smoother than others.
- Note the path of movement: is it as expected, or does it deviate?

These qualities may vary considerably from one part of the range of motion to another.

Test once, believe your hands. Test once, perhaps twice, only rarely more.

- Repeated testing will often mobilize tissue, so the results or range of motion tests will change with successive tests, leading to confusion.
- Repeated testing may irritate tissue, and/or annoy your client.

While carrying out your planned assessment, stay open to additional information. As you assess, stay on task. Unless a contraindication arises, collect the information you are looking for. At the same time, stay alert to other kinds of information. For example, in checking range of motion at the elbow, we usually test the range of motion at both elbows for comparison. Examining both elbows may lead to noticing one arm is cooler than the other, or a marked difference in muscle bulk between the two arms. Such observations were not the intended goal of the movement testing but may point to fruitful lines of investigation. *Focus both narrow and broad.* As you assess a particular body part, stay alert to the rest of the person.

- Does any part of the client's body guard against your testing?
- Does a distant body part move in a surprising way in response to your test?
- Does the person's breathing rate or breathing pattern change?
- Does any part of the client's skin color change?
- Are there changes in facial expression?
- Do muscles elsewhere in the body relax or tighten?

Break contact gently and respectfully. As you complete a test assist the body parts tested to a comfortable position. If there is any doubt, ask the client if the position is comfortable. Break contact in a measured way designed to increase both the client's bodily comfort and the client's confidence in you as a practitioner.

Connect the dots. Immediately consider the results of the test.

- What new information has been gathered?
- In what ways does the new information from this test support hypotheses or answer questions previously posed?
- In what ways does information from this test not support hypotheses previously made, or fail to answer questions posed?
- What new hypotheses or questions do the results of the test suggest?
- By what means can these new hypotheses or questions be tested?

Dynamic stabilization during mobility testing

During passive mobility testing we move one body part relative to a neighboring body part. To accomplish this, we usually stabilize one body part with our hands as a platform on which to move another body part. As an example, to examine the mobility of a finger joint we stabilize a proximal phalanx and move a middle phalanx on the stabilized proximal phalanx.

There is more than one way to stabilize a body part and the way a body part is stabilized strongly influences the results of mobility testing. There is a large contrast between the results of:

- a strong clamping stabilization of a body part preventing any movement, and
- a less forceful dynamic stabilization where any tendency of the stabilized body part to move is met with just enough back force to prevent movement. The amount of back force and the exact direction of back force will

vary substantially through the range of motion. This requires constant monitoring and sensitive adjustment of force.

Lack of awareness of and attention to this distinction is a reason interrater reliability for mobility testing has sometimes been reported as low.

Compared to a dynamic stabilization, a static stabilization which is insensitive to the dynamics of the movement will give a mobility test result of much less total range and less ease of movement within range.

Because a dynamic stabilization is more like the normal mechanics of the body as we go through life, the larger range of motion demonstrated by using dynamic stabilization during testing provides more realistic results. Therefore, all mobility testing should be done with dynamic stabilization.

Dynamic stabilization requires a constant alertness by the therapist for any tendency of the gently stabilized part to move. The therapist applies an ever shifting back load just preventing movement of the stabilized part. This back load varies from moment to moment in both direction of load and force of load.

The therapist must maintain constant, moment by moment detailed awareness of:

- any tendency of the stabilized part to move
- effort required to move the mobile part
- smoothness of movement of the mobile part
- range of motion of the mobile part in a succession of directions
- slightest signs of distress from the client.

One awareness cannot be sacrificed for another; all must be constantly monitored.

Assessment method 14: yes–no questions (applied kinesiology and a variant)

Origin
Created by George J. Goodheart, Jr. DC and variant by Jean-Pierre Barral DO.

Concept
It is possible to obtain answers to questions that can be clearly stated to have *yes* or *no* answers by asking the client's body. There are many ways to do this. Two methods are described here.

Classic applied kinesiology
Test the strength of any muscle by asking the person to resist your applied force.

Before the test is made, the therapist formulates a question with certain characteristics.

1. It must be clearly answerable *yes* or *no*. Think carefully about any ambiguities.
2. It must address a concrete quality of the body of the person being treated. This method is ineffective both for intangibles and for things outside the person's body.

The therapist holds this question in mind while testing the strength of the muscle. A strong muscle means yes, a weak muscle means no.

Example: The client's arm can be held straight forward from the shoulder, with the hand in a loose fist. A downward force on the forearm applied by the therapist tests the strength of the anterior deltoid muscle.

Example: The client holds the tip of the thumb and second finger of one hand together. The therapist uses his hands to try to pull the fingers apart as the client resists.

Later developments

1. The therapist places their hand lightly on top of the client's head. The question is asked internally. A tissue pull forward or forward-and-right on the top of the head means yes; either a backwards motion or no motion means no.
2. The therapist touches any part of the body and then internally poses a question. A tissue pull toward superiorly, or for the upper limbs proximally, means yes; inferiorly, or for the upper limbs distal, means no. This can be multitasked while treating.

Ask the body

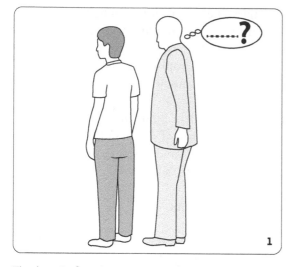

The therapist formulates a question about concrete or tangible qualities of the client's body, which can be clearly answered *yes* or *no*.

Holding that question in mind, the therapist places the palm of their hand centered on the top of the client's head.

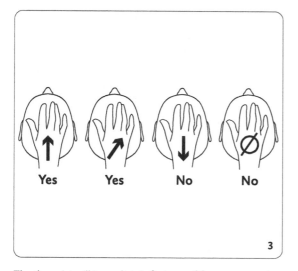

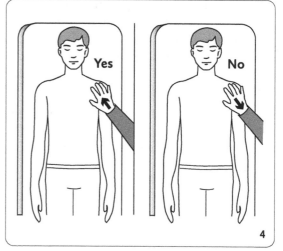

The therapist will immediately feel one of four responses in the tissue on top of the client's head.

- A straightforward tissue pull means yes.
- A right anterior tissue pull means yes.
- A posterior pull means no.
- No tissue pull means no.

The same kinds of questions can be asked through hand contact anywhere on the body.

A tissue pull superior, or for the upper limb proximal, means yes. A tissue pull inferior, or for the upper limb distal, means no. As for the top of the head, no tissue pull means no.

The tissue pull will vary in strength from moderate to very small. The strength of the pull has no meaning. If the tissue pull is not felt within five seconds, that either means no or the tissue pull was missed. After five seconds, an unwind may begin which has a similar feel to the answer to the question but is not an answer to the question. If in doubt, break contact and start over.

Assessment method 15: developing intuition

Origin
Osteopathic discoverer Andrew Taylor Still MD cultivated intuition equally with his cultivation of sensory awareness. He valued both ways of gathering information and developed both to an extraordinary high level.

Concept
Swiss psychologist Carl Jung distinguishes intuition from sensation in the following way.

Sensation means conscious perception through the sense organs. It is always possible to say by what sensory pathway the information arrived. For example:

- "I saw it with my eyes."
- "I felt it on my shoulder."
- "I heard it with my ears."
- "I smelled it with my nose."

Intuition is an experience that is immediately given to consciousness through no perceptible physical pathway. We cannot say we saw it with our eyes, heard it with our ears, or smelled it with our nose. Intuition is a hunch, a gut-level feeling, or an extra-sensory-perception experience.

Both intuition and sensation provide valuable information. Both can be incorrect. Both sensation and intuition can be trained to provide correct information more often. Both can also be trained to provide information more completely and quickly. The two keys to improving each of these ways of gathering information are:

1. Feedback on performance.
2. Expressions of gratitude.

INTUITION IS UNIQUE IN EACH PERSON
Intuition expresses itself in many ways. Get several of your colleagues and/or friends together for a round table on tuition. Ask them each to say:

- How intuitive do you feel you are?
- How does intuition work for you?

The diversity of responses to these questions is large and fascinating. How intuitive each person believes they are is often incorrect. How intuition is experienced by each person is as unique as snowflakes, varying over wide ranging spectra. Books on the variability of intuition include:

- *Jung and Intuition: On the Centrality and Variety of Forms of Intuition in Jung and Post-Jungians* by Nathalie Pilard.
- *The Science of Intuition: How to Access the Inner-net of Intuitive Knowledge* by Nora Truscello and Heidi Sutherlin.

Get to know your own intuition. In what ways do you as an individual perceive without your senses? How can you best cultivate this?

Andrew Taylor Still MD, discoverer of osteopathy, actively cultivated both sensation and intuition throughout his life, mastering both. He is a worthy role model in many ways.

Method
Start paying attention to those little moments from day to day when you get a perception you cannot account for with your senses.

As you notice these events investigate them. Look for sensory information both to support, and to disprove, these nonsensory perceptions. This is one of the strongest ways to grow your intuition.

A common error is to look only for information that confirms intuition. Be sure to look also for sensory information that weighs against intuition. Your intuition likes to do a good job. Give it accurate feedback on its performance.

Similarly, cross check your sensory perceptions. If you seem to see something, how else can you examine it? Can you look at it from another angle? Is it possible to hear it? Can it be felt with your hand? Our sensory perceptions can be correct or not. Our intuitions can be correct or not. Train your senses as well as your intuition.

As you notice nonsensory impressions, cautiously act on these impressions, and observe the results. Be sensible about what you act on and how. What were the qualities of the perceptions you had, and what were the results of acting on these impressions? Correlating details of your perception with the results of your actions based on those perceptions will inform and train your intuition.

Your intuition likes to be appreciated. Let your intuitive faculty know you are interested in it. Thank it for trying. Give it kudos for doing well. Ask how it likes to be nurtured.

For a period of months keep a written log of:

- correlations, positive and negative, between intuition and sensory information
- results of acting on intuition.

Like any skill, intuition comes more easily to some people than to others. Anyone can increase their intuition. With intuition, as with any skill, practice leads to improvement.

Hints:

- Take time for mindfulness meditation. There are many benefits to meditation including increased intuition. Just as you observe external phenomena, watch your mind in action.

- Sometimes information which we seem to get intuitively is at least partially coming to us through a sensory channel. When you get what seems to be an intuitive insight, look for what sensory information may have informed that. In this way use seeming intuition to cultivate sensation and to distinguish between sensation and intuition.

- We learn some things in a way that we can easily describe in words. It is easy to tell another person about it or to teach it. This is called explicit learning. We learn other things by unconscious association or by trial-and-error processes that do not utilize language. We can perform these tasks but find it difficult to describe the process in words or teach such processes to another person. This is called implicit learning. Some but not all actions we seem to perform intuitively are the result of implicit learning. If you find yourself doing something that you have difficulty explaining, take the time and effort to formulate the language for it. There are usually gems there.

Assessment method 16: introduction to use of the craniosacral rhythm as an assessment tool

Origin

Early osteopathic methods following the work of W. G. Sutherland DO.

History and physiology

The craniosacral rhythm (CSR) is a small-scale rhythmic expansion and contraction in all parts of the body. This rhythm was first noted by William Garner Sutherland DO (1873–1954). Sutherland recognized that most humans of all ages have slightly mobile joints between the bones that make up the skull.

Following the principle that structure and function are related, Sutherland hypothesized there must be movements in the joints of the skull. Sutherland experimented with applying forces to move the bones of the skull, much as we would mobility test any joint. He also observed closely to feel for any naturally occurring movement between the bones of the skull, such as occurs at the costovertebral joints with breath. He noted a slow regular movement of the bones of the skull which varied from person to person, and from time to time for each person. The briefest description of this movement is an expansion of the skull for 3–7 seconds followed by a return or contraction of the skull for the same amount of time. Details of what each bone of the skull does are intricate and worthy of study.

Soon after, Sutherland observed that the same rhythm was observable at the sacrum as a flexion and extension movement. The sacral movement paralleled the movement of the occiput and was precisely in synch with it. From this observation, he coined the term craniosacral rhythm (CSR).

Later, Sutherland noticed that this same rhythm was observable everywhere on the body. As the skull expands the limbs roll subtly out, as do the left and right halves of the torso.

Sutherland developed therapeutic methods utilizing this rhythm. Other workers in the field

since Sutherland have continued to expand the repertoire of therapeutic methods utilizing the CSR.

Sutherland noted that the joints between the parietal bones and the temporal squama resemble fish gills. He hypothesized that the CSR was therefore a respiratory mechanism more primary to the body than pulmonary or other rhythms. He renamed this rhythm the primary respiratory mechanism (PRM).

Sutherland believed that the CSR, i.e., PRM, originated in the joint between the basilar portions of the sphenoid bone and the occipital bone. He saw the similar rhythmic movement palpable at the sacrum and everywhere else on the body as driven from the spheno-basilar joint (SBJ). This has since been disproven. There are no contractile or other motor units in the SBJ. By age 25, the SBJ naturally fuses. Those of us older than 25 do not have a sphenoid bone and an occiput; as such we have what might be called a spheniput. After age 25, apparent movement between the greater wings of the sphenoid and the occipital squama represent elasticity of the bone rather than movement between the bones.

What is the craniosacral rhythm (CSR)?

If the craniosacral rhythm is not driven by the spheno-basilar junction, what does drive it?

The short and true answer is, we don't know. That said, here is a tantalizing bit of research.

German researchers Ludwig Traube, Ewald Hering, and Siegmund Mayer measured blood pressure at each heartbeat and observed that blood pressure is not constant, it fluctuates up and down over a few heart beats at about a 6–14 second period. These are known as Traube-Hering-Mayer (THM) waves.

Subsequent research has demonstrated that THM waves correlate well with the CRS. Although several theories have been advanced, the source of both the CSR and the THM rhythms have not yet been confirmed. Both the CSR and the THM have not been confirmed to originate in any part of the body but are physiologic features of all parts of the body.

Variability of the CSR

The CSR varies in rate from person to person and from time to time. Unlike breath and heart rate, CSR rate does not change with exercise. Very fast rates may reflect numerous mechanical restrictions in the body, as if the movement cannot go very far before it must turn around. Occasionally one part of the body will be observed to contract while other parts are expanding. This is viewed as undesirable and there are means to correct these local phase aberrations.

The CSR varies in amplitude or intensity from person to person and from time to time, and from one part of the body to another. Variability from one part of the body to another usually reflects mechanical restriction at the area of amplitude transition. There are means to correct this, so the amplitude is uniform throughout the body.

The CSR is frequently observed to be unequal between the expansion and the contraction phase. In this situation, there is a felt sense that the body is expanding more than it is contracting or vice versa. *This cannot be literally true.* If each expansion phase went farther than each contraction phase over time the body would become progressively larger with each expansion. Since there are 3,155,760 ten-second periods in a year, a 1 percent increase per period would result in the body being at least 30,000 times larger by the end of a year. What is happening is the movement is more effortful in one direction than the other. This is seen as undesirable and there are means to correct this.

The movement of the CSR should be smooth in all parts of the body. Either globally or locally the CSR is frequently observed to be rough or ratcheting in at least part of its range. This is viewed as undesirable and there are means to correct it.

Uses of the CSR as a diagnostic tool

There are many ways to use the CSR as a diagnostic tool. Here I present three of these ways. Details are on the following pages.

1. The primary restriction in the body can be found by feeling for the location of changes in the CSR at many locations in the body, followed up with use of local listening and inhibition to make pairwise comparison of primacy between these several areas. This method is too slow for practical use in the treatment room. However, it is a useful learning exercise to develop skill in a) feeling variations in CSR from one place to another, and b) local listening and inhibition.

2. The skills used in step 1 can be used efficiently on a local basis. To do this, the neighborhood of a primary restriction is located using one or more of the general assessment methods, usually with follow up using local methods. General knowledge of the location of the primary restriction can then be refined to a highly specific location by observing changes in CSR locally.

3. In the head, the CSR may be within normal parameters in all ways. More often it is not. Mechanical restrictions distorting the CSR in the head may be in the head. More often the restrictions distorting movement in the head are in the thorax, pulling up through the neck to distort the head, including the expression of the CSR in the head. There is a way to find out if the restrictions distorting the expression of the CSR are in the head, in the thorax, or in both.

Use of the CSR to locate a primary lesion

Origin

Finding variations in the CSR—William Garner Sutherland.

Comparing pairs of lesions using local listening and inhibition to find relative primacy—traditional osteopathic technique, exact origin lost.

Combining finding changes in CSR with the use of local listening and inhibition—Jeffrey Burch.

Concept

It is possible to find the location of a primary restriction using only the variations in PRM from one part of the body to another and inhibition. This assessment is done by feeling the CSR at many locations of the body, each area requiring at least 30 seconds to evaluate. As soon as two areas of change in CSR characteristics are discovered, those two areas can be compared with local listening and inhibition to find which of the two is the relative primary. By this process of discovery and pairwise comparison, a primary restriction can be found.

Method

Starting at the head and progressing inferiorly, feel the CSR in various parts of the body in a systematic pattern. As soon as two areas where the CSR changes are discovered, compare these two areas with local listening and inhibition to find which of the two is the relative primary. As a third area of change is discovered, compare it to the previously found relative primary. Continue to compare each new disturbance found to that last known relative primary until the most primary restriction in the body is found.

So that the whole body is accessible, start with the client seated on a bench or stool. As you approach the waist, have the client stand. Move around as needed to access various parts of the body working from the sides and behind. For the lower legs and feet, you may want to have the client lie down.

The description below starts out in more detail, and then as you progress through various parts of the body, it is shortened to avoid unnecessary repetition. The elements of the process are the same throughout the body.

1. First put a hand on each side of the head. Notice the PRM. Is it symmetrical? If it is not symmetrical, shift your hands to look for the line of demarcation between the two qualities on the sides. It may not be down the middle.
2. Place a hand gently on each side of the neck. Is the rhythm in the neck the same as in the head? Is it the same left to right when any discrepancy is noted?
3. Place the hands on the upper shoulders, again feeling for differences left to right and from what was felt above.
4. Feel at the elbows.
5. Feel the hands.
6. Feel the upper lateral chest.
7. Feel the lower chest.
8. Feel the sides of the abdomen.
9. Feel the hips.
10. Feel the knees.
11. Feel the ankles.
12. Feel the toes.

This process requires about 30 seconds at each station to make the initial assessment of the CSR. Homing in on differences in CSR requires more 30-second increments. Over the whole body this adds up to too much time to be practical for use in clinical practice. It is useful as a skill building exercise, learning to feel the CSR focally in the body and learning to do local listening and inhibition.

Use of the CSR to further localize a lesion

Origin

Further development of the work of W. G. Sutherland DO. Discoverer unknown.

ASSESSMENT METHOD 16

Concept

The general assessment methods give us the general area of a primary restriction. We still have work to do to precisely locate and characterize the restriction. In the previous section, a tedious process to find the primary restriction in the body was described. Now we will look at an efficient local use of this same assessment pattern to locate a primary restriction more precisely.

Method

Once a primary restriction is found using one, two, or three of the general assessment methods, place a hand gently a little proximal to but not precisely on the area believed to be primary. Note the qualities of the craniosacral rhythm:

- rate
- amplitude
- balance of expansion and contraction
- smoothness.

Then move your hand a short distance to the distal side of the area believed to be the primary restriction. Again, note the qualities of the CSR. How are these like the qualities of the tissue just proximal to the primary restriction and how are they different?

Now feel the CSR a little closer to the primary restriction. In small increments, move closer, feeling the qualities of the rhythm at each area. When the qualities shift to those found proximal to the primary you have passed the primary.

By this process you have precisely located the primary restriction. Confirm this with a manual thermal sweep which will also show you the size and shape of the primary restriction. How congruent are these two different methods of locating the primary restriction?

Proceed with layer listening and with questions about tissue type to further locate and characterize the primary restriction.

Use of the CSR to distinguish between sources of cranial distortion

Origin

Jeffrey Burch.

Concept

The CSR may have all the same characteristics in all areas of the head or there may be variations in different parts of the head, commonly between the left and right halves of the head. See the previous section for a description of the CSR.

The local differences in CSR characteristics observed in the head may be created entirely by the fibrosities in the head. More commonly some of the fibrosities disturbing the CSR in the head lie elsewhere in the body, pulling through the neck into the head. Most commonly there are some CSR disturbing fibrosities in the head and others elsewhere in the body.

When a source of observed CSR distortion *at* the head is not *in* the head, the distortion is most commonly in the thorax, though it may be more inferior and occasionally in the upper limbs.

Distortions in the thorax are commonly transferred to the head by structures passing through the neck including:

- Tension in the esophagus and/or trachea through the pharynx which attaches to both bones of the spheno-basilar junction.
- Vasculature, more commonly arterial than venous. This can be in the carotid arteries and/or vertebral arteries.
- Nerves, commonly the vagus nerves.
- Dural tube.

Method

With the client supine on the table, sit comfortably at the head end of the table. Use a classic craniosacral monitoring position pioneered by W. G. Sutherland DO. Gently contact the head with your two hands. Place the pads of the thumbs just posterior to the lateral margins of the orbits so they overlie the greater wings of the sphenoid bone. At the same time, wrap your relaxed hands around the head so the pads of at least your fifth digits contact the squamous portion of the occiput.

With your relaxed hands in this position maintain butterfly wing light contact on the head. Notice the craniosacral rhythm. On expansion the greater wings of the sphenoid will roll inferior and anterior, and the occiput will roll inferior and posterior. On the contraction phase the bones move in the opposite directions. Note if the CSR is balanced in terms of:

- expansion and contraction (also called CSR flexion and extension)
- smoothness throughout its range, at a reasonable rate 6–14 times per minute
- amplitude within normal range.

Are the characteristics of the rhythm the same on both sides of the head, left and right?

If any feature of the CSR is not as it should be, use the palms of your hands more superiorly on the head to gently push the head a little inferior, giving slack to the neck. Neither flex nor extend the neck, make this a straight inferior load. Approach this test maneuver cautiously to stay within comfortable ranges for the client. Do not do this if cervical disk bulges are known or suspected. With the head gently held inferior in this fashion, again observe all the characteristics of the CSR described in the last paragraph. If any feature or features of the CSR improve that means some of the fibrosity creating these aberrations in the expression of the CSR in the head lie in the thorax. The greater the degree of correction in any feature, and the greater the number of features corrected, the higher the proportion of the distortion creating the cranial distortion lying in the thorax.

To locate this pull from the thorax, use an application of ultraslow mobility testing. Very slowly reduce the pressure down on the top of the head. As the slack in the neck is slowly reduced, feel for precisely the first line of pull felt through and beyond the neck. Given its location, hypothesize anatomy. Further investigate this line of pull with local listening, manual thermal assessment, local tap, possibly other assessment methods, and ultimately mobility testing to fully localize and characterize this fibrosity.

If all the fibrosity distorting the CSR in the head appears to be in the thorax, proceed to treatment of the fibrosity you have found in the thorax.

More commonly there will be some fibrosity both in the head and in the thorax contributing to the distortion of the CSR in the head. In this case, localize the restrictions in the head using manual thermal assessment, local listening, layer listening, local tap, and possibly other methods. If two or more areas of fibrosity are found in the head, compare these with local listening and inhibition to find the relative primary within the head. Then use the same process to compare the most primary area in the head with the area discovered in the thorax. Use local listening and inhibition to compare the relative primacy of the most primary component of the distortion found in the head, with the most primary component of the cranial distortion found in the thorax. Treat the more primary of these two.

Then resume the classical monitoring hold on the head to learn how much correction of the CSR has been achieved. If the cranial distortion is not fully corrected, again slack the neck to see if there is a component of the distortion in the thorax. If slacking the neck fully restores the CSR in the head, treat the thorax. If slacking the neck partially corrects the head, then follow the procedure above to find the most primary area within the head and compare this to the area of fibrosity in the thorax that is distorting the cranium. Treat the more primary of these two areas. If slacking the neck makes no correction in the craniosacral rhythm, then the next issue to treat is in the head.

ASSESSMENT
METHOD 16

You may be able to continue to cycle this until the CSR in the head is substantially corrected. However, ask questions at each cycle to see if this process should be continued at this time or if it is better to return to general assessment.

EXTENDED ASSESSMENT METHODS

Once a primary restriction has been located, a treatment method chosen, and treatment initiated, it frequently happens that a tissue pull is felt from the area being treated to another area. We call this tissue pull from an area being treated an extended listening. If a tissue pull from the primary restriction to another area of the body is not spontaneous there are ways to "fish" for these tissue pulls.

This "extended listening" can be used either to enhance treatment at the site being treated, or to include the secondary site found, or both. This process can be extended from the secondary site to further sites.

These extended assessments are detailed in this section. Complex treatment methods built on this assessment are described in the treatment section as the Laughlin Method.

ASSESSMENT
METHOD 16

Assessment method 17: extended listening

Origin
Earliest osteopaths. Used by George Laughlin DO and likely by Andrew Taylor Still MD.

Principles

- There are no purely local phenomena in the body.
- Restrictions in the body are always big patterns that, at any moment, we perceive in part.
- The body is continuously remodeling this restriction network.
- Our job is to assist the body to remodel its restriction patterns more effectively and efficiently.
- It is sometimes most useful to work on a small part of the pattern and often useful to work on larger components of the pattern.

Actions
As you engage tissue to begin a treatment, stay alert for tissue pulls to other areas. They are almost always present. When you observe such a tissue pull, there are several ways in which to enhance treatment. All of these include continuing what you are doing locally while managing the continuity to another area in a range of ways, including:

1. Move the tissue you are working on to slack the connection to another area.
2. Move the tissue you are working on to adjust the tension between it and the distant one to a first barrier. This may mean moving away or toward.
3. If practical, shift one hand to the other perceived area. Set up a treatment locally at the other location *and* adjust the tension between the two areas being treated to a useful level which facilitates tissue change. The tension level established between the two areas may be anywhere on the continuum from zero tension through first barrier to mid barrier.
4. To accomplish any of the above, remember the table (or bench or floor) as your third hand.
5. Have the client gently move one or more body parts to a different position to establish useful force levels which facilitate change.
6. Position the client differently to achieve useful force levels:
   a. Move limbs
   b. Rotate torso
   c. Prop with pillow
   d. Shift to another position on table, supine, side-lying, etc.
   e. Shift from lying to seated or standing.

Extended listening can lead directly into the use of long lever treatment, mixed long and short lever treatment, and/or Laughlin technique.

Extended listening

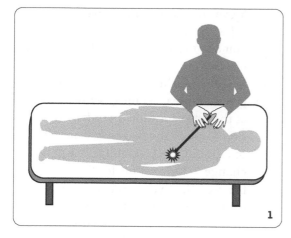

As you set up a treatment on a local area, stay alert to the possibility of tissue pulls to another area.

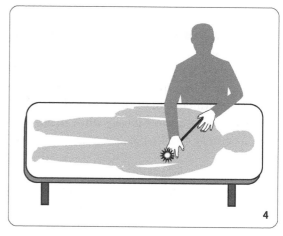

One way to work with such a tissue pull to another area is to gently move the area you are treating toward or away from the other area to adjust the tension between the two areas to a level that facilitates change in the area you are treating.

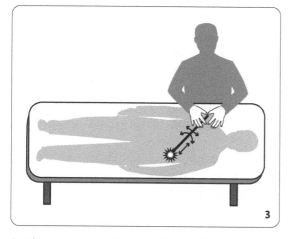

Another way to work with such a tissue pull is to use the area you are treating as a long lever to set up a treatment on the tissue at the other end of the line of pull. This may be the same treatment method as you are using at the primary area or a different method.

If the treatment setup at the primary area can be maintained with one hand, and if the distance to reach is practical, you can move a hand to the other area to set up a treatment, and at the same time manage the tension between the two areas to facilitate release.

ASSESSMENT
METHOD 17

Extended listening (*cont.*)

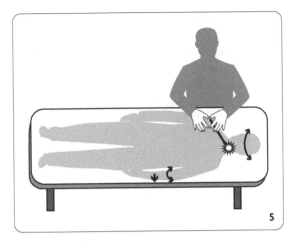

5

As you maintain your treatment setup at the primary area you can ask the client to move very slowly in specific directions to find positions that facilitate treatment and engage the second area.

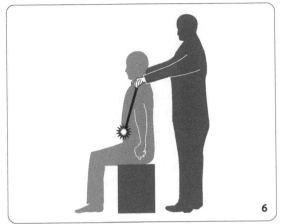

6

If you are treating a seated or standing client, you can move the client gently over their base of support to find positions that facilitate change in both the primary area and the one found with extended listening. You can also ask the client to move. For example, you might tilt the client's torso slightly right, and rotate their torso slightly left, then ask the client to rotate their head gently to each side fishing for the best position.

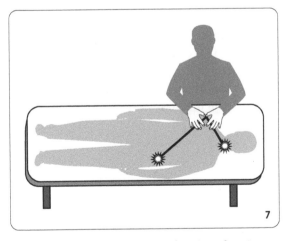

7

Occasionally, you may feel more than one line of tension from the primary area you are treating. In some instances, it is practical to organize treatment along more than one line using the above methods.

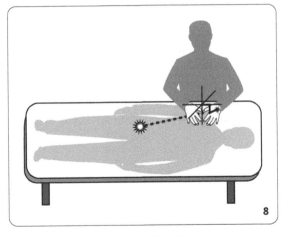

8

If you do not notice a tissue pull from the primary area you are treating and you wish to utilize this method, keep the treatment setup you have, and at the same time move the area you are treating slowly in a succession of directions until a line of pull is felt to another area.

When you have set up a treatment on a primary lesion you will often but not always feel a line of tension to another area. This is an opportunity to treat more than one part of the lesional chain. There are several methods to engage the additional component(s) of the lesional chain. These methods can be used singly or in combination.

Assessment method 18: listening from a symptomatic area

Origin
Early osteopaths, exact origin unknown.

Concept
Each restriction in the body is connected to several other restrictions. At any given moment some of these restrictions will be better entry points to affect the whole system than others, i.e., more primary. When a relatively primary restriction is treated, not only will it change but several other restrictions will change also. Usually, we cannot predict which other restrictions will change. However, there is a way to direct part of the benefit of changing a primary restriction to a particular (often symptomatic) part of the body.

This is beneficial in two ways. It maintains relationship with the client as they feel something is being done to directly address their symptoms. The symptoms may improve sooner than purely following a series of primary restrictions. The trade-off is this is not the most efficient way to normalize the person's whole system.

This method should be used sparingly, and always in the middle of a treatment session. Stepping outside the sequence of primary restrictions will to some degree rock the person's boat. Honor the primaries presented by the person's system at the beginning of the treatment session. In the middle of a treatment session sometimes do a move or two organized by listening from a symptomatic area. Leave time later in the treatment session to do several more moves directed by the person's system to clean up any messes you made by not fully honoring the person's primaries.

Method

1. Use general assessment methods and then local assessment methods to find and characterize the person's current primary restriction.
2. Load tissue at the symptomatic area. Observe any extended listenings from this area.
3. Load the area of extended listening found in step 2 to find a further extended listening.
4. Repeat step 3 until an extended listening arrives at the primary restriction.
5. Position the client and apply load at both the primary restriction and the symptomatic area engaging the segmented line of tension between the two.
6. Treat along this line using suitable functional methods.

Listening from a symptomatic area

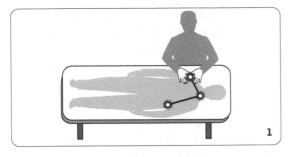

Begin as for Laughlin technique. Find a primary lesion, and as you engage the tissue at the primary with your hands, feel for extended listening. Continue this to find a Laughlin line.

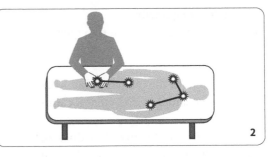

Move your hands to a symptomatic area. From this area, find an extended listening as the beginning of another Laughlin line.

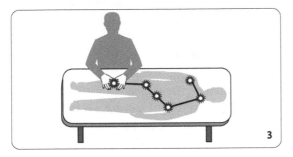

Extend the Laughlin line from the symptomatic area until it connects to the Laughlin line from the primary lesion.

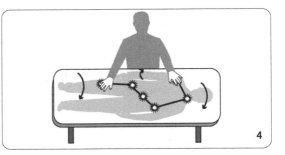

If practical, put one hand at the primary lesion and the other hand at the symptomatic area. Organize a treatment at each of those points and Laughlin treatments along the lines and points between these two areas. As needed, instruct the client to make small slow movements of body parts to engage these lines and points.

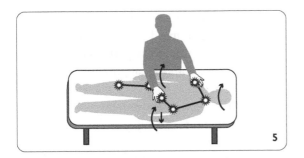

In some situations, it may be more practical to have a hand on one end of the double Laughlin line, and the other hand at another point along the line. As needed, instruct the client to make small slow movements of body parts to engage these lines and points.

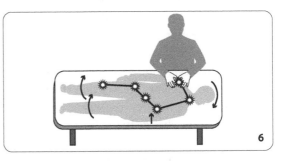

If necessary to organize the treatment, use both hands on one point, usually at an end of the line, and instruct the client to make small slow movements of body parts to engage these lines and points.

An advantage of this method is it maintains relationship with your client by directly addressing their areas of complaint. This may not be the most effective or efficient way to organize the whole body. Use this method sparingly, and always in the middle of a treatment session, not at the beginning or end.

ASSESSMENT METHOD 18

Assessment method 19: assessment algorithm

Rationale and guidelines

In therapeutic assessment, two questions must be answered:

1. Where in the body should I work?
2. What should I do in that location?

This therapeutic localization does not mean that the effect of treatment is only local. On the contrary, changing anything will change many things. Some of this change will be immediate, other elements of change will appear over a period of weeks.

Here is a useful paraphrase of this. As therapists, we must perpetually have in our minds the question: To make the most positive change for the whole person, where can I work on this person and what can I do from that location?

We use several assessment methods to answer these questions. No single assessment method can show everything. One assessment method may show issues another assessment will miss. Two or more assessment methods may confirm each other's findings.

This book describes several assessment methods that provide useful answers to our perpetual questions. Typically, there is not a single answer, but rather a cluster of solutions that could be useful. Among this cluster of useful solutions however, one may be a more effective and/or more efficient intervention than others. We always seek efficiency: the way to provide the greatest positive change in the least time and for the least effort.

Certain attitudes or mindsets are useful as we apply any assessment methods.

- Openness to experience—I am open to new and surprising things.
- Vibrant curiosity—Every aspect of the universe intrigues me.
- Complete suspension of expectations—I approach my client without expectations. I observe accurately what is.
- Genuine compassion—As Buddha put it, "During our myriad lifetimes all beings have been my mother, so I treat all beings with equally deep caring and respect."
- Excellent boundaries in every sense including this doublethink—There is a precise and knowable set of boundaries between my client and me. It is beneficial to all concerned to discover and live on the right side of those boundaries.

Inquiry and testing

- Listen on the phone.
- Have the client submit an intake form well before the first appointment.
  - Read the intake.
  - Formulate follow up questions.
- Watch movement and posture as the person walks in.
- Start with open questions.
- Follow up with more closed questions.
- Recognize risk factors.
  - Consider safely proceeding.
  - Keep in mind things not to do.
- Consider tests to be performed.
- Observe standing alignment front, side, and back.
- Observe active movement.
- Perform standing passive movement testing.
- As needed, do seated or lying down passive movement testing.
- Do orthopedic testing as indicated.
- Have the client stand again.
- Ask yes–no questions if it is safe and beneficial to treat.
- Apply selected tests starting general and

moving to specific. Always include mobility testing as a late step.

- Perform an initial treatment method to the most primary lesion you can find.

- Return to assessment to locate what has now become the next primary restriction.
- Cycle through assessment and treatment until the body signals it has had enough treatment for today.

PART 3

Treatment Methods

INTRODUCTION TO TREATMENT TECHNIQUES

Andrew Taylor Still MD was deeply insightful and highly creative in developing treatment techniques. Still's biographer John Lewis DO describes Still as lying awake at night thinking up new ways to do things, and never doing something the same way twice. Still assumed his students should enjoy the same exercise of creativity, so he taught anatomy thoroughly but with little technique. While none of his followers were as prolific as Still collectively, they have developed a wealth of new treatment methods. The following chapters detail many of these methods.

It is possible to practice using only one or a very few methods. Greater effectiveness and efficiency in practice is achieved by knowing and using many treatment methods, selecting the best for each situation.

The least easy component of treatment methods to describe in writing is qualities of touch. While this book can serve as a training manual, beginners are strongly advised to take closely supervised classes to learn the qualities of touch. After several methods have been learned, it may be possible to learn additional methods from this and other books.

Six factors have been described to categorize these treatment methods. These factors or features are described in the introduction to this book. The treatment methods to follow are organized using two of these six features: 1) whether tissue engagement is made by the therapist, or by the client's tissue, and 2) whether unwinding is used or not.

In the previous chapter, an additional feature is described which may be used with many of the treatment methods. This is the leverage used. It is possible to treat directly in contact with the lesioned structure or leverage may be applied from a short distance away, or from a longer distance away. In some instances, anatomy requires the use of longer levers. In other situations, a longer lever simply works better.

At the end of the chapters describing treatment methods, the use of leverage is used the other way around and taking it a step farther. Once a treatment is set up on a particular structure, leverage can then be exerted from that area to treat additional areas, creating a chain amplifying the treatment.

The treatment methods are presented in an order generally from simpler to more complex and from least directive to more directive. Learning the methods in the order presented has been found to work well. Take your time. Learn each method well before proceeding to the next.

The description of each treatment method is followed by three examples of use of that method on a diversity of body parts and tissue types.

These must not be taken as specific recipes for using this technique. Many other methods will be effective on these same tissues.

Prior to the description of the techniques there is a section clarifying certain terms used to describe treatment methods.

Bon voyage.

A proposal for clear terminology

In the literature and verbal communication of manual therapists the terms functional direct technique, often abbreviated simply as direct, and functional indirect technique, similarly often abbreviated as indirect, are used in highly inconsistent ways. This inconsistent use of terms has deteriorated to a point where when someone uses one of these terms the listener is obliged, as an early step to comprehension, to ferret out which definition of the term is in use. To add to the confusion, writers and speakers sometimes seem to be not clear in their own minds what they mean by these terms.

Below I list some of the alternative meanings of these terms. I then propose two steps to clarity of communication in this arena. The first is a recommendation for choices among certain synonymous terms by writers and speakers. Second, at the risk of adding to the babel, I propose two new terms which are highly descriptive of physical treatment methods and thereby hopefully less susceptible to wandering off meaning.

Meanings of terms currently in use

Direct	Indirect
Working right at the site of the lesion	Working on a lesion from a distance
Synonymous with short lever technique	Synonymous with long lever technique
Treat forcefully	Treat gently
Work in a highly directive way requiring the tissue to do specific things	Listen to the inherent movement in tissue and follow that inherent tissue movement

Work in direction of effort* (see below for further disambiguation)	Work in direction of ease* (see below for further disambiguation)
Move body part away from direction of perceived positional displacement	Move body part further into the direction of perceived positional displacement

Direction of ease and direction of effort are assessed with mobility testing. The tissue is moved first in one direction, allowed to relax back to neutral, then moved in the opposite direction. The direction which can be moved farther before resistance is felt is referred to as direction of ease. However, some therapists assess this by moving the tissue to a first barrier, other therapists assess it by moving the tissue to end-feel. Which direction shows the shorter distance to first barrier is uncorrelated with which direction shows the shorter distance to end-feel; the same is true of the farther distance.

I propose two steps to disambiguation.

1. Among some but not all practitioners, the term "direct" is understood as synonymous with short lever treatment. Similarly, "indirect" is understood as synonymous with long lever treatment. A problem comes when such practitioners communicate with other practitioners whose concept of direct and indirect has other meanings. Since short lever treatment may be understood to mean either direct treatment or indirect treatment, I suggest using the more descriptive terms short lever and long lever rather than direct and indirect to describe this feature of treatment.

2. The terms "direction of ease" and "direction of effort" are widely understood as reflecting which direction one feels tissue resistance sooner versus later when mobility testing; however, as indicated above, even this can have reversed meaning. At the risk of adding to the babel of terminology, I propose two new terms which are clearly descriptive of physical findings to express the meaning often attributed to the terms direction of effort and direction of ease. If tissue is moved

slowly first in one direction to a first barrier, then allowed to rest to neutral, and then moved slowly in the opposite direction, the distance from neutral to one of these first barriers will be shorter and the distance to the opposite first barrier will be longer. This descriptive difference is captured in two new terms:

Term	Meaning
Near first barrier	The first barrier found by moving tissue the shorter distance.
Far first barrier	The first barrier found by moving tissue the longer distance.

I will use these two new terms consistently through the rest of this book.

Humor during treatment

Include humor in your communication with your client. If your client spontaneously laughs while you are treating, their tissue will usually release much faster. To be effective, the client's laughter must be spontaneous. Telling the client to laugh won't work. Tell a joke. Make a humorous comment.

Introduction to treatment method examples

For each of the treatment methods in this book I give three examples of how to use this method on a range of body parts and tissue types.

These examples are a few of the thousands of possible applications for each treatment method. These examples must not be taken as the only places or even the best places to use these methods. Even after more than 40 years of practice it is a rare week that I do not encounter something to work on that I have not seen before.

Most treatment methods can be used on most tissues and most body areas. However, for each client at each moment, some treatment methods will be more effective and more efficient than other treatment methods. I always seek to work in the way that achieves the best result for my client, with the most comfort, in the least time. In the assessment portion of this book, I described how to find out which treatment methods will be the most effective and efficient in each moment.

There are a few exclusions of certain treatment methods on some body parts for safety reasons. These exclusions are described in the description of those treatment methods. There are also a few situations where certain methods are more likely to be used for physical convenience.

It often happens that the same treatment method must be applied to a tissue two or more times to achieve full results. Think of a wall that requires more than one coat of paint, or a vegetable patch that must be watered several times before a crop is ready to harvest.

Frequently, a succession of two or more treatment methods must be used on the same tissue, one after the other for best results. There is a protocol to determine whether a tissue needs more treatment and which treatment method to use next. This protocol is given here and referred to toward the end of the descriptions of each treatment method.

Completion of treatment protocol

Each treatment session will include several treatment moments. Each treatment moment will focus on a particular bodily area or issue for a period of time ranging from seconds to minutes. At the conclusion of each treatment moment, we must answer these questions:

- Is treatment of this tissue complete for now? (At a later time or later date there might be more treatment.)
- If treatment is not complete for this moment, what treatment method should I use next?

When the treatment episode is complete, for

example if unwinding is used, when the unwinding stops, or if the Reconstructed Still technique is used, after the circumduction at the end of the procedure:

- Post treatment mobility test the area using the local tests.
- Ask if this area is sufficiently treated.

The results of these inquiries may be:

- If the mobility is now normal and the person's system says it is sufficiently treated, you are done; return to general assessment to find the next primary lesion.
- If mobility testing is improved but still somewhat limited and yes–no questioning says that area is sufficiently treated, you are done with this area for now. Return to the beginning of the assessment to find the next primary. You may find yourself directed to this area again either later in the same session, or in a later session. However, if at the end of a treatment session mobility is improved by less than 50 percent, make a note to recheck this area at the next treatment.
- If mobility testing shows improvement but is still somewhat limited and the person's system says the area is not sufficiently treated, then ask, "Is the best treatment method to use now the same one just used?" If the answer is yes, use the same treatment method again. If the yes–no questioning says no, then inquire further to learn what is the best treatment method to use next.

Whether the next treatment episode for this area is the same as the most recently used or another method, follow this second treatment with mobility testing and questioning about completeness of treatment for this area for now. Any number of treatment episodes and/or treatment methods may be used but it is unusual for there to be more than four treatment episodes.

When the person's system says this area is sufficiently treated for the moment:

- Ask your client what they notice. Redo all local and larger scale mobility tests. Tell the client what you observe. Assist the client to feel or see what you see and feel. Do this with the understanding that you and the client will be able to perceive some of the same things, and each of you will be able to perceive some things the other person cannot.
- If mobility is improved by less than 50 percent, make a note to recheck this area at the next treatment.
- Return to general assessment to find the next primary dysfunction.

This protocol for the completion of each treatment moment will be used in each of the treatment examples described below.

TREATMENT METHODS IN WHICH THERAPEUTIC ENGAGEMENT IS MADE BY THE CLIENT'S SYSTEM AND UNWINDING IS USED

Treatment method 1: classic unwinding

Origin
Early osteopathic technique. Original discoverer unknown.

Pretest

- Ask the client what they feel in their body.
- Observe alignment in the person's body both locally and globally.
- Observe active movement patterns locally and globally.
- Test ranges of motion in the area to be treated and in related areas.
- Point out to the client what you see and feel. Assist them to see and feel this.

Therapeutic method
Approach the person's body with soft flexible hands. As you make contact allow the inherent movements in the person's tissue to move your hands.

Whatever motions the person's body makes follow these, neither accentuating nor retarding the movement. It is like listening to your friend who needs to talk. Listen to the story compassionately and without judgment or comment. Go along for the ride.

Completion
When the movement comes to a stop and there is a sense of peace or rest in the tissue, this therapeutic episode is over. Return to assessment.

Post test
Observe alignment and test ranges of motion. It is often useful to point the change out to the client. The treatment method is so gentle, many clients will feel that nothing is happening. This lack of awareness is a sign you are successful in not engaging defense mechanisms.

Classical unwinding

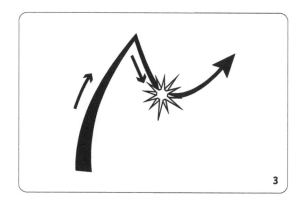

Touch the body softly. Tissue begins to move.

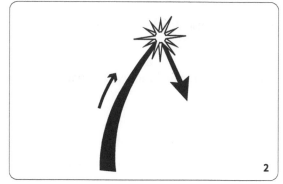

A release happens, followed by tissue moving in a new direction.

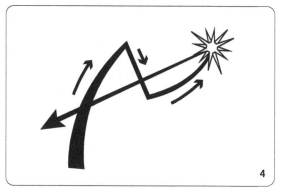

Then another release, followed by a different, new direction of movement.

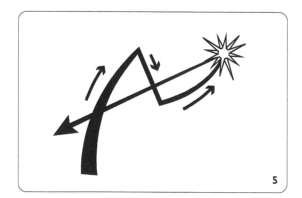

And another release, followed by yet another new direction.

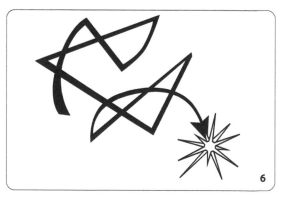

Any number of releases, followed by new directions.

Eventually a larger, more general release happens. Then the tissue stops moving. This treatment episode is complete. Take your hands off. Return to assessment to find the next piece to treat.

Special situations

There are two special situations where you will actively intervene in unwinding.

- Repeated patterns of unwinding.
- Too fast movement.

REPEATED PATTERNS

When the tissue being treated changes direction, continue to follow unless the tissue under treatment falls into a repeated pattern.

When a repeated pattern appears, observe it until you can discern the features of the whole pattern. The pattern may be simple or complex. Choose a relatively tight turn in the repeated pattern. Exert just enough counterforce to stop the tissue movement in the tight turn. Wait. Eventually, the tissue will begin to move in a new direction outside the repeated pattern. Once this new direction begins, resume simply following.

What to do when a repeated pattern happens during unwinding

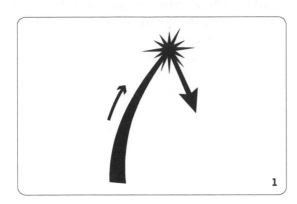

An unwind begins (see Classic unwinding)...

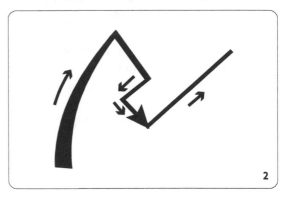

...and goes through any number of legs.

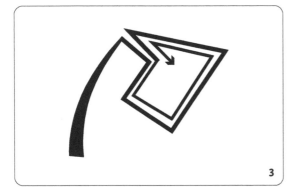

You notice a repeating pattern of movement.

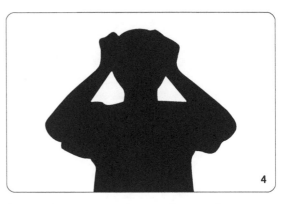

A repeated pattern means the person's system does not know how to release this particular issue.

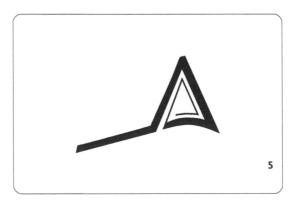

The repeated pattern may be simple...

What to do when a repeated pattern happens during unwinding (*cont.*)

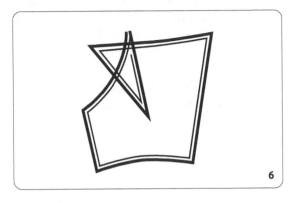

6

...or complex...

7

To facilitate release from a repeated pattern, follow the tissue to a relatively tight corner in the repeated pattern. At that corner, exert just enough back pressure to prevent the repeated pattern from continuing.

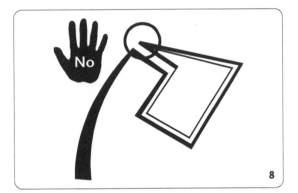

8

Body—you may not proceed in the old pattern. Choose any new direction.

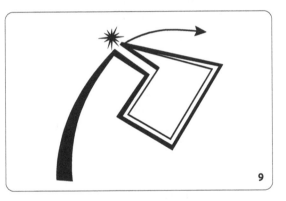

9

After a little time, the tissue will release in a new direction. At this point, fully release your back pressure. Allow the unwinding to continue until the usual expansive quiet endpoint is felt. Then remove your hands and return to assessment.

A new repeated pattern could happen. Continue to be vigilant.

TOO FAST MOVEMENT

Speed of movement in the tissue will vary from one person to another, from one body part to another, and over time. Follow the natural pace of the tissue being treated unless quick movement is observed. If you feel like you are being jerked around by the person's tissue, it is too quick. Too quick movement does not allow time for change. In this situation, slow the natural movement down by exerting a very gentle counter-load to slow but not stop the movement. Change the direction of your counter-load to match each new leg of the unwind.

Six factor model: Classic unwinding

TISSUE ENGAGEMENT

Tissue engagement is achieved by gradually applying light force into the body with a relaxed hand, just until the client's tissue pulls the therapist's hand.

FORCE

Just enough pressure into the body is used to form tissue engagement. If the tissue to be treated is near the surface of the body, pressure from the therapist's hand will be quite light. If the tissue being treated is deeper, the pressure at the surface will be somewhat greater to deliver a light force deeper.

Two special situations require the use of additional light force:

1. If a repeated pattern is observed, then a minimum force required to stop movement at a relatively tight corner in the pattern is exerted.
2. If the tissue moves too fast, a minimum counterforce is used to slow the movement to a productive range.

See below for detail on these two situations.

SPEED

The speed of the therapist's hand normally exactly matches the speed of the movements in the client's body. In this method, the therapist never makes the tissue move faster than it wants to.

If a repeated pattern is observed, the movement is brought to a stop at a tight corner.

If the client's tissue moves too quickly so the therapist feels rushed by it, then the therapist slows the tissue.

CONSTRAINT

Normally the tissue is not prevented from moving in any direction.

If a repeated pattern is observed, then tissue is prevented from moving along its familiar path until it moves in a new direction.

DIRECTIVENESS

Normally, tissue is not directed to move in any specific direction.

If the tissue moves too fast, it is directed to move more slowly.

RELATIONSHIP TO EFFORT BARRIERS

Effort barriers are not observed or utilized in this method. Forces normally used in this method are distinctly less than first barrier. When repeated movement is stopped at a corner, or too fast movement is slowed, sufficient force is used to achieve the desired effect without reference to force barriers.

Classic unwinding example 1

GENERAL ASSESSMENT

General assessment points to a primary dysfunction which is posterior, midline near the cervico-thoracic junction. Local listening, layer listening, and tissue type questions refine this as the superficial fascia overlying the vertebra prominens. Manual thermal assessment shows it to be an irregular shape about 10 cm² in area with its centroid approximately overlying the spinous process of C6.

CLIENT INQUIRY

Ask about the client's awareness of their body:

- in general and
- at the base of the neck.

LARGER AREA MOBILITY TESTING

- Active range of motion: With the client seated or standing, ask the client to successively move the head, left rotation, right rotation, left side bending, right side bending, extension, and flexion.
- Passive range of motion: With the client supine, instruct the client to allow you to move their head, neither resisting nor assisting. Place both hands under the back of the head. Move the head gently and slowly to a soft stop in left rotation, right rotation, left side bending, right side bending, extension, and flexion.

FOCAL MOBILITY TESTING

Superficial fascia is an elastic layer of connective tissue lying just deep to the skin which allows skin to move over deeper layers, giving the appearance of skin gliding. This is not a true lubricated glide plane but rather stretch in the superficial fascia which is just deep to the skin. Stiff superficial fascia prevents skin from moving well on underlying tissues. Therefore, a local mobility test is to engage the skin and attempt to move it in several directions on what lies under it. Non-moving skin can be distinguished from skin which will move over tissue under it. The margins of the fibrosed area of superficial fascia can be cleanly defined by testing the movement of skin in adjacent areas. It is important to test skin movement in several directions as one direction may be more limited than other directions.

With the client seated or in a side-lying position, contact the skin at the vertebra prominens and attempt to move the skin over the tissue under it in several directions, superior, inferior, left, right, and diagonals. Move your contact a finger width inferior and try this again. Try a finger width superior to the original location, a finger width left, a finger width right, testing skin movement in each location. By incrementally expanding the area tested, the edges of the area of limited skin movement can be found. Test each direction once and move on. Repeated testing may mobilize the stiff tissue and the results of testing will change with repetition leading to confusion.

For both focal and larger area mobility testing, note the results of the testing and point out the results of the testing to the client. Guide them to feel this from the inside.

TREATMENT

Place the client in a convenient position, usually seated, or side-lying. Prone may be used if a face cradle is provided so the head is not lying in a rotated position, nor in extension nor flexion.

Gently contact the skin over the fibrosed area of superficial fascia. Use a contact appropriate to the size of the area to be treated: a fingertip, two or more fingertips, part of the palm of the hand, the whole palm of the hand. With your hand, sink to the depth of the superficial fascia. Allow an unwind to begin. Follow the procedure for classic unwinding, described above.

POST TREATMENT TESTING (ALSO MENTIONED IN THE PREVIOUS CLASSIC UNWINDING SECTION)

When the unwinding movement stops:

- Post treatment mobility test the area using all the same tests as above.
- Use yes–no questioning to ask if this area of superficial fascia is sufficiently treated.

The results of these inquiries may be:

- If the mobility is now normal and the person's system says it is sufficiently treated, you are done; return to general assessment to find the next primary.
- If mobility testing is improved but still somewhat limited and the person's system says that area is sufficiently treated, you are done with that area for now. Return to general assessment to find the next primary. However, if mobility is improved by less than 50 percent, make a note to recheck this area at the next treatment.
- If mobility testing shows improvement but is still somewhat limited and the person's system says the area is not sufficiently treated, then ask, "Is the best treatment method to use now pure unwinding?" If the answer is yes, use pure unwinding again. If the person's system says no, then inquire further to learn what is the best treatment method to use next. Whether the next treatment episode for this area is pure unwinding or another method, follow this with mobility testing and questioning about completeness of treatment for this area for now. Any number of treatment episodes and/ or treatment methods may be used but it is unusual for there to be more than three treatment episodes. When the person's system says this area is sufficiently treated for the moment, return to general assessment to find the next primary dysfunction. However, if mobility is improved by less than 50 percent, make a note to recheck this area at the next treatment.

Point out the results of the mobility testing to the client. Guide the client to feel the results of this testing and how it is different from the pretest results.

Classic unwinding example 2

GENERAL ASSESSMENT

General assessment points to a primary dysfunction which is near the inferior margin of the left side of the thorax anterior–laterally. Local listening, layer listening, and tissue type questions refine this as the cartilage of the left costal arch. Manual thermal assessment shows a gently curved stripe consistent with the left costal arch from rib 8 to rib 10.

MOBILITY TESTING

Mobility test this area. Note the results and point them out to the client.

ACTIVE LARGE SCALE MOBILITY TESTING

- Observe the client make a full inhale and a full exhale. Observe the client rotating the trunk to the left and to the right.

PASSIVE FOCAL MOBILITY TESTING

With both hands, grasp the right costal arch. Gently bend the whole of it a little. Make smaller grips to bend a succession of focal areas of the arch. With both hands grasp the left costal arch; gently bend it a little. Make smaller grips to bend a succession of focal portions of it. Compare flexibility of the two sides, left and right with each other. Compare the flexibility of focal areas within each side. Compare all of this to your store of memories of other costal arches you have tested in the past.

Point out the results of the large- and small-scale mobility testing to the client and assist them to feel it from the inside.

If the left costal arch is not uniformly stiff use yes–no questioning to ask if it is best to treat a portion of the costal arch rather than the whole costal arch. If the answer is yes, use local listening and inhibition to compare stiff areas to find the most primary area to treat. Remember that the stiffest area is seldom the most primary.

TREATMENT

Contact the area to be treated with the fingers of one or two hands as appropriate to the size of the area of costal arch to be treated. Gently sink into the depth of the costal arch. Allow an unwind to begin at that tissue depth. Follow each leg of the unwind, neither inhibiting nor increasing the movement. A release will be felt at each change in the unwind direction. After seconds to minutes, a larger release will be felt and unwinding will stop. At that moment, remove your hands.

POST TREATMENT TESTING AND INQUIRY

Use the standard post treatment procedure for mobility testing and question asking detailed in the introduction to treatment methods section. Either treat this same area further, as indicated by this inquiry, or return to general assessment.

Classic unwinding example 3

ASSESSMENT

General listening is a forward and slightly right lean from low in the lower limb. General lift and general tap point to this same area.

Inhibitory contact at the right greater trochanter witness point for the lower limb establishes this primary restriction as existing in the right lower limb.

Inhibitory contact at the right lateral malleolus witness point for the ankle and foot establishes this primary restriction as existing in the right foot or ankle.

Ask the client to lie on the table with heels just off the end of the table. A manual thermal sweep of the right foot and ankle shows thermal variation at:

- medial malleolus
- medial part of the subtalar joint complex
- talonavicular joint
- first tarso-metatarsal joint
- second metatarso-phalangeal joint.

Pairwise inhibition among these areas establishes the talonavicular joint as the most primary.

Yes–no question asking establishes the primary restriction as describable by a single tissue type. Asking about a succession of tissue types establishes the primary restriction as existing in the joint capsule, which supports the earlier findings.

MOBILITY TESTING

Note all test results. Point out all test results to the client and assist them to feel it from the inside.

LARGE SCALE ACTIVE MOBILITY ASSESSMENT

- Watch the client walk, particularly observing movement through the foot, at the ankle, at each knee, and in each hip. (Problems with ankle, knee hip, and low back all refer symptoms to the other members of this group.)
- Ask the client to lie supine on the treatment table with heels just off the end of the table.
- Ask the client to slowly plantarflex both feet and all toes. Compare movement in the two feet. Repeat this with dorsiflexion of the feet and all toes.

ADJACENT AREA PASSIVE MOBILITY TESTS

- Using the distal femur as a handle internally rotate, then externally rotate each hip joint. During this test, place your other hand on the anterior ilium to limit the movement to the femero-acetabular joint rather than allowing the pelvis to roll on the table.
- Test the mobility of both talocrural joints. The directions given here are for the right ankle. Trade the hand positions for the left ankle. With the left hand, grasp

the distal tibia and fibula at the malleoli to make a dynamic stabilization. With the right hand, put the web of the thumb on the anterior talus and grasp the talus with your thumb and index fingers. Your two hands will be adjacent, touching each other. Use the hand on the talus to fully dorsiflex the talus on the lower leg. Let it return to neutral. Then fully plantarflex the talus on the lower leg. Note the ranges and ease of motion, comparing the two ankles to each other and to your store of memories of other ankles you have tested.

LOCAL PASSIVE MOBILITY TESTS

Test the talonavicular joint mobility. These directions are for the right foot; shift your hands so your left hand now approaches the talus anteriorly and grasping it to make a dynamic stabilization of the talus. Place the web of your right thumb adjacent to this on the navicular bone and grasp the navicular with the bases of your thumb and index fingers. Circumduct the navicular clockwise on the dynamically stabilized talus. Then circumduct the navicular counterclockwise on the dynamically stabilized talus. Next make an A-P axis rotation of the talus on the navicular first clockwise, then counterclockwise.

Repeat all this on the other foot. Compare the results between the feet and to your store of memories of other similar joints you have tested. Note and point out the results to your client.

TREATMENT

Using holds on the talus and navicular bones as for the mobility testing to control the bones, subtly compact the bones toward each other to sink into the joint capsule material with a slightly long lever until an unwind starts. Stay at this depth as the unwinding proceeds, simply following each leg of unwind, neither encouraging nor limiting each movement. A release will be felt at each change of direction. After seconds to minutes a larger release will be felt and the unwind will stop. Remove your hands.

POST TREATMENT TESTING AND INQUIRY

Use the standard post treatment procedure for mobility testing and question asking detailed in the introduction to treatment methods section. Either treat this same area further, as indicated by this inquiry, or return to general assessment. This will include:

- Post mobility test the talonavicular joint as above.
- Use yes–no questioning to ask if treatment of the talonavicular joint is sufficiently complete for now.

Treatment method 2: augmented unwinding

Origin
Early osteopathic technique. Original discoverer unknown.

Concept
In unwinding, the client's tissue spontaneously moves in a succession of unpredictable directions, with a softening or release at each turn or corner from one leg of unwind to the next. Sometimes the therapeutic effect can be increased by a brief gentle push each time the tissue tries to change direction. The gentle push takes the tissue slightly farther in the direction it had been traveling before the change of direction.

Therapeutic method
Pretest in the usual way utilizing local, global, active, and passive tests.

Then, to initiate the treatment, approach the person's body with soft flexible hands. Allow the person's inherent tissue movements to move your hands.

Whatever motions the person's body makes, follow this to the end of each leg of movement. When the tissue starts to change direction, do not immediately allow this change, but rather for about one second direct the tissue a little further along the path it was on. After this brief augmentation, release the tissue to follow what path it will. The new path may be different than the direction change noted before the augmentation load was applied because the augmentation load changes the tissue.

Repeated patterns are less common with augmented unwinding than with pure unwinding. When a repeated pattern appears, use the standard procedure to break the repeated pattern. See earlier section on repeated patterns.

Pace
Follow the natural pace of the tissue being treated unless quick movement is observed.

Too quick movement is much less common with augmented unwinding than with pure unwinding. In the unlikely event that too quick a movement occurs, follow the standard procedure to break this pattern (see earlier section on too quick movement). Even though you are slowing the movement, you will still encourage the movement in terms of range each time it tries to change direction. This requires a change in direction of load you apply at the moment the tissue starts to change direction.

Completion
When the movement comes to a stop and there is a sense of peace or rest in the tissue, this therapeutic episode is over. Return to assessment.

Post treatment testing and inquiry
Use the standard post treatment procedure for mobility testing and question asking detailed in the introduction to treatment methods section. Either treat this same area further, as indicated by this inquiry, or return to general assessment.

Six factor model: Augmented unwinding
TISSUE ENGAGEMENT
Approach the person's body with soft, flexible hands. Allow the person's inherent tissue movements to move your hands. Tissue engagement is made by the client's tissue.

FORCE
Just enough pressure into the body is used to form tissue engagement. If the tissue to be treated is near the surface of the body, pressure from the therapist's hand will be quite light. If the tissue being treated is deeper, the pressure at the surface will be somewhat greater to deliver a light force deeper.

In the moments of augmentation, the force used is at or below first barrier; however, effort barriers are not specifically assessed.

Two special situations require the use of additional light force:

1. If a repeated pattern is observed, then a minimum force required to stop movement at a relatively tight corner in the pattern is exerted.
2. If the tissue moves too fast, a minimum counter force is used to slow the movement to a productive range.

SPEED

While following the natural movement of an unwind, the speed of the therapist's hand normally exactly matches the speed of the movements in the client's body. In this method, the therapist never makes the tissue move faster than it wants to.

In the augmentation portion of each leg of movement, speed will be like or a bit less than the natural movement of that leg of movement.

If a repeated pattern is observed, the movement is brought to a stop at a tight corner.

If the client's tissue moves too quickly so the therapist feels rushed by it, then the therapist slows the tissue. In this case, the augmentation also proceeds at a similarly reduced rate.

CONSTRAINT

Normally, the tissue is not prevented from moving in any direction.

If a repeated pattern is observed, then tissue is prevented from moving along its familiar path, until it moves in a new direction.

DIRECTIVENESS

When following the natural movement of the tissue any movement direction is allowed.

At the end of each leg of natural movement, the therapist directs the tissue to move a little further in that same direction for 1–2 seconds.

If the tissue moves too fast, it is directed to move more slowly.

RELATIONSHIP TO EFFORT BARRIERS

Effort barriers are not assessed or utilized in this method. Forces normally used are distinctly less than the first barrier. When repeated movement is stopped at a corner, or too fast movement is slowed, sufficient force is used to achieve the desired effect without reference to force barriers.

Augmented unwinding

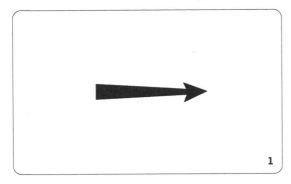

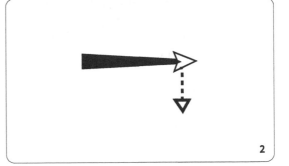

As you touch tissue gently with a soft hand, it begins to move.

At the first hint of a change of direction, just for a second gently push the tissue a little further along its first path. Then let it go where it wants to.

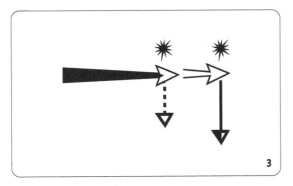

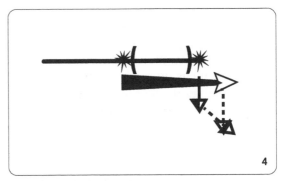

This will often (but not always) increase the amount of release.

As usual with unwinding, the tissue will soon try to move in another direction.

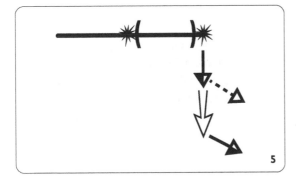

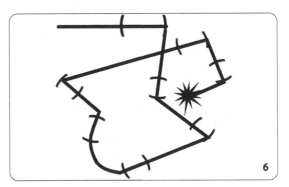

Again, ask the tissue to go further very briefly in the direction it was going just before this change of direction.

Augment each leg of the unwind in this way until there is a larger, more general release followed by the tissue movement stopping.

This treatment episode is over. Remove your hands. Return to assessment to find the next piece to work on.
Repeated patterns are much less common with augmented unwinding than with classic unwinding but stay alert to this possibility.

Augmented unwinding example 1

Assessment methods lead to the intermuscular septum between the right gastrocnemius and soleus muscles as the current primary.

Place the client supine on the table with heels off the end of the table.

MOBILITY TESTS

- Gently lift the left heel to assess knee extension. Put the left heel down and do the same thing with the right heel.
- For the right ankle, stand at the client's right side. Place the web of the left thumb over the distal left lower leg bones and the thumb and forefinger on the malleoli to provide a dynamic stabilization of the distal crura. Place the right hand under the heel to grasp the calcaneus. Draw the calcaneus inferior and anterior to both dorsiflex the foot on the crura, to ask for length in the Achilles tendon and associated muscles. Set up a mirror image of this to test the left side.
- For the right side, sit or stand at the client's right side facing the lower leg. Place the left hand under the belly of the gastrocnemius muscles. Place the right hand over the upper half of the tibia with the thumb aligned vertically just posterior to the tibia, and the tips of fingers 2–5 touching just posterior to the medial aspect of the tibia, these to control the sartorius muscle. Make a gentle shearing mobility test bringing the gastrocnemius toward you and the soleus and tibia away from you. Let this rest to neutral, then reverse directions to bring the tibia and sartorius toward you and the gastrocnemius away from you. Note apparent movement between the two muscles. Set up the mirror image of this to test the other leg.

TREATMENT

Place your hands on the right lower leg as for the mobility test. Sink gently in between the two hands to arrive at the intermuscular septum between the gastrocnemius and sartorius muscles. Let an unwind begin. Each time the tissue tries to change directions give it a gentle brief, less than one second, push in the direction it was going before it tried to change directions. After seconds to minutes, a larger release will be felt and the tissue will stop unwinding.

When the unwind stops, use your hands, already in this position, to reassess lateral glide between these two muscles. Use the standard post treatment procedure for mobility testing and question asking detailed in the introduction to treatment methods section. Either treat this same area further, as indicated by this inquiry, or return to general assessment.

Augmented unwinding example 2

General assessment methods followed by local assessment methods lead to a primary lesion of a focal area of parietal pleura contracture deep to angles of right ribs 6, 7, and 8.

MOBILITY TESTING
Active

- With the client standing ask the client to make a full inhale, and a full exhale. Observe what areas of the chest fill easily and which not.
- Ask the client to make trunk motions:
  - Flexion
  - Extension
  - Left side bending
  - Right side bending
  - Right rotation
  - Left rotation.

Passive

- Have the client lie in a side-lying position with the right side up, and knees and hips comfortably flexed. Place pillows under their head, and in front of the torso with their arm on that pillow, and if the client wishes, a pillow between knees.

Use ribs as handles to attempt vertical stretch of portions of the right half of the chest wall. Start distal to the area indicated by assessment. Incrementally test several areas to define the area of stiff chest wall. This will usually be an irregularly shaped area.

Also sink into this area and try to glide the chest wall on the lung deep to it. Try this in the area of reduced mobility and in other areas. This discriminates whether there is pleural adhesion as well as pleural contracture in this area. The two often but not always occur together. If there is both adhesion of the visceral to parietal pleura and parietal pleura contracture it is usually more productive to restore the glide plane first before attempting to restore the elasticity of the parietal pleura, but not always. If a visceral–parietal pleura adhesion is discovered ask if it is better to release the adhesion first. If the answer is yes, it is better to release the adhesion first; this seems to contradict the earlier assessment that the primary is a contracture. This is an example of the fact that any assessment method can give a false answer. If this is the situation, we don't know which is more primary, the adhesion or the contracture, as we have contradictory information about this. However, both the adhesion and the contracture are likely high on the primacy list.

TREATMENT

To treat the contracture with augmented unwinding, make a contact in this area of a size reasonable to the size and shape of the area of contracture discovered. This may be anything from a fingertip to both hands. Sink into the level of the parietal pleura. As you arrive at this depth let an unwinding begin. At each change of direction, gently and briefly push the tissue a little farther in the direction it was going before it tried to change direction. Then allow the direction change.

When the unwinding stops, ask if this pleural fibrosity remobility tests both stretch and glide of the parietal pleura in this area. Use the standard post treatment procedure for mobility testing and question asking detailed in the introduction to treatment methods section. Either treat this same area further, as indicated by this inquiry, or return to general assessment.

Augmented unwinding example 3

Assessment leads to bone in the left patella as the currently most primary lesion.

ALIGNMENT AND MOBILITY TESTING
Active

- Observe the client standing, then walking.

Passive

- Place the client supine on the table. With both hands on the right patella, gently try to bend bone in the patella in several directions. Do the same with the left patella. Compare the flexibility of bone in the two patellae, and to your store of memories of patellae you have tested before.
- Place a hand behind the right knee and the other hand on the patella. Providing dynamic stabilization with the posterior hand for the distal femur and proximal tibia, gently move the patella in a succession of directions, medial, lateral, superior, inferior, and diagonals between these cardinal directions. Do the same with the other knee. Compare the mobility of the two patellae and compare both to your

store of memories of other patellae you have mobility tested.

- Place the client in a side-lying position with the left side up. Provide a pillow under the head and a pillow in front of the torso to rest the left arm on and to provide stability. Arrange the client in a comfortable position with the right leg more fully extended and the left leg somewhat flexed at both knee and hip with a pillow under the leg to limit adduction.

- Stand beside the table behind the client. With your right hand, provide a dynamic stabilization of the distal left femur. With the left hand, control the distal lower leg to gently fully extend the knee, then fully flex the knee. Note ease and range of motion. Report your observations to the client.

TREATMENT

Return the client to a supine position. With the fingers of one hand laterally on the patella and the other hand medially on the patella, sink gently into the bone with both hands until an unwind begins. The excursions of each leg of unwinding within bone will usually be small. Each time the unwind starts to change direction, briefly and gently push it a little farther in the direction it was going before it started to change direction. After seconds to a few minutes, the bone will stop unwinding. Remove your hands.

POST TREATMENT TESTING AND INQUIRY

When the unwinding stops ask if this is sufficiently treated and try the local bending tests of the patella again. Use the standard post treatment procedure for mobility testing and question asking detailed in the introduction to treatment methods section. Either treat this same area further, as indicated by this inquiry, or return to general assessment.

Eventually, when questions say it is sufficiently treated, redo all mobility tests active and passive, draw the client out on their awareness, and point out what you see. Note for future review if the improvement is less than 50 percent. Return to basic assessment to find the next primary lesion.

Treatment method 3: alternate interrupt unwinding

Origin
Created by Jeffrey Burch and named by Carol Gray.

Concept
Alternate interrupt treatment techniques is an expansion of the method used to break a repeated pattern. Instead of blocking just a repeated pattern, every second movement is blocked. A way of conceptualizing how alternate interrupt unwinding works is that the frequent blocking makes the person's system think outside its box to find new solutions.

Alternate interrupt is both an independent variant of unwinding treatment technique, and an element that can be added to any functional methods that utilize unwinding. This technique component can be added to any functional method that utilizes pure unwinding, augmented unwinding, stacking techniques, and those scraping the walls and pendulum techniques that use the unwinding phenomenon.

Pretest
Pretest by looking at alignment and mobility, locally and globally, in the usual ways.

Method
Treatment steps

1. Initiate an unwind.
2. Allow the first movement of unwinding.
3. When the tissue tries to change direction at the end of the first leg of the unwind, do not allow this attempted second movement. Give just enough directed back pressure to prevent it.
4. Soon the tissue will try a different direction of movement; allow this new movement.
5. Return to step 3. Cycle steps 3 and 4 dynamically preventing every-other movement until movement stops and there is an expansive softening indicating the end of treatment.

Repeated patterns cannot happen with the alternate interrupt methods.

Movement which is too fast has not yet been reported with the alternate interrupt unwind treatment method.

Post test
Use the standard post treatment procedure for mobility testing and question asking detailed in the introduction to treatment methods section. Either treat this same area further, as indicated by this inquiry, or return to general assessment.

Six factor model: Alternate interrupt unwinding

TISSUE ENGAGEMENT
The initiation of treatment tissue engagement is made by the client's system as in pure unwinding. At the moments of pattern interruption, the therapist briefly takes the lead.

FORCE
Force used is low to moderately low. The amount of force used to initiate the unwind varies with the base technique to which this additional element is added, always first barrier or less. The force used to block movement is only the minimum required. If excessive force is used, it will not be possible to feel the new direction of movement. The force used to block the changes in the unwind direction are not intimately related to the first barrier, or other specific barrier, rather it is the minimum necessary to stop the movement of unwinding.

SPEED
Speed used is the low speed consistent with any method utilizing the unwind phenomenon.

TREATMENT
METHOD 3

CONSTRAINT

Although force is low, constraint is intermittently high, alternating with episodes of no constraint. Specifically, constraint is high when the specific vector of every other movement is forbidden, but all other movements are allowed.

DIRECTIVENESS

There is no directiveness. No specific movements are required.

RELATIONSHIP TO EFFORT BARRIERS

The force required to stop movement is not related to first, second, or other barriers. The force is gauged as only the minimum to stop the movement.

Alternate interrupt, unwinding variant

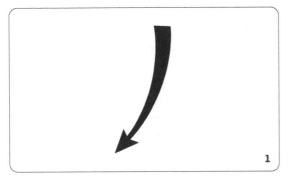

Contact the area to be treated gently with a soft hand. Tissue begins to move (see Classic unwinding).

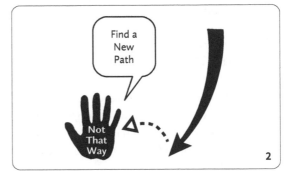

As soon as the tissue tries to change direction, exert just enough back pressure to prevent only that particular movement.

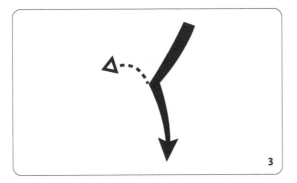

Fully allow movement in the new direction. Release your back pressure.

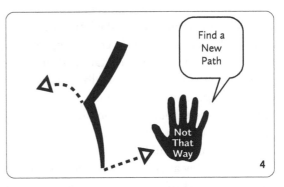

At the next corner, again offer just enough back pressure to prevent only the new direction of movement but...

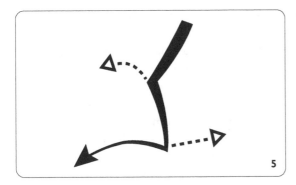

...allow the second movement the person's system offers and release your back pressure.

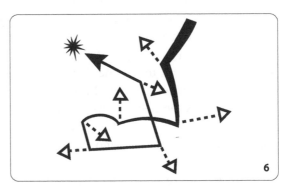

Continue this process at each corner. Eventually there will be a larger, more general release. This treatment episode is complete. Take your hands off. Return to assessment to find the next piece to treat.

This method redirects release at every turn by the same method used to open repeated patterns.
Repeated patterns have not been reported with this method.

Alternate interrupt unwinding example 1
Assessment has led to a primary lesion in the right olecranon bursa.

POSITIONAL OBSERVATION
Observe the client standing. *Note:*

- Shoulder position on each side, elevation, depression, protraction/retraction.
- How does the arm hang?
- Positional fullness of rib cage on each side.

MOBILITY TESTING
Perform a circumduction test of each gleno-humeral joint. Stand behind the client. For the right gleno-humeral joint, place the left hand on the top of the shoulder girdle contacting scapula and clavicle for a dynamic stabilization. With the right hand, contact the elbow to control both the humerus and the ulna so the humerus can be moved through a circumduction without the elbow flexing. Move the humerus on the scapula in mixed mild flexion and adduction to end range. Stay at end range as you continue to flex and adduct the humerus; on the scapula do not internally or externally rotate it. Proceed from here to make a full circumduction of the gleno-humeral joint, noting any irregularities. Repeat for the other shoulder.

Ask the client to lie supine. For the right arm place the left hand under the distal humerus and with the right hand control the right wrist. Slowly fully flex the elbow noting end range and ease of movement. Next, fully extend the elbow noting end range and ease of movement through the range. Repeat for the other arm. Compare the two elbows with each other and with your store of memories of other elbows you have tested.

With the client still supine, place a finger over the tip of the olecranon process. Sink almost to the bone. Contact the olecranon bursa and attempt to glide it medial and lateral. Repeat for the other arm. Compare the two elbows with each other and with your store of memories of other elbows you have tested.

TREATMENT
Using the same contact as for local assessment of glide in the olecranon bursa, sink to the level of the bursa; allow an unwind to start. The first time the tissue tries to change direction, use just enough back pressure to prevent the new direction. In a few seconds, the tissue will try to move in a different direction; allow this movement. The next time the tissue tries to change directions, again use minimal dynamic force to prevent the new direction. Then when the tissue moves in a different new direction, allow that movement. Proceed in this way, allowing every other movement, until the unwind stops. Remove your hands.

POST TREATMENT TESTING
When the unwind stops, use the standard post treatment procedure for mobility testing and question asking detailed in the introduction to treatment methods section. Either treat this same area further, as indicated by this inquiry, or return to general assessment.

Alternate interrupt unwinding example 2
Skin overlying approximately the middle third of the left vastus lateralis muscle.

MOBILITY TESTING AND POSITIONAL OBSERVATION
Active and postural

- Observe the client standing. View, front, back, and from the left side. Note particularly knee extension in standing, and apparent pelvic tilt.
- Observe the client walking. How is mobility at both hips and both knees?

Passive

- Have the client lie supine on the table.
- Stand at the client's right side. Place your

left hand on the right anterior superior iliac spine (ASIS) and your right hand on the distal right femur. Use the right hand to make a dynamic stabilization of the right femur so the distal femur does not come off the table. With the left hand, attempt to rock the left ilium posteriorly, making an extension of the hip.

- Still standing at the client's right side, place your left hand under the distal right thigh and your right hand on the client's ankle. Instruct the client to neither resist nor assist as you move the leg. Flex the knee and hip, seeing how close the heel will come to the ischial tuberosity. As the knee flexion proceeds, rotate your hand out and laterally so your hand is not a limiting factor to knee flexion. Return the knee to the table.

- With your hands, gently stretch the skin on the anterior right thigh in several directions.

- Step to the left side of the table and reproduce all this on the left side. Expect to find reduced skin stretch over the middle part of the left vastus lateralis. The shape of the stiff skin area is usually irregular and can be any size. Any other mobility limitation may also be observed in either leg.

TREATMENT

Depending on the size and shape of the area of skin-stretch limitation; place a portion of your hand, the whole hand, or both hands on the area of stiff skin. Allow an unwind to begin. When the tissue tries to change direction of movement, offer just enough back force to prevent the new movement. In a short time, the tissue will begin to move in a different direction. Allow that second new direction of movement. The next time the tissue tries to change direction, use minimal force to dynamically prevent the new direction of movement. Soon the tissue will begin to move in a different new direction. Allow this movement.

Continue in this way, preventing every other movement. In seconds to minutes, the unwinding will stop. Remove your hands.

When the unwind stops, follow the Completion of treatment protocol (page 95).

Alternate interrupt unwinding example 3

ASSESSMENT

The primary restriction is found to be focal area of stiffness in liver tissue.

TREATMENT TYPE INQUIRY

Yes–no inquiry into treatment method recommends a first barrier stack to near first barriers with alternate interrupt.

POSTURAL OBSERVATION

Observe the client standing, with particular attention to shoulder position and rib cage position. Look from the front, back, left side, and right side.

RANGE OF MOTION

Active

- Request a full deep breath followed by a full exhale. Note breath excursion, particularly any differences between the left and right sides.
- Ask the client to swing both arms up laterally (abduction) so their hands meet above their head. Note any differences in shoulder movement range and ease.
- Ask the client to walk. How well does movement flow through the thorax and abdomen?

Passive

- Either current liver pathology or liver fibrosity from historical events will reliably refer right shoulder pain and/or stiffness (see Goodman and Snyder 2000).
- Stand behind the client. Examine scapular glide on each side. For the left shoulder,

put your left hand on the top of the right shoulder girdle with the thumb against the lateral aspect of T1. Use your hand to grasp the upper thorax, creating a dynamic stabilization. Place your left hand more laterally on your client's left shoulder so you can control the scapular position. Protract the scapula over the rib cage. Allow the scapula to return to neutral, then retract the scapula. Shift your left hand to the proximal end of the left humerus. With your left hand, lift the left scapula, then allow it to settle down again.

- Shift your position and contact to a mirror image of this to examine right scapular protraction, retraction, and elevation.
- Compare the mobility of the two shoulder girdles and compare each side to your store of memories of other shoulder girdles you have tested.
- Ask the client to lie supine. Support the knees and lower legs on pillows to give the abdominal wall some slack. The use of pillows for this is preferable to the client holding their knees up, as the use of pillows avoids the client's use of muscular effort. Sit or stand at your client's right side. Place your left hand on the right lower rib cage. Glide some skin on the thorax inferiorly to give more slack to the abdominal wall and maintain it there, anchoring your left thumb on the inferior surface of the right costal arch. Ask your client to tell you if there is the slightest discomfort. Place your right hand flat on the upper right abdomen. Gently move your right hand toward supination so the palm of the hand faces the liver. Does the liver feel hot? Ask your client about any discomfort. If the liver is hot, and/or is uncomfortable to touch, abort this test procedure. The liver or portions of it may

also be hard. Hard by itself may reflect fibrosity from historical events and this is something you can work on. If the liver is hot and/or uncomfortable to touch, there may be current pathology. Jaundice, a yellowing of the whites of the eyes or skin, is a warning sign of liver problems. Pain in the right shoulder, right side of the neck, and possibly right side of head is a potential sign of liver or gall bladder inflammation. If the liver is hard, as well as hot and painful, this is a red flag. How many warning signs you see shapes how urgently you will recommend your client see a medical doctor.

TREATMENT

Assuming the liver is not hot and/or painful, note any stiffness in the liver. Sink gently into the liver. Stack the tissue to a near first barrier in three planes. Allow an unwind to begin. While maintaining the first barrier load direction developed in the first barrier stack, manage the unwind as an alternate interrupt. The first time the tissue starts to change direction, exert just enough back force to dynamically prevent the direction change. Soon the liver tissue will begin to move in a different direction; allow this movement. Then when the liver tissue next tries to change direction of unwind, exert minimal force to prevent the new direction of movement. Soon the tissue will begin to move in a different direction. Allow this new movement. Proceed in this fashion, preventing movement at each corner until a different direction of movement begins which you will allow. After seconds to minutes, the unwind will stop. Remove your hands.

COMPLETION OF TREATMENT

When the unwind stops, follow the Completion of treatment protocol (page 95).

TREATMENT TECHNIQUES IN WHICH TISSUE ENGAGEMENT IS MADE BY THE THERAPIST AND UNWINDING IS USED

Introduction to first barrier stacking techniques

Concept

The unwinding treatment techniques in the previous section all utilized client-initiated tissue engagement. Next, we will look at a set of techniques where the tissue engagement is made by the therapist followed by unwinding initiated by the client's tissue.

In this set of techniques, the therapist precisely assesses certain mobility qualities of the tissue and uses this information to establish a first barrier directional load. This load is maintained throughout the unwinding treatment.

This unwind may be managed in a simple unwind fashion, or with augmentation, or as an alternate interrupt.

In later sections of this book, other ways of initiating an unwind will be presented. Several treatment methods will also be presented in which unwinding is not used or even forbidden.

Terminology

If tissue is mobility tested in a succession of opposite directions just to a first barrier, the first barrier in one direction is always found to be farther from neutral than the other. I call the first barrier found at the shorter distance the near first barrier, and the first barrier found at the longer distance the far first barrier.

It is important to know that the first barrier found at the shorter distance is not related to which end range is at a shorter distance. The same thing applies to farther first barriers and farther end ranges.

See the larger discussion of this on page 119.

Treatment method 4: near first barrier stack

Origin

Early functional technique, following the work of H. V. Hoover DO. Original discoverer not known.

Concept

In the previous section, unwinding treatments were initiated by a tissue engagement from the client. Stacking techniques are among the several techniques where the tissue engagement is made by the therapist. The therapist taking the lead in this way gives a different flavor to the treatment and is often but not always more productive.

The central feature of stacking techniques is local mobility testing of tissue to first barriers in a succession of opposite, cardinal, or physiologic movement axes. The tissue is then loaded to several selected first barriers that were found in this way. An unwind then begins and continues, while the directional load established by the therapist is dynamically maintained.

Pretest

Look at standing alignment.

Mobility test in both of two different ways:

1. Test and note the end range. If the anatomy of the area is known, test each established physiologic axis. Where applicable, circumduction should also be tested. If the anatomy is not known, simply mobility test the tissue in three cardinal dimensions.
2. Test and note first barriers on both ends of each range of motion in two or more dimensions. These dimensions can be cardinal planes such as distal–proximal,

or physiologic motions such as flexion and extension. For each dimension, one direction will present a first barrier sooner (after a shorter excursion) than the other direction; note these differences.

Directions of near first barrier and far first barrier

Find first barriers in both directions of each of at least three dimensions. These directions may be cardinal and/or physiologic axes. In each dimension, you will find that a first barrier is discovered at a greater distance in one direction and at a shorter distance in the opposite direction. The direction which presents a first barrier at less distance is called the near first barrier. The direction that presents a first barrier after the relatively greater distance is called the far first barrier.

Nomenclature

Near first barrier is more commonly called direction of effort. Far first barrier is more frequently called direction of ease. While less common, the terms near first barrier and far first barrier are more descriptive, and therefore less prone to confusion.

Treatment method

For the near first barrier treatment, mobility test tissue to first barriers in several pairs of opposite directions. As you work through this succession of low force mobility tests, apply and accumulate first barrier load at each of the near first barriers. Soon a tissue release will follow. This release will change the tissue qualities. Continue to maintain your original direction of load to a first barrier; however, the position is likely to change. Usually, your hand will move slightly farther with each release as the tissue expands. If during a release you lose the sense of where the first barrier is, then retest the first barriers and stack again in direction of ease.

Note—In the setup of first barrier treatments, it is possible to test each dimension separately, remember the results, and then stack the several dimensions to the near barriers. This utilizes substantial memory and more time. It is a good shortcut to test one dimension and maintain the tissue at the near first barrier in that dimension, and then test a second dimension. Also, maintain the tissue at a first barrier load in this second dimension of effort. Two dimensions are now concurrently loaded in direction of effort. Then test the first barrier of the third dimension and add this dimension of first barrier load in the direction of effort. This method saves time and memory compared to testing each dimension separately, remembering all their directions and then stacking all three again.

Optional additional features

Augmentation or alternate interrupt may be added to the basics of this treatment. Practice and become comfortable with the stacking technique before adding additional dimensions.

Movement which is repeated or too fast

Unwinding movement in repeated patterns or movement which is too fast is quite rare with stacking techniques. Stay alert to these possibilities and manage them in the usual way if they do occur.

Post treatment testing and inquiry

Use the standard post treatment procedure for mobility testing and question asking detailed in the introduction to treatment methods section. Either treat this same area further, as indicated by this inquiry, or return to general assessment.

Near first barrier stack (direction of effort)

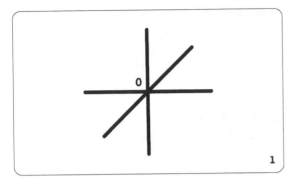

1

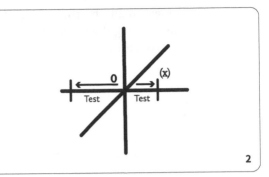

2

Consider axes of movement for the given tissue; these may be either cardinal planes or physiologic axes.

Along one of these axes, successively mobility test the tissue to a first barrier load first in one direction, then in the opposite direction.

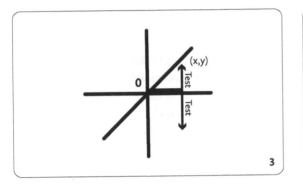

3

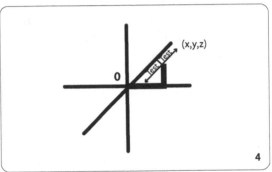

4

Maintain the tissue at a first barrier load in the shorter direction; from this new starting point mobility test the tissue to a first barrier load in each direction along a second axis.

Having found the second dimension of first barrier, maintain the tissue at the shorter distance first barrier in both of the dimensions tested. From this starting place, mobility test to a first barrier in a third dimension.

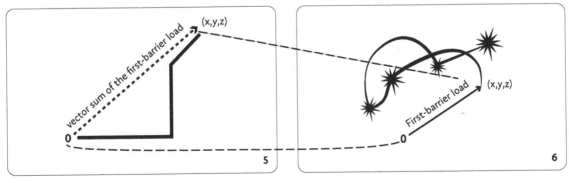

5

6

Note the vector sum of the three loads applied. Maintain a first barrier load in this combined direction.

While maintaining this combined direction of load, allow an unwinding. The usual small releases will be felt at each corner, and a larger, more general release at the end followed by the unwind stopping. Release the load applied to the tissue and return to assessment.

Six factor model: Near first barrier stack

TISSUE ENGAGEMENT

Tissue engagement made by the therapist is accomplished by stacking the tissue to near first barriers (direction of effort).

FORCE

First barrier only.

SPEED

Follow the speed of tissue movement, unless:

1. The movement is too fast; in which case, slow it down.
2. A repeated pattern is observed. When this happens, exert the minimum counterforce to prevent that movement. However, allow the next movement and then continue.

(These two phenomena are rare with this technique.)

CONSTRAINT

This technique uses no constraint unless a repeated pattern is noted; in which case, minimum force is used to stop the movement in a tight corner.

DIRECTIVENESS

The initial multidimensional load is mildly directive. This is a static load. No specific movement is required. The only directiveness is the rare need to slow a too fast movement.

RELATIONSHIP TO EFFORT BARRIERS

Treatment is accomplished at a first barrier load. The only time more force may be used is the minimum necessary to stop a repeated pattern. The only time less than first barrier force may be used is in slowing down a too fast movement.

Near first barrier stack example 1

GENERAL ASSESSMENT

General assessment points to a primary dysfunction in the right upper limb. Manual thermal assessment, local listening, layer listening, and tissue type questions refine this as the right annular ligament.

CLIENT INQUIRY

Ask about the client's awareness of their body:

- in general, and
- at the right upper limb in general and elbow and wrist in particular.

LARGER AREA MOBILITY TESTING

Active

- With the client seated or standing, ask the client to successively flex the right elbow and then fully extend it. Then request the client to turn the right hand palm down, and then palm up.

Passive

- With the client supine, instruct the client to allow you to move their right upper limb, neither resisting nor assisting. Sitting or standing at the client's right side, place your left hand under the client's right elbow. With your right hand, support the client's wrist so you can flex and extend the elbow while maintaining the wrist in a relaxed neutral position. Slowly fully flex and then fully extend the right elbow, noting range and ease of movement.
- Focal passive range of motion testing:
  - With your left hand still under the extended right elbow, use your right

hand at the wrist to first pronate then supinate the hand. Note range and ease of movement.

- – With the client's forearm on the table and your left hand still under the elbow, provide dynamic stabilization of the proximal ulna. Move your right hand to the radial head. Glide the radial head, first medial and then lateral on the ulna. Note range and excursion. Excursion should be small but nearly even medial vs lateral.

TREATMENT

With the client still supine, leave your hands in the position of the last focal passive range of motion test, that is, the left hand controlling the proximal ulna and the fingers of the right hand controlling the proximal end of the radius.

Again, glide the radial head medial and lateral on the ulna assessing near and far first barriers. Load the radial head to the near first barrier in this dimension. Then mobility test the motion of the radial head on the ulna distal versus proximal glide. Load this dimension also to a near first barrier. Then using the base of the palm of your hand to control a more distal portion of the radius, test pronation and supination of the hand which is also an internal and external roll of the proximal radius. Load this dimension to a near first barrier.

While maintaining the vector sum of these three loads, follow an unwind of the tissue in the vicinity of the proximal radio-ulnar joint. Be watchful for repeated patterns or for too fast movement. When the unwinding stops proceed to post treatment testing.

POST TREATMENT TESTING AND INQUIRY

Use the standard post treatment procedure for mobility testing and question asking detailed in the introduction to treatment methods section. Either treat this same area further, as indicated by this inquiry, or return to general assessment.

Near first barrier stack example 2

GENERAL ASSESSMENT

General assessment points to a primary dysfunction in the left lower limb. Manual thermal assessment, local listening, layer listening, and tissue type questions refine this to the left hip joint capsule.

CLIENT INQUIRY

Ask about the client's awareness of their body:

- in general, and
- at the left hip.

LARGER AREA MOBILITY TESTING

Active

- Ask the client to walk.
- Ask the client to squat down and then stand up again.

Passive

- With the client supine on the table, stand at the right side of the client facing their right thigh. Instruct the client to adjust their body on the table so it is diagonal on the table with the right hip at the edge of the table and the right leg off the edge of the table. Support the client's leg on your right hand at mid-calf. Place your left hand on the client's anterior ilium to provide dynamic stabilization. Instruct the client to allow you to move their leg without either assisting or resisting. Move the client's leg medially and slightly flexed so it is in front of the left leg at end range. Perform a circumduction of the leg maintaining the hip at end range throughout the circumduction. The path should be a smooth curve. Note where there are limitations in movement and deviation from a smooth curve. Point this out to the client.

Ask the client to return to lying centered on the table.

TREATMENT

Maintain your right hand in its position mid-calf. Place your left hand to control the right greater trochanter. Gravity will provide stabilization of the pelvis on the table. Using your two hands, explore first barrier ranges of motion at the hip joint: 1) internal–external rotation, 2) adduction abduction, 3) compaction–decompaction. For each dimension, load the tissue to a first barrier in the shorter direction. While maintaining the vector sum of these three loads, follow an unwind of the tissue at the hip joint. Follow directions for near barrier unwind (page 119).

Be watchful for repeated patterns or for too fast movement. When the unwinding stops proceed to post treatment testing.

POST TREATMENT TESTING AND INQUIRY

Use the standard post treatment procedure for mobility testing and question asking detailed in the introduction to treatment methods section. Either treat this same area further, as indicated by this inquiry, or return to general assessment.

Near first barrier stack example 3

GENERAL ASSESSMENT

General assessment points to a primary dysfunction in the right superior quadrant of the abdomen. Manual thermal assessment, local listening, layer listening, and tissue type questions refine this as an adhesion between loops of small intestine and the inferior surface of a portion of the transverse colon and its mesentery about halfway between the midline of the body and the right body wall.

CLIENT INQUIRY

Ask about the client's awareness of their body:

- in general, and
- at the abdomen.

LARGER AREA MOBILITY TESTING
Active

With the client seated or standing, ask the client to:

- take a deep breath
- extend their torso
- side bend their torso left, then right
- rotate their torso left, then right.

Focal passive

- With the client supine, instruct the client to allow you to explore their abdomen, neither resisting nor assisting. Sitting or standing at the client's right side, use your two hands to locate the transverse colon. Map its course from right to left across the abdomen. With your left hand, contact the transverse colon where it first becomes palpable as it emerges from under the costal arch. Gently grasp the colon with your thumb and fingers. With your right hand, gently sink in just inferior to this to the depth of the small intestines. Individual loops of the small intestine cannot be palpated in the same way as the large intestine, they are too soft. Gently grasp a portion of small intestine immediately inferior to your hold on the transverse colon. Between your two hands make a medial–lateral counter movement to assess glide between the transverse colon and adjacent loops of small intestine. Release your hold and move a hand width more medial.
- Repeat the same glide test in this new location. Continue this glide testing across the length of the transverse colon until it disappears under the left costal arch. Note areas where there is good glide and where there is not. Areas other than what you found as primary may be found

to be adhered. Treat what is primary, not what is just stiff. If there is more than one area that appears adhered, you may wish to use local listening and inhibition to confirm the most primary area of transverse colon adhesion (page 45).

TREATMENT

With the client still supine, return your hands to the most primary area of adhesion between the transverse colon and loops of the small intestine. Mobility test for first barriers between these two structures: 1) medial–lateral, 2) anterior–posterior, 3) clockwise–counterclockwise as viewed from superiorly, and 4) compaction–decompaction. For each dimension, maintain a first barrier load at the shorter distance observed. While maintaining the vector sum of these three or four loads, follow an unwind of the tissue in this intestinal adhesion. Follow directions for near barrier unwind on page 119. Be watchful for repeated patterns or for too fast movement. When the unwinding stops, proceed to post treatment testing.

POST TREATMENT TESTING AND INQUIRY

Use the standard post treatment procedure for mobility testing and question asking detailed in the introduction to treatment methods section. Either treat this same area further, as indicated by this inquiry, or return to general assessment.

TREATMENT
METHOD 4

Treatment method 5: far first barrier stack

Origin

Early functional technique, following the work of H. V. Hoover DO. Original discoverer not known.

Concept

In the previous method, tissue was mobility tested to first barriers in opposite directions and the first barriers closer to the starting equilibrium were chosen for the treatment stack. For the present method, the far first barriers are chosen instead.

Method

Mobility test in different ways:

1. For each dimension tested, test and note the end range. Testing may simply be in three cardinal planes. If the anatomy of the area is known, testing may be in physiologic axes.

2. Test and note first barriers on both ends of each of the same ranges of motion tested for end range. For each dimension, one direction will present a first barrier sooner (after a shorter excursion) than the other direction; note these differences. The direction of each pair that presents a first barrier at a greater distance is called the far first barrier. This is also known as the direction of ease.

3. In the direction of ease (far barrier), successively apply and accumulate first barrier load to each of the dimensions discovered by first barrier mobility testing.

4. Soon a tissue release will follow. As each successive release occurs, maintain the original stack direction load. If during a release you lose the sense of where the first barrier is, then retest the first barriers and stack again in direction of ease.

Note—It is possible to test each dimension separately; remember the results and then stack the several dimensions to the far barriers. This requires memory and more time. It is a good shortcut to test one dimension and maintain the tissue at the far first barrier in that dimension, and then test a second dimension. Also, maintain the tissue at a first barrier load in this additional longer dimension. Two dimensions are now concurrently loaded in direction of ease. Then test the first barrier of the third dimension and add this dimension of first barrier load to the longer dimension. This method saves time and memory compared to testing each dimension separately, remembering all their directions, and then stacking all three again.

During the sequence of releases, if a repeated pattern is detected, apply minimally adequate force to stop the tissue movement in a relatively tight corner. Wait for the tissue to release in a new direction. Repeated patterns will be found much less commonly than with pure or augmented unwinding. Similarly, too fast movement is rare with this unwinding method.

END OF TREATMENT

Several releases will be felt. Eventually, there may be a larger or more general release, after which the sequence of releases will stop, and the tissue will feel quiet.

POST TREATMENT TESTING AND INQUIRY

Use the standard post treatment procedure for mobility testing and question asking detailed in the introduction to treatment methods section. Either treat this same area further, as indicated by this inquiry, or return to general assessment.

Far first barrier stack (direction of ease)

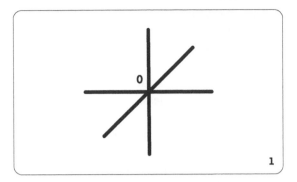

Consider axes of movement for the given tissue; these may be either cardinal planes or physiologic axes.

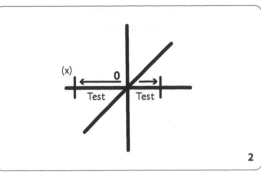

Along one of these axes, successively mobility test the tissue to a first barrier load first in one direction, then in the opposite direction.

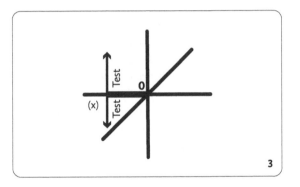

Maintain the tissue at a first barrier load in the longer direction; from this new starting point, mobility test the tissue to a first barrier load in each direction along a second axis.

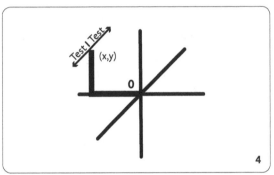

Having found the second dimension of first barrier, maintain the tissue at the longer distance first barrier in both of the dimensions tested. From this starting place, mobility test to a first barrier in a third dimension.

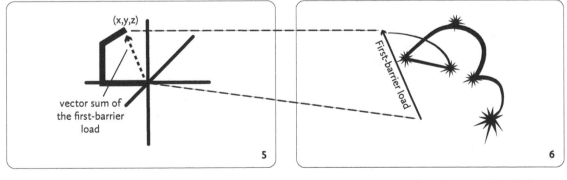

Note the vector sum of the three loads applied. Maintain a first barrier load in this combined direction.

While maintaining this combined direction of load, allow an unwinding.

The usual small releases will be felt at each corner, and a larger, more general release at the end followed by the unwind stopping. Release the load applied to the tissue, break contact, and return to assessment.

Six factor model: Far first barrier stack

TISSUE ENGAGEMENT

Tissue engagement is accomplished by stacking the tissue to far first barriers (direction of ease).

FORCE

First barrier only.

SPEED

Follow the speed of tissue movement, unless:

1. The movement is too fast; in which case, slow it down.
2. A repeated pattern is observed. When this happens, exert the minimum counterforce to prevent that movement. However, allow the next movement and then continue.

(These two phenomena are rare with this technique.)

CONSTRAINT

This technique uses no constraint unless a repeated pattern is noted; in which case, minimum force is used to stop the movement in a tight corner. The tissue loading in a particular direction can be viewed as a constraint as it will be difficult for tissue to unwind in a direction opposite this load.

DIRECTIVENESS

No specific movement is required. Tissue movement is directed to slow down in the rare need to slow a too fast movement.

RELATIONSHIP TO EFFORT BARRIERS

Treatment is accomplished at a first barrier load. The only time more force may be used is the minimum necessary to stop a repeated pattern. The only time less than first barrier force may be used is in slowing down a too fast movement.

Far first barrier stack example 1

ASSESSMENT

Assessment leads to the middle one-third of the sagittal suture.

MOBILITY TESTING

Rule out adjacent structures and define the area of cranial suture stiffness.

1. Move skin in this area over underlying tissue, compare mobility to adjacent areas.
2. Test skin elasticity in this area, compare mobility to adjacent areas.
3. Starting at the anterior end of the sagittal suture, contact the two parietal bones in fingertip size areas adjacent to the sagittal suture. Attempt to distract the two bones away from each other laterally. Work your way posteriorly, finger widths at a time, to define the stiff area of suture. This area may or may not fully correspond to the area found by other assessment methods. There may be additional adjacent or non-adjacent portions of the sagittal suture which are stiff, but not primary.

TREATMENT

1. Situate the client in a comfortable position. Supine, side-lying, or seated may serve well. Seek comfort for the client and convenience for you as a therapist.
2. Place the pad(s) of a finger or fingers of one hand on the parietal bone immediately adjacent to the stiff and primary area of sagittal suture. Place the pad(s) of a finger or fingers of the other hand on the other parietal bone also immediately adjacent to the stiff and primary area of sagittal suture. The fingertips of one hand will lightly touch the tips of the fingers of the other hand.
3. With the fingers of both hands, sink into the level of the bone. Gently move the

bones opposite each other in a succession of directions. Stack as you go at far first barriers:

a. Proximal–lateral
b. Anterior–posterior
c. Gently press in versus release pressure out
d. Counter rocking or teeter-totter around a transverse axis.

4. Maintain the directional vector sum of these dimensions dynamically loaded to a far first barrier as the tissue unwinds.

POST TREATMENT TESTING AND INQUIRY

Use the standard post treatment procedure for mobility testing and question asking detailed in the introduction to treatment methods section. Mobility testing will include all the same tests as in the pretests including skin and all parts of the sagittal suture. Either treat this same area further, as indicated by this inquiry, or return to general assessment.

Far first barrier stack example 2

ASSESSMENT

Assessment methods lead to an adhesion between the visceral peritoneum of the lateral aspect of the first leg of the sigmoid colon and the parietal peritoneum overlying the left iliacus muscle. This is a common finding which impairs the iliacus muscle in its role as a hip flexor and external rotator in open kinetic chain, and control of anterior–posterior tilt of the ilium in closed kinetic chain.

After general and local assessment methods have localized the primary restriction to this area, specifically test the integrity of the glide plane between the second leg of the sigmoid colon and the adjacent iliac fossa. This is done by gently and slowly sinking the tips of the fingers of one hand into this potential glide plane. With the client supine on the table and the knees supported on pillows to give slack to the abdomen, stand at the client's right side. Explain the procedure to the client. Place your left hand flat on the lower left quadrant of the abdomen and slack it laterally. Have the fingers of the right hand straight but relaxed. With the tips of the right fingers arranged in a superior–inferior direction just medial to the left ilium, slowly sink in. How well are you able to sink in between the second leg of the sigmoid colon and the lateral body wall? Is the full depth of the cleft available? Is the full vertical dimension of the cleft available?

TREATMENT

Positioned as for the above assessment, place the fingers of one of your hands palm sides facing the medial aspect of the first leg of the sigmoid colon. With your other hand, gently control the anterior part of the left ilium. Make gentle counter movement between these two structures. Most of the movement will be made for the first leg of the sigmoid colon; however, a counter-load will always be applied to the ilium. Move these two structures opposite each other in three directions:

1. Superior–inferior
2. Anterior–posterior
3. Clockwise–counterclockwise around a non-physiologic transverse axis.

Note first barriers in each pair of opposite directions. Accumulate far first barriers as you go into a stack.

As an unwind begins, dynamically maintain the same directional vector sum load between the first leg of the sigmoid colon and the ilium. Proceed through a succession of releases until there is a larger, more general release and the tissue then ceases to unwind.

POST TREATMENT TESTING AND INQUIRY

Use the standard post treatment procedure for mobility testing and question asking detailed in the introduction to treatment methods section. Either treat this same area further, as indicated by this inquiry, or return to general assessment.

Far first barrier stack example 3

ASSESSMENT

General and local assessment methods lead to the right patellar bursa.

GLOBAL MOBILITY TEST

With the client supine on the table, support the right knee with one hand and place the other hand on the right ankle. At a moderate pace, lift and flex the right knee. As you approach full flexion, slide the knee hand out from behind the knee, so it supports the knee laterally rather than interfering with flexion in a posterior position. Note both range and ease of movement. Similarly, lower and straighten the knee again. As the knee arrives at the table, remove your knee hand to allow full extension.

FOCAL MOBILITY TEST

With the client supine on the table, place both of your thumbs adjacent to each other on the lateral aspect of the patellar tendon. At the same time, place your index fingers adjacent to each other on the medial aspect of the patellar tendon. Providing dynamic stabilization of the proximal tibia with the palms of both hands and with your other fingers, attempt to move the patellar tendon first medial with respect to the tibia and then medial with respect to the tibia. With dynamic stabilization, do not allow the tibia to roll or displace medial or lateral. This process assesses glide in the patellar bursa. Do the same test for the other patellar tendon and patellar bursa. Note the results and discuss them with your client.

TREATMENT

Standing at the right side of the table, place one hand under the proximal tibia. With the thumb and forefinger of the other hand, gently grasp the patellar tendon. Make counter movement between the patellar tendon and the proximal tibia. Almost all the movement will be of the patellar tendon, and there will always be a dynamic counter-load applied to the proximal tibia with the other hand. Test, medial–lateral, superior–inferior, and counter rotated around an anteroposterior axis. Load to far first barriers, accumulating these as you test.

An unwind will begin. Allow the unwind to continue as it will while you keep a dynamic first barrier loan applied in the vector sum direction arrived at by stacking in far first barrier axes.

When the unwinding stops, proceed to post treatment testing and inquiry.

POST TREATMENT TESTING AND INQUIRY

Use the standard post treatment procedure for mobility testing and question asking detailed in the introduction to treatment methods section. Either treat this same area further, as indicated by this inquiry, or return to general assessment.

Treatment method 6: mixed directions of near and far first barrier stack

Origin

Early functional technique, following the work of H. V. Hoover DO. The original discoverer is not known.

Concept

There is another possibility in addition to stacking in directions far first barrier or near first barrier. It is sometimes more effective and efficient to stack some dimensions to a far first barrier and other dimensions to a near first barrier, all in the same stack. Sometimes tissue will change more readily in response to this mixed stack.

Pretest

Observe alignment in the person's body both locally and globally.

Test range of motion in the tissue to be treated.

1. Find and note the end range of motion in at least three dimensions. If the anatomy of the area is known, test each established physiologic axis. Where applicable, circumduction should also be tested. If the anatomy is not known, simply mobility test the tissue in three cardinal dimensions.
2. Test the available ranges of motion and note first barriers on both ends of each range of motion. Examples include flexion–extension, superior–inferior, proximal–distal, clockwise–counterclockwise.

First barriers, near and far

In mobility testing, the direction which presents a first barrier after the shorter excursion is called the direction near first barrier. The direction that presents a first barrier after the relatively greater excursion is called the direction far first barrier.

Treatment method

Apply a far first barrier load to one or two of the three dimensions. Then apply a near first barrier load to the remaining dimension or dimensions. To accomplish this, first move the tissue in one dimension in its direction of ease; stop when the first increase of effort required to move the tissue is felt. Maintain this first barrier load while you test a second dimension and then concurrently load the tissue in a second dimension in its direction of ease to the first barrier. Maintaining both directions of ease, load a third axis to a first barrier in direction of effort. In the instructions given here, two dimensions are loaded to near first barrier, and one dimension to far first barrier. Any count of some dimensions loaded to near and others to far will work.

If physiologic axes are used or included, the total number of axes may be more than three. In that situation, load some of the dimensions at near first barrier, and the others at far first barrier. The exact count of barrier types, and order or barrier type choice, is usually not important. What matters is that there are some of each in the stack. However, if the tissue is not changing easily, try a different combination.

Repeated patterns or too fast movement are quite rare with this method, but remain alert.

End of treatment

Several releases will be felt. Eventually there will be a larger or more general release, after which the sequence of releases will stop, and the tissue will feel quieter, more relaxed, and more at ease.

Post treatment testing and inquiry

Use the standard post treatment procedure for mobility testing and question asking detailed in the introduction to treatment methods section. Either treat this same area further, as indicated by this inquiry, or return to general assessment.

Six factor model: Mixed near and far first barrier stack

TISSUE ENGAGEMENT

Tissue is engaged at only a first barrier at each of the three or more dimensions.

FORCE

Treatment is carried out at a first barrier load. No greater or lesser force is used in this method.

With this treatment method, it is quite rare for tissue to fall either into a repeated unwinding pattern or to move too quickly. On the rare occasions when either of these unwinding characteristics occur, manage them in the usual way.

SPEED

Follow the natural speed of tissue movement in the body.

With this treatment method, tissue moving too quickly is quite rare. When tissue does move too rapidly, slow it down in the usual way.

CONSTRAINT

No direction of movement is forbidden.

The only exception is the very rare, repeated pattern; in which case, the tissue is held at a tight corner in the usual way.

DIRECTIVENESS

No specific movement is required.

The only exception is the very rare occurrence of tissue moving too fast; in which case, the tissue is directed to move more slowly.

RELATIONSHIP TO EFFORT BARRIERS

The mixed ease and effort treatment method is carried out at first barrier force.

The only exception is in the very rare circumstance in which there is a repeated pattern. To break this pattern, the tissue is constrained in a tight corner of its pattern; the force used to constrain it is not gauged by effort barriers, but is the minimum force required to stop the movement at the corner.

Mixed near and far first barrier stack

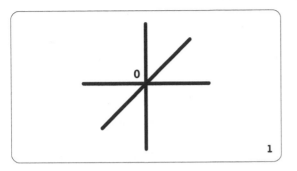

1

Consider axes of movement for the given tissue; these may be either cardinal planes or physiologic axes.

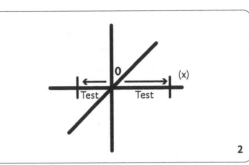

2

Along one of these axes, successively mobility test the tissue to a first barrier load first in one direction, then in the opposite direction.

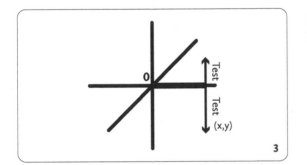

3

Maintain the tissue at a first barrier load in the longer direction. From this new starting point, mobility test the tissue to a first barrier load in each direction along a second axis.

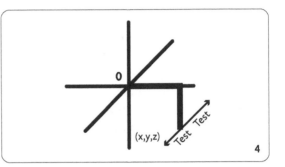

4

Having found the first barriers in the second dimension, maintain the tissue at the longer distance first barrier in both of the dimensions tested. From this starting place, mobility test to a first barrier in a third dimension.

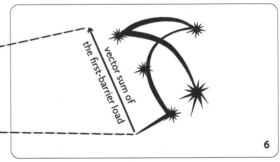

5

Having found the first barriers in the third dimension, maintain the tissue at the shorter distance in this third dimension as well as the longer distance in the first two dimensions.

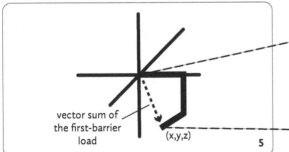

6

An unwind will now proceed in the usual way until a more generalized release happens and the unwind stops. Release the stack loading, break contact, and return to assessment.

The description is for a mixed near and far barrier stack with the first two dimensions held in far barrier, and the third dimension held in near barrier (far–far–near). Any other sequence of near and far barriers may be used, i.e., far–near–far, near–far–far, near–far–near, near–near–far, or far–near–near.

Mixed near and far first barrier stack example 1
Caution—This treatment and the associated testing must not be done on clients known to have osteoporosis or who have risk factors for osteoporosis but have not been recently tested for osteoporosis. Any other condition known to cause bone fragility is also a contraindication.

ASSESSMENT
General and local assessment leads to intraosseous strain in the right lamina of the fifth thoracic vertebra (T5).

MOBILITY TESTING
Global active

- Ask the client to sit on a stool or bench. Ask the client to roll down through their spine starting with their head, unstacking the spine segmentally from the top, then ask the client to return to upright stacking the spine from the bottom.
- Look for groups of vertebrae that do not move well on each other. Observe spinal motion first during flexion and then during extension of the spine. Note the behavior of all parts of the spine with particular focus on the upper thorax.

Global passive

- Standing or sitting behind your seated client, place your hands on the top of the thorax left and right of the base of the neck. This hand placement will contact elements of the shoulder girdle, but more importantly for this test, contact the upper ribs both in front and in back.
- Instruct the client to allow you to move their body without the client either helping or resisting. With your hands, rotate the torso first to the left to a soft end-feel. Rest back to neutral.

- Then rotate the thorax to the right. Note total range of motion and ease with range of motion. Note particularly the behavior of the upper thoracic spine.

Local passive

- Ask the client to lie in a side-lying position with the right side up, and the hips and knees comfortably flexed. Provide pillows under the client's head, in front of the torso for the right arm to rest on, and if the client wishes, also between the knees.
- Sit behind the client. With the thumb and fingers of the left hand, gently and securely grasp the spinous process of T3. With the thumb and fingers of the right hand, gently and securely grasp the right transverse process of T3. Slowly spring these two prominences apart, taking the spinous process a little left, and swinging the right transverse process anterior. This process tests the flexibility of the bony lamina spanning between these two vertebral processes.
- Repeat this test process on T4, T5, T6, and T7. Compare the flexibility of these five vertebral laminae, both to each other and to your store of memories of other laminae you have tested. T5 will likely be stiffer than usual and may or may not be stiffer than neighboring vertebrae. Neighboring laminae may also be stiff, but less primary than the T5 lamina.

TREATMENT
Test the first barrier flexibility of the lamina of T5 in three dimensions. Make choices about utilizing near and far first barriers to create a stack as you go.

1. Spring the spinous and transverse processes away from each other, let them

settle to neutral, then approximate the two processes toward each other.

2. Take the tip of the spinous process superior at the same time as you move the tip of the transverse process inferior, let the processes settle to neutral, then take the spinous process inferior and the transverse process inferior.

3. Picture an oblique axis between the spinous process and the transverse process. Counter-rotate the tips of the two processes opposite each other on this imagined axis, first in one direction and then in the other direction.

Once the stack is established, an unwind will begin. Maintain the final vector sum load of these three dimensions throughout the unwind. When there is a larger, more general release, followed by the tissue ceasing to unwind, this treatment episode is complete.

POST TREATMENT TESTING AND INQUIRY

Use the standard post treatment procedure for mobility testing and question asking detailed in the introduction to treatment methods section. Either treat this same area further, as indicated by this inquiry, or return to general assessment.

Mixed near and far first barrier stack example 2
ASSESSMENT

Global and local assessment leads to a primary lesion in an adhesion of an anterior–lateral portion of the left talocrural joint capsule to the periosteum of the distal tibia.

MOBILITY TESTING

Active

- Ask the client to dorsiflex the foot and then to plantarflex the foot.

Passive

- Ask the client to lie supine on the table with heels just off the end. Instruct the client to allow you to move the foot with the client neither resisting nor assisting. One at a time, test the range of motion of each ankle.

- For the right ankle, stand at the client's right side facing the ankle. With your left hand, place the web of the left thumb over the distal end of the tibia and fibula and use the thumb and fingers to grip the lateral and medial malleoli for dynamic stabilization. Place the web of the right thumb anteriorly on the talus adjacent to the left hand. Grasp the talus and calcaneus with the thumb and fingers of the right hand. Plantarflex the talus on the crura. Allow the foot to return to neutral. Dorsiflex the talus on the crura. Note total range of motion and the ease within the range of motion. Reverse these directions for the left ankle. Compare mobility between the two ankles and to your store of memories of the talocrural joints you have previously tested.

CAPSULAR GLIDE

The joint capsule of the talocrural joint, like the capsule for most synovial joints, attaches to bone, not right at the joint line but some distance back on the bone. Stabilizing the bones of the lower leg (crura) with the left hand, use the tip of the index finger to sink to the depth of the joint capsule on the anterior portion of the distal tibia. Engage the capsular material and attempt to glide it medially and laterally on the distal 5 mm of the tibia. Shift your contact a finger width lateral and again engage the capsule and attempt to drag it medial and lateral. Continue this pattern to incrementally test your way posterior–laterally around the distal tibia. In this fashion, you can define the area of joint capsule which is adhered to the periosteum too close to the joint line. This identifies the primary area of reduced capsular glide.

TREATMENT

Dynamically stabilize the distal lower leg with the left hand. With the tip of the right index finger, sink to the depth of the adhesion between the joint capsule and the periosteum. Make a series of movements in opposite directions of that area of joint capsule with counter-loads to the distal tibia. There will be little movement with this adhesion. The distance traveled for both near first barrier and far first barrier will be quite small, yet these two distances will be distinguishable.

Attempt to glide the joint capsule over the bone.

1. Medial–lateral
2. Superior–inferior
3. Clockwise rotation–counterclockwise rotation.

Stack all three of these dimensions to a first barrier load. Stack at least one to near first barrier. Stack at least one to a far first barrier.

As an unwind begins, maintain the dynamic load of the vector sum of these three dimensions. The distance loaded will likely increase a little as the succession of releases during treatment proceed but keep the direction of force and first barrier sense unchanged until the final release.

When a larger and more general release occurs followed by the tissue ceasing to unwind, this treatment episode is over. Release your contact and proceed to post treatment testing and inquiry, including doing all the same pretreatment testing again.

POST TREATMENT TESTING AND INQUIRY

Use the standard post treatment procedure for mobility testing and question asking detailed in the introduction to treatment methods section. Either treat this same area further, as indicated by this inquiry, or return to general assessment.

Mixed near and far first barrier stack example 3

ASSESSMENT

General and local assessment leads to the median ligament. This bladder support ligament lies in the anterior midline laminated between the linea alba and the anterior portion of the parietal peritoneum.

POSTURE ASSESSMENT

Observe the client standing and sitting. Are there signs of anterior abdominal wall vertical shortness, which can lead to a kyphotic appearance?

Check the relative position of the anterior and posterior superior iliac spine (ASIS and PSIS) on each side as measures of anterior or posterior pelvic tilt. A tight median ligament would tend to hold the front of the pelvis up, biasing the pelvis toward a posterior tilt. The position of the pelvis has many influences. This examination is more useful to monitor change from pretreatment testing to post treatment testing.

MOBILITY TESTING

Active

- Ask the client to take a deep breath. To what extent does the front of the body wall lengthen vertically? To what extent is there a sense of shortness or tethering down near the anterior midline?
- Ask the client to sit on a bench or stool. Ask the client to extend their trunk. What limitations are there to extension? Is the lower abdomen able to lengthen vertically with extension?

Passive

- Explain to the client the anatomy of the median ligament. Use illustrations and anatomic models. State the purpose of testing the length and elasticity of the ligament and describe the procedure to test it. Ask the client to lie supine on the table. Stand at the client's right side. Ask the client to find and touch the superior surface of the pubic symphysis. Place the pads of the second, third, and fourth fingers of your right hand on the superior surface of the pubic symphysis. With the fingers of your other hand, grasp the umbilicus. While you dynamically stabilize the medial portions of the two pubic bones with one hand, use your other hand to move the other hand superiorly, thereby testing the length and span of the median ligament.

- Return the umbilicus to its original position. Similarly, test the left medial ligament by moving the umbilicus superior–laterally toward the middle of the right clavicle. Return this to neutral. In the same fashion, test the span of the right medial ligament by moving the umbilicus superior–laterally toward the middle of the left clavicle. Return the umbilicus to neutral.

TREATMENT

Test the median ligament to first barriers in three dimensions.

1. Torsion around a vertical axis.
2. Side bending, bowing it to the left then to the right in a frontal plane.
3. Side bending, bowing it in and out in a mid-sagittal plane.

Stack to three first barriers as you work through this with at least one dimension to far first barrier, and at least one dimension near first barrier.

As an unwind begins, maintain the dynamic load of the vector sum of these three dimensions. The distance loaded will likely increase a little as the succession of releases during treatment proceed but keep the direction of force and first barrier sense unchanged until the final release.

When a larger and more general release occurs followed by the tissue ceasing to unwind this treatment episode is over. Release your contact and proceed to post treatment testing and inquiry, including doing all the same pretreatment testing again.

POST TREATMENT TESTING AND INQUIRY

Use the standard post treatment procedure for mobility testing and question asking detailed in the introduction to treatment methods section. Either treat this same area further, as indicated by this inquiry, or return to general assessment.

Treatment method 7: stack–restack: a sequence of single release stacks

Origin
Jeffrey Burch.

Concept
During an unwind, return to neutral after each single release. Remobility test the first barriers and stack according to the new findings which will often have changed from even the first release. An advantage of this technique is it keeps the stack precisely oriented. With a succession of releases, the tissue characteristics progressively change so the stack direction becomes incrementally less accurate. The wall scrubbing techniques described later are yet another way of achieving a more continuously accurate first barrier load.

The stack–restack oscillation concept leads to a cluster of related techniques which may utilize a single dimension of first barrier load, two dimensions, three dimensions, or more. However, many dimensions are used; loading may be to near first barriers, far first barriers, or mixed near and far first barriers.

Pretest

1. Observe and note standing alignment locally and globally.
2. Test and note the end range as a pretest.
3. Test and note first barriers on both ends of each range of motion, e.g., flexion–extension, superior–inferior, and clockwise–counterclockwise.

You may also wish to test the range of motion at distant sites in the body. Treatment effects typically propagate considerable distances in the body quickly; point these out to the client.

Treatment method—single dimension, one direction
Choose a particular axis of mobility. Along this axis, apply a first barrier load in the direction of either ease or effort. Soon a tissue release will be felt. Allow the tissue to return to neutral, then immediately reload the tissue on the same axis as before and in the same direction as before; however, the distance to the first barrier will usually have changed.

Treatment method—single dimension, alternating directions
Choose a particular axis of mobility. Along this axis, apply a first barrier load in the direction of either ease or effort. Soon a tissue release will be felt. Allow the tissue to return to neutral, then immediately reload the tissue to the other barrier. If near first barrier was first used, now load to far first barrier. Again, wait for a release; follow the release at its natural pace, and then at the end of the release, return to neutral and proceed immediately to the opposite barrier.

Continue to oscillate between opposite direction barriers in the chosen dimension until a larger, more general release is felt. With each release, the position of the barriers will change, usually in a more expansive direction.

Treatment method—multidimensional stacking, single first barrier direction
Apply a first barrier load to two or more of the dimensions discovered by first barrier testing. Once the dimensions are all loaded to a first barrier near, far, or mixed, wait for a release. After the release, let the tissue settle to neutral. Remobility test to first barriers and stack again with the same choice of direction as before.

Treatment method—multidimensional stacking, with mixed direction of first barrier
Apply a first barrier load to two or more of the dimensions discovered by first barrier testing. Once the dimensions are all loaded to a first barrier near, far, or mixed, wait for a release. Allow the tissue to settle to neutral. Remobility

test first barriers, then stack again but change the direction of the stack. Usually if near first barriers were first used, now stack to far first barriers or vice versa. If mixed near and far barriers are used, the possibilities for re-stacking multiply.

Allow one release at each set of stacked first barriers, before changing to a different barrier stack.

Treatment method—combined unilateral and bidirectional oscillation

Maintain one or more dimensions consistently in either near first barrier or far first barrier. For an additional dimension or dimensions, oscillate near first barrier or far first barrier, waiting for a release at each.

A FACTOR WHICH MAY BE COMBINED WITH ANY OF THESE VARIATIONS

Augmentation may be added to any of the above variations. As the tissue releases, ask it briefly to go a little farther in the direction of the release than it would on its own, before returning to neutral. See augmented unwinding, page 107.

Treatment completion

There will be a larger release with an expansive feeling followed by quiet in the tissue.

Post treatment testing and inquiry

Use the standard post treatment procedure for mobility testing and question asking detailed in the introduction to treatment methods section. Either treat this same area further, as indicated by this inquiry, or return to general assessment.

Succession of single release stacks

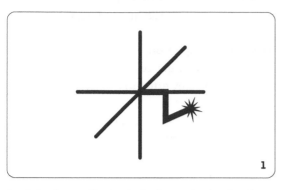

1

Stack the tissue to first barrier in the near barrier direction. Allow one tissue release, then release your stack.

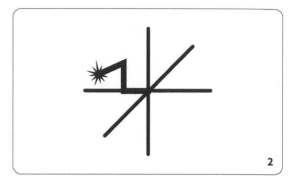

2

Next stack the tissue again, this time to far barriers. Allow one tissue release, then release your stack.

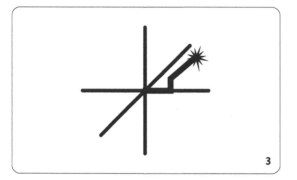

3

Stack the tissue again to near first barrier. The location of the stack will usually be different than it was the first time because the tissue has changed with the treatment.

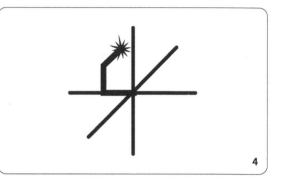

4

Stack the tissue again to a far first. Allow one tissue release, then release your stack.

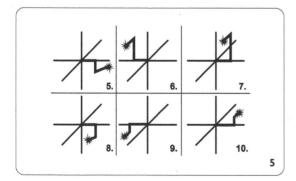

5

Continue to alternate stacks in opposite directions allowing one release for each stack. Position of the stack will continue to shift as the treatment chapters progressively change the tissue.

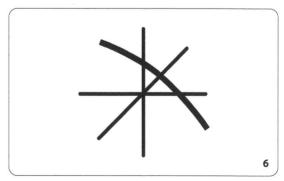

6

Eventually there will be a larger, more general release. This treatment episode is now complete. Return to assessment.

These directions are for alternate stacking beginning with a near first barrier stack. You may also a) begin alternate stacking with far first barrier, b) make all stacks near barrier, c) make all stacks far barrier, and d) include mixed stacks, either consistently or alternated with near and far stacks.

Six factor model: Stack–restack

TISSUE ENGAGEMENT

Tissue is engaged by the therapist and only at a first barrier load. In this method, there is no possibility of a repeated pattern, so alternative force level to break a repeated pattern is not a consideration.

FORCE

First barrier only.

SPEED

Transition between near first barrier to far first barrier is done at slow to moderate speed. Release follows the body's natural pace, which is usually at a slow to moderate pace.

CONSTRAINT

In the set-up phase of each move the tissue is held to a first barrier in one or several dimensions. In the release phase, any movement is allowed.

DIRECTIVENESS

In the release phase of each setup, any movement is allowed, none is required. If augmentation is used, then each release is briefly exaggerated by the therapist. This is a mild directiveness saying, "Do more of what you were doing."

RELATIONSHIP TO EFFORT BARRIERS

- Setup: first barrier
- Following the release: no barrier
- Augmentation encouragement at the end of the release: first barrier

Stack–restack example 1

Assessment leads to the right second finger proximal interphalangeal joint.

Standing observation:

- How do the client's upper limbs hang?
- How similar are the two?

Active range of motion:

- Ask the client to slowly make a fist with each hand, one at a time.
- Ask the client to slowly extend all fingers on each hand, one at a time.
- Ask the client to slowly extend each wrist, one at a time.
- Ask the client to slowly flex each wrist, one at a time.
- Ask the client to slowly circumduct each shoulder, one at a time.

PASSIVE ROM

Sit across a table from your client. Ask your client to rest their hands and forearms on the table. Arrange the hands so the wrists are near neutral, i.e., neither flat palm on the table nor palm up, but the thumb a bit up in the air but not fully straight up. Assess the range of motion in each of their eight proximal interphalangeal joints. Ignore the thumb for the moment. To assess a joint, use two hands. For a given finger, make one contact on the proximal phalanx near the proximal interphalangeal (PIP) joint where you will make a dynamic stabilization. Using the fingers of your other hand, control the middle phalanx of the same finger also near the PIP joint. Slowly move the middle phalanx on the proximal phalanx to full extension, let it rest back to neutral, then move it to full flexion, then let it rest back to neutral. Repeat this with the other seven fingers. Note how the ease and range of these joints compare to each other and to your store of memories of other similar joints you have tested in the past.

TREATMENT

Using the same contact on the right second proximal and middle phalanges that you did for mobility testing, gently begin to mobility test between the two bones in dimensions to establish your barrier stack. You can use flexion–extension, left and right side bending, long axis rotation, or compaction–decompaction. Stack all four dimensions to a near first barrier. After the first therapeutic release, break contact. Remobility test the joint in all dimensions. Compared to the earlier testing, the distances to first barriers will now be different, and the direction of near versus far barriers may be different in at least some dimensions. Restack all dimensions of this joint to the new first near barriers. After one release, break contact. Mobility test to end-feel. If the joint is sufficiently released, the treatment is complete. If it is not sufficiently mobile, again mobility test to first barriers and establish a new near barrier stack. Repeat this cycle until either the joint has sufficient mobility, or you feel a slight edema.

COMPLETION OF TREATMENT

Follow the instructions in the completion of treatment protocol described in the introduction.

Stack–restack example 2

Assessment leads to the intermuscular septum between the long and short heads of the left biceps brachii muscle.

CLIENT INQUIRY

Ask about the client's awareness of their body:

- in general, and
- at the left arm and shoulder.

MOBILITY TESTING

Global active

- Observe the client walking, noting particularly arm and shoulder movement with gait.
- Ask the client to stand and then make a circumduction of first the right arm and then the left.
- Ask the client to flex the left elbow, then, with the elbow flexed, bring the hand to the top of the shoulder, then to return the arm and hand to neutral, hanging at the side.

Global passive

- With the client standing, stand behind the client slightly left of center. Place your right hand on top of the client's left shoulder girdle to stabilize the scapula and clavicle. With your left hand, grasp the distal left upper arm and extend the arm back, allowing the elbow to naturally flex. Note the range and ease of movement. Return the arm to hanging neutral.
- Shift your left hand distal to control the elbow, so you can again extend the shoulder while maintaining the elbow in full extension. Note how the shoulder movement appears different from the previous test.
- Make the same two active tests on the other arm for comparison.

Focal passive

- Ask the client to lie supine on the table. Sit at the client's left side facing the upper arm. Place your right hand under the middle of the client's upper arm to control both the humerus and the short head of the biceps brachii. Place your left hand on the middle of the front of the upper arm to control the long head of the biceps brachii muscle. Make medial and lateral counter movements of the long and short heads of the biceps brachii muscles to assess mobility between them, which is an expression of the flexibility of the intermuscular septum between the two.
- Make the same assessment on the other arm for comparison.

TREATMENT

Treat with a far first barrier stack and augment each release.

Using the same hand holds as for the focal passive assessment, mobility test to first barriers.

1. Medial–lateral
2. Superior–inferior
3. Compaction–decompaction.

Stack all dimensions to far first barriers. As a release happens, note the direction of the tissue movement at release; immediately at the end of this release gently push the tissue a little farther in the direction of release for less than one second. Break contact. Mobility test the joint to end-feel. If it is sufficiently mobilized, the treatment is done. If not, mobility test again to first barriers, and again stack to the new far first barriers. As the first release happens, note the direction of the tissue movement at release; immediately at the end of this release gently push the tissue a little farther in the direction of release for less than one second. Break contact. Mobility test the joint to end-feel. If it is sufficiently mobilized, the treatment is done. If not, mobility test again to first barriers, and again stack to the new far first barriers. Repeat this cycle until either joint mobility is sufficient or a slight edema appears in the tissue.

POST TREATMENT TESTING AND INQUIRY

Use the standard post treatment procedure for mobility testing and question asking detailed in the introduction to treatment methods section. Either treat this same area further, as indicated by this inquiry, or return to general assessment.

Stack–restack example 3

Assessment leads to the ligamentous continuity of the round ligament of the liver and the ligamentum venosum. These are two portions of the same organ support structure developmentally derived from the umbilical vein. The round ligament of the liver portion runs superiorly from the scar tissue of the umbilicus superiorly behind the linea alba to where it approaches the liver. From there, it swings posteriorly, lying in the groove on the inferior side of the liver which demarcates the left and right lobes of the liver. Posteriorly, it

attaches either directly to the portal vein or more commonly a short distance from the portal vein on the hepatic vein.

CLIENT INQUIRY

Ask about the client's awareness of their body:

*   in general
*   at upper abdomen, and
*   at lower thoracic spine.

MOBILITY TESTING

Global active

*   Observe the client walking, noting particularly mobility in the upper abdomen and lumbodorsal hinge area.
*   Ask the client to sit on a bench or stool, and then to make a slow extension of the spine, return to neutral, and then roll down through the spine starting with the head. Observe upper abdominal and lumbodorsal hinge area movement.

Focal passive

*   Ask the client to lie supine on the table. Sit at the client's right side facing the middle of the torso. Place your left hand under the client's lower thoracic spine to control vertebral movement in that area. Use the thumb and fingers of your right hand to gently grasp the umbilicus. At a moderate pace, move the umbilicus superiorly. Do any of the lower thoracic vertebrae move in response to your moving the umbilicus? If present, the response will be immediate as you move the umbilicus. Holding the umbilicus superior will produce no further movement. While maintaining contact with the umbilicus, let the umbilicus rest to its natural position. At a moderate pace, traction the umbilicus inferiorly. How soon do lower thoracic vertebrae

move? How much elasticity does there appear to be in the former umbilical vein?

TREATMENT

Treat with alternating near and far first barrier stack–restack.

Use the same hand holds as for the focal passive mobility tests. Starting from the natural resting point, mobility test for first barriers:

- Superior–inferiorly
- Rotate clockwise, counterclockwise viewed from superiorly
- Bow the round ligament of the liver left then right in a frontal plane.

For a mixed near–far first barrier stack, the dimension of length along the ligamentous continuity from umbilicus to lower thoracic vertebrae will always be in tension, as compacting the length of this structure is not practical. For this reason, we do not know if the first barrier of stretch is near or far first barrier. For the other two dimensions, longitudinal torsion and side bending, both the near and far first barriers are available. Since we do not know whether the ligament stretch axis is far or near, to create a mixed near–far stack, one of these other two axes must be loaded at near first barrier, and the other to far first barrier.

Using the same hand holds as for previous mobility testing of this structure, lower thoracic vertebrae, and umbilicus, move the umbilicus superior, slacking the ligament. In so doing, feel for one or more thoracic vertebrae that are felt to move. As it moves, continue to move the

umbilicus superior past where the vertebra stops moving. Then gradually allow the umbilicus to spring back inferiorly until the first hint of vertebral movement is felt again. At this point, you are at a first barrier stretch on this ligamentous continuity. Maintain this superior–inferior umbilicus position as you rotate the umbilicus first clockwise then counterclockwise around a cardinal superior–inferior axis, noting near and far first barriers. Load this dimension to near first barrier, maintaining it stacked with the first barrier stretch on the ligament. Next, concurrently rotate the umbilicus clockwise around an anteroposterior axis and sweep it a little to the right. Note the first barrier. Relax only this dimension to neutral, then rotate the umbilicus counterclockwise around an anteroposterior axis and slightly sweep the umbilicus to the left. Note the first barrier, comparing its distance to the prior mirror image movement. Load this dimension to far first barrier. Allow one release to happen. Soften your contact, releasing the loads. Re-test the end-feel stretch of the ligament. If it is sufficiently elastic, the treatment is done. If not, repeat the testing to first barriers, using that information to establish a new mixed near–far stack at the new first barrier positions, and allow one more release. Repeat this cycle until the ligament has sufficient elasticity.

POST TREATMENT TESTING AND INQUIRY

Use the standard post treatment procedure for mobility testing and question asking detailed in the introduction to treatment methods section. Either treat this same area further, as indicated by this inquiry, or return to general assessment.

Treatment method 8: walking through the spectrum of barriers

Origin

Early osteopathic method. Discoverer unknown.

Concept

Often, we treat at a first barrier; however, other later barriers can be used and are sometimes more effective. In addition, in any single treatment, more than one effort barrier can be successively used with good effect.

Pretest

Assess alignment and mobility in the usual ways.

Method

1. Sink into the tissue to a first barrier level of compression. Wait for a release.

2. As soon as the release has occurred, sink slowly deeper until the next barrier is found; wait there for another release.

3. Continue to sink incrementally deeper, pausing at each effort barrier for a release.

4. When you have either reached end-feel or client discomfort, begin to back out one barrier at a time, pausing at each for a release.

5. Cycle steps 1–4 until a generalized softening and larger release of the tissue is felt.

Post test

Assess alignment and mobility in the usual ways. Illustrations for this technique are on the following page.

TREATMENT
METHOD 8

Walking through the spectrum of barriers

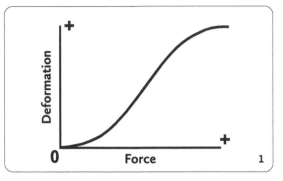

For an object made of a single substance with uniform texture, forces applied to it will change its shape in a regular way with a force deformation curve similar to this one with a nearly linear central section.

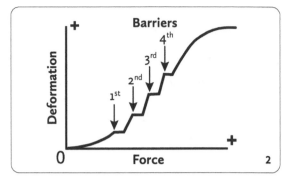

However, if the object is made of a composite material, the force deformation curve will have a succession of steps as each component material, and interface between materials is encountered. Human tissue is quite mixed in its composition.

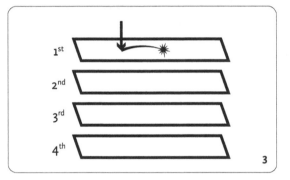

In this diagram, the force barriers are visualized as a succession of planes at various depths from the surface. A force exerted at a first barrier level will initiate an unwind. The first release is shown in this diagram.

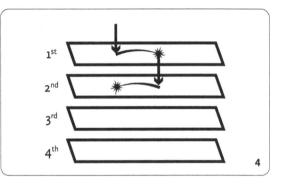

After the first release, increase your pressure until the second barrier is reached. Allow one leg of unwind with one release at this second force barrier.

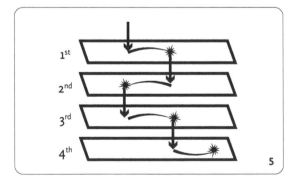

Proceed down through the succession of force barriers, allowing only one release at each barrier, then proceeding to the next.

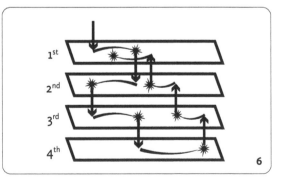

Continue through the succession of barriers to the last barrier at which an unwind will happen. Then incrementally lighten your force to allow one release at each force barrier on the way out.

Six factor model: Walking through the spectrum of barriers

TISSUE ENGAGEMENT

Tissue engagement occurs by pressure loading at each of a succession of barriers.

FORCE

Force varies incrementally from first barrier to near end-feel.

SPEED

Speed must be considered for two separate aspects of this method.

- The speed of sinking into the tissue is very slow and incremental, with pauses at each barrier. The return from higher pressure toward first barrier is similarly quite slow and incremental.
- While pausing at each force barrier, movement matches inherent movement of the tissue. If augmentation is used, the movement is like the movement that the person's tissue demonstrated moving toward the release.

CONSTRAINT

None. No movement is prevented.

Too fast movement has not been reported with this method, so there has been no need to slow movement.

DIRECTIVENESS

None. No specific movement is required at any of the force barriers encountered.

RELATIONSHIP TO EFFORT BARRIERS

All treatment occurs at effort barriers. During the treatment, all or most barriers from first barrier to end-feel are given an opportunity to show a release. At each episode of the treatment, one specific force barrier is maintained.

Walking through the spectrum of barriers example 1

General assessment leads to the left lower limb, not to include the foot or ankle. Local assessment methods including local listening, manual thermal assessment, inhibition, local lift, local tap, and applied kinesiology localize this as a stiff portion of the left fibula.

Place the client supine on the table with heels off the end of the table.

GENERAL MOBILITY TESTS

Active

- Ask the client their awareness of their lower legs.
- Ask the client to walk. Observe gait. Note and point out to the client what you see.
- Ask the client to lie supine on the table with heels off the end of the table. Then ask the client to dorsiflex their foot, return it to neutral, then plantarflex it. Compare to the other leg and to your store of memories of other legs you have observed.

Passive

- For the right ankle, stand at the client's right side. Place the web of the left thumb over the distal left lower leg bones and the thumb and forefinger on the malleoli to provide a dynamic stabilization of the distal crura. Place the right hand under the heel to grasp the calcaneus. Draw the calcaneus inferior and anterior to both dorsiflex the foot on the crura and ask for length in the Achilles tendon and associated muscles. Set up a mirror image of this to test the left side.
- For the right knee, sit or stand at the client's right side facing the lower leg. Place your left hand under the knee. With the right hand, control the ankle.

At a moderate pace, flex the knee. As you approach full flexion, swing your knee hand out to the side, so it does not interfere with end range. Return the leg to the table. Lift the ankle to test extension end range. Reverse directions and repeat this for the other leg.

- **Specific passive mobility test**
  *Do **not** do this if osteoporosis is known or suspected.*

  With your two hands, grasp the two ends of the left fibula.
  - Gently bend it, bowing it in a sagittal plane.
  - Gently bend it, bowing it in a frontal plane.
  - Gently torsion the fibula along its length around a vertical axis.

  Repeat the above tests on the fibula of the other leg for comparison.

  Move your hands so they are adjacent to each other near the distal end of the fibula. Make gentle focal bends of the fibula at this area. Shift your hands a short distance superior and repeat the same bends, comparing elasticity of the two portions of the bone. Continue this process along the length of the bone identifying stiff portions of the bone.

- **Focal primacy test**
  Use local listening and inhibition to determine the relative primary stiffness among the stiff areas of the fibula.

TREATMENT

Place your hands on the most primary portion of the left fibula as for the focal mobility test. Slowly and gently compact the bone between your two hands to a first barrier load. Allow only one leg of unwind to occur. Compact gently again to the second barrier. Allow one more leg of unwind to occur at this second barrier. Again, compact gently between your two hands to a third barrier. Let one leg of unwind occur. Continue in this fashion through a succession of force barriers, allowing one leg of unwind at each until either end-feel is reached or a barrier is reached where no unwind occurs. Then gently begin to release the vertical compaction in the bone, reversing the process you used on the way in, now pausing for one release at each barrier on the way out.

POST TREATMENT TESTING AND INQUIRY

Use the standard post treatment procedure for mobility testing and question asking detailed in the introduction to treatment methods section. Either treat this same area further, as indicated by this inquiry, or return to general assessment.

Walking through the spectrum of barriers example 2

General assessment leads to the right side of the neck. Local assessment, including local listening, manual thermal assessment, and layer listening, leads to an irregularly shaped area of superficial fascia of about 12 cm² overlying the middle portion of the left lateral part of the neck.

GENERAL MOBILITY TESTS

Active

- Ask the client their awareness of their neck.
- Ask the client to move their head, left then right rotation, left then right side bending, flexion, and extension.

General passive

- Ask the client to lie supine on the table with their head near one end of the table. Ask the client to allow you to move their head without either helping or resisting. Assure them you will move their head slowly and carefully. Sit at the client's head. Cradle the client's head in your hands. Move it slowly and gently in left rotation, right rotation, left side bending, right side bending, flexion, and extension.

- Focal passive mobility test
  - Touch the skin near but not on the area indicated as primary. Move the skin superior, inferior, anterior, and posterior on the underlying tissue. Now do the same thing on the area indicated as primary. Try this on several areas to define the area of superficial fascia stiffness. Test each area only once. Repeated testing of the same area may mobilize the superficial fascia, confusing your results.

TREATMENT

Place pads of fingers on the area of reduced skin movement. Use several fingers and placement of fingers corresponding to the size and shape of the stiff area. Support the other side of the neck with your hand. Sink in gently to a first barrier, allow one leg of unwind to occur. Compact gently again to the second barrier. Allow one more leg of unwind to occur at this second barrier. Again, compact to a third barrier. Let one leg of unwind occur. Continue in this fashion through a succession of force barriers, allowing one leg of unwind at each until either a comfortable end-feel is reached, or a barrier is reached where no unwind occurs. Then gently begin to release the compaction, reversing the process you used on the way in, now pausing for one release at each barrier on the way out.

POST TREATMENT TESTING AND INQUIRY

Use the standard post treatment procedure for mobility testing and question asking detailed in the introduction to treatment methods section. Either treat this same area further, as indicated by this inquiry, or return to general assessment.

Walking through the spectrum of barriers example 3

ASSESSMENT

General assessment leads to the posterior aspect of the right lower leg.

Local assessment methods, including local listening, manual thermal assessment, layer listening, and yes–no questioning, led to the intermuscular septum between the right gastrocnemius and soleus muscles as the current primary.

CLIENT INQUIRY

Ask the client:

- how they have been feeling in general, and
- of their awareness of knees, lower leg, ankles, including any differences between their legs.

MOBILITY TESTS

Large scale active

- Ask the client to walk. Observe gait, particularly ankle and knee movement.
- Ask the client to squat down to a comfortable degree and stand again.

Focal active

Place the client supine on the table with heels off the end of the table. Ask the client to:

- plantarflex both feet, and
- dorsiflex both feet.

Passive focal

- Gently lift the left heel to assess knee extension. Put the left heel down and do the same thing with the right heel.

- For the right ankle, stand at the client's right side. Place the web of the left thumb over the distal left lower leg bones and the thumb and forefinger on the malleoli to provide a dynamic stabilization of the distal crura. Place the right hand under the heel to grasp the calcaneus. Draw the calcaneus inferior and anterior to both dorsiflex the foot on the crura and ask for length in the calf muscles. Set up a mirror image of this to test the left side.

- For the right side, sit or stand at the client's right side facing the lower leg. Place the left hand under the belly of the gastrocnemius muscles. Place the right hand over the upper half of the tibia with the thumb aligned vertically just posterior to the tibia, and the tips of fingers 2–5 touching just posterior to the medial aspect of the tibia, these to control the sartorius muscle. Make a gentle medial–lateral shearing mobility test, bringing the gastrocnemius toward you and the soleus and tibia away from you. Let this rest to neutral, then reverse directions to bring the tibia and sartorius toward you and the gastrocnemius away from you. Note apparent movement between the two muscles. Set up the mirror image of this to test the other leg.

TREATMENT

Place your hands on the right lower leg as for the mobility test. Sink gently in between the two hands to arrive at the intermuscular septum between the gastrocnemius and soleus muscles to find a first barrier. Let only the first leg of unwind happen at this first barrier, then promptly sink in to the second barrier. Allow one leg of unwinding to occur here. Sink to the third barrier and allow one leg of unwinding to occur. Continue this process, sinking in through a succession of barriers until either end-feel is approached or no unwinding occurs. Then incrementally back out, pausing at each force barrier, allowing one leg of unwind.

POST TREATMENT TESTING AND INQUIRY

Use the standard post treatment procedure for mobility testing and question asking detailed in the introduction to treatment methods section. Either treat this same area further, as indicated by this inquiry, or return to general assessment.

Treatment method 9: stack and borrow

Origin
Method by Jeffrey Burch, named by Wayne Still.

Concept
Tissue is stacked first to a far barrier. Then a single dimension is restacked to a near first barrier. After this, an attempt is made to concurrently restack the remaining dimensions to a near barrier, but there will be almost no movement available as most of the slack in the system was used up by reloading the first barrier. A near barrier stack has now been created but around a very different centroid than if the stack had been made from neutral for each dimension.

Pretreatment tests
Observe postural alignment in the person's body both locally and globally. Test ranges of motion in the area to be treated.

Treatment method

1. Mobility test the tissue to be treated to first barriers and stack the tissue slightly beyond a far first barrier. Tissue is initially stacked slightly beyond a first barrier, so it will not yet begin to release. Release is allowed only after additional steps of setup.

2. Maintain all but one dimension a little beyond first barrier in direction of far first barrier. Move a single dimension to just beyond a first barrier in direction near first barrier. As this first dimension of tissue mobility is moved toward the near first barrier it will now move farther than when it was originally tested. This greater movement happens because the slack gathered from the other dimensions by stacking them at far first barriers

is borrowed for this single dimension of effort.

3. All together at the same time, move all the remaining dimensions originally stacked to far first barrier ease across to the near first barrier. It will be found that these remaining dimensions can move only a very short distance before encountering the near first barrier. This happens because most of the slack in the system has already been used up to move the tissue in the first dimension that was transitioned from far first barrier to near first barrier.

4. Slightly slacken the first dimension transitioned toward near first barrier down to a first barrier. It was initially held at slightly more than first barrier so tissue would not begin to unwind until the other dimensions were also transitioned to be near first barrier. The resulting stack is near first barrier; however, the position achieved is very different than if near first barrier had been approached directly from neutral.

5. It is unlikely the tissue would ever have arrived at this position in the ordinary course of life. The resulting cascade of information from the stretch receptors in the tissue to the central nervous system will be quite novel. This is a strong wake up call for the proprioceptive system.

6. While continuously maintaining the near first barrier stack, follow releases of unwind which may or may not occur.

7. Completion. Several steps of unwind release will sometimes but not always be felt. If so, there will be a final more general normalizing of tissue tone, usually a softening, after which unwinding will

TREATMENT
METHOD 9

stop. Alternatively, if unwinding does not occur, there may be only a single large release followed by quiet, reminiscent of the process in Hoover's centralizing technique.

Post treatment tests
Test physiologic or cardinal range of motion in the area treated. Observe postural alignment in the person's body both locally and globally.

Stack and borrow

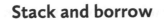

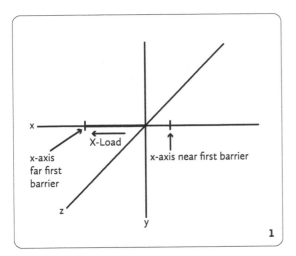

1

Assess the mobility of the tissue to be treated. Then assess the location of the near and far first barriers in one dimension. Load the tissue to the far first barrier, also known as the direction of ease. The Z axis in these illustrations is actually perpendicular to the plane of the page. It is drawn here as diagonal, giving a perspective view to represent three dimensions on a two-dimensional page.

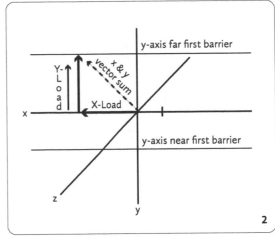

2

Maintaining the far first barrier load established in the first step, now assess the location of the near and far first barriers in a second dimension. Load the tissue to the far first barrier in this second dimension. Two dimensions are now stacked.

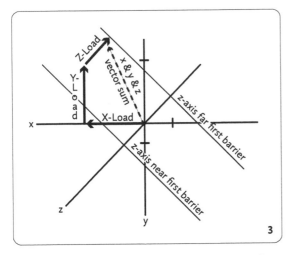

3

Maintaining the far first barrier loads established in the first two dimensions, now assess the location of the near and far first barriers in a third dimension. Load the tissue to the first barrier in this third dimension. Three dimensions are now stacked to far first barrier loads.

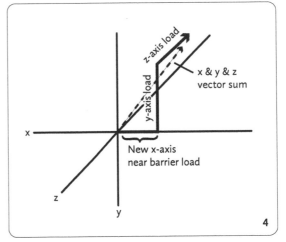

4

Choosing any one of the three dimensions, change the load in that single dimension to near first barrier. The distance traveled from neutral to this new near first barrier will be greater than when originally tested.

Stack and borrow (*cont.*)

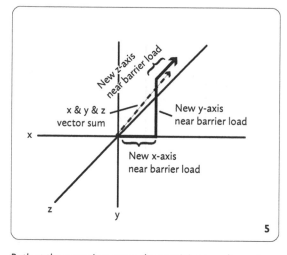

5

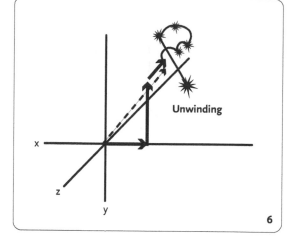

6

Both at the same time, move the remaining two dimensions to near first barrier. It will be found there is very little distance to travel as most of the slack in the system was used up by moving the first dimension to near first barrier. A near first barrier stack has now been established, but because this near first barrier stack was arrived at by a different path than usual, the position will be quite different than if a plain near first barrier stack was created.

Maintain the sum vector load created in the first five steps as you allow an unwind to proceed. This may be a plain unwind, or augmented, or alternate interrupt. Once a larger more general release is felt, and the unwind stops, remove your hands. Post mobility test the tissue to learn what change has occurred. Make a choice to further treat this area with either the same or another technique, or to return to general assessment.

Six factor model: Stack and borrow

TISSUE ENGAGEMENT

Tissue engagement is achieved by first barrier loading.

FORCE

Low. During portions of the setup phase, a little more than first barrier force is used. In the treatment phase, first barrier forces are used.

SPEED

Slow to moderate during the setup phase. Slow for the treatment phase, following physiologic movement.

Tissue moving too fast is rare with this method but remain watchful for too rapid movement and slow the tissue down if this occurs. Similarly, repeated patterns of unwind are rare, but remain watchful for repeated patterns and assist the body to move out of this pattern in the way described for unwinding.

CONSTRAINT

Moderate. Tissue is stacked to a first barrier and maintained there. Other movements are allowed, but given the level of constraint, there is limited possibility for unwind. Often the release occurs all at once as with centralizing technique.

DIRECTIVENESS

None. No specific movements are demanded.

RELATIONSHIP TO EFFORT BARRIERS

All therapeutic loads applied in this technique are at a first barrier.

STACK AND BORROW EXAMPLE 1

Caution—Do not do this on a person known to have osteoporosis or who has any risk factors for osteoporosis but has not been tested for osteoporosis. Do not do this on a person who has or might have any other sources of bone fragility.

ASSESSMENT

General assessment points to the right hip area. The witness point at the greater trochanter rules out the leg. Seated general listening also rules out the leg.

Local assessment, including a gliding local listening, manual thermal assessment, layer listening, and applied kinesiology questions, leads to strain in bone in the right ilium.

CLIENT INQUIRY

Ask the client:

- about awareness of their body in general,
- and at the hips, particularly any differences between the left and right hip areas.

MOBILITY TESTING

Global active

- Observe the client walking.
- Ask the standing client to:
  - touch their toes without bending their knees, and
  - with a wider stance, weight shift left, return to center, then to the right.

Global passive

- With the client standing, sit behind the client.
- Find and assess positions of the ASIS and PSIS to evaluate pelvic tilt and torsion between the two halves of the pelvis.
- With a hand broadly on each iliac crest, attempt to gently rock one side anterior while rocking the other side posterior. Avoid rotation of any part of the pelvis around vertical axes. Let this settle to neutral, then rock the ilia in the opposite direction.

Local passive

- Ask the client to lie supine on the table.
- Stand or sit on the side of the client to be tested.
- Place your two hands on the right iliac crest, one in front of the other. Gently bend the bone:
  - bowed in a sagittal plane
  - bowed in a transverse plane
  - spiraled around an A–P axis.
- Test the flexibility of bone in the other ilium in the same way.

TREATMENT

Place your hands in the position on the right iliac crest used for the last mobility test.

Mobility test to first barriers, both directions spiraling the bone around an A–P axis. Load the bone to a first barrier in far first barrier. Maintain this load as you:

- Bow the ilium in a transverse plane. Note first barriers in each direction. Load the bone to a first barrier in the far first barrier direction.
- Maintain these two dimensions of load as you bow the ilium in a sagittal plane in each direction. Load the bone to a first barrier in the far first barrier direction.
- Maintain the first barrier loads in the A–P torsion dimension and the transverse plane bowing. Change the direction of the sagittal plane load to near first barrier load. The distance to the first barrier will usually be significantly greater than when first tested.
- Maintaining the new sagittal plane load, concurrently change the transverse plane load and the A–P spiral load to the opposite (near) first barrier load. Usually, it will be found there is now very little excursion to this barrier. All this establishes a near

first barrier stack but with a very different final vector than if the stacking was done right into near first barrier.

- As you maintain the new near first barrier stack load, the tissue may or may not unwind. If it does unwind, dynamically maintain the new final vector load. Whether or not an unwind occurs, there will eventually be a larger, more general feeling of softening or release in the bone.

POST TREATMENT TESTING AND INQUIRY

Use the standard post treatment procedure for mobility testing and question asking detailed in the introduction to treatment methods section. Either treat this same area further, as indicated by this inquiry, or return to general assessment.

Stack and borrow example 2

ASSESSMENT

General assessment points to the upper right limb, confirmed by an inhibitory contact at the right olecranon process.

Local assessment, including a gliding local listening, manual thermal assessment, layer listening, and applied kinesiology questions, leads to an adhesion in the right olecranon bursa.

MOBILITY TESTING

Global active

- Ask the standing client to make several movements of each arm, one arm at a time.
  - Elbow flexion.
  - Elbow extension.
  - Forward flexion of the arm at the shoulder while maintaining the elbow extended.
  - Bring the hand to the shoulder flexing the elbow, and maintaining this flexion, now forward flex the shoulder.

Global passive

- With the client standing, stand facing your client's right side. Ask your client to allow you to move their arm without either resisting or assisting.
- Perform all the same tests as in the active test list above.

Local passive

- With your client supine, sit or stand comfortably at your client's right side. Internally rotate the client's right arm to a comfortable extent to make the olecranon process accessible. Place the tip of your left index or middle finger of your left hand on the olecranon process. Place your right hand on the opposite side of the elbow providing dynamic stabilization.
- With the finger over the olecranon process, sink into the depth of the olecranon bursa. Attempt to glide its outer wall successively medial, lateral, proximal, and distal to comfortable end-feel.
- In the same way, test the olecranon bursa of the left arm for comparison.

TREATMENT

Place your hands on the right elbow in the same positions as for the passive mobility test. Sink into the depth of the olecranon bursa. Mobility test glide of the outer wall of the bursae to first barriers medial and lateral. Load the tissue to a far first barrier. Maintain this medial or lateral first barrier load as you mobility test the bursal tissue gliding proximal and distal. Load this second dimension to far first barrier. Maintaining these first two dimensions of the far first barrier stack, rotate the bursal tissue clockwise and then counterclockwise to locate the first barriers. Add this third dimension of rotation to your now three dimensional far first barrier stack. Select any one of the dimensions and transition it to a near first barrier. Then concurrently transition the remaining two dimensions to a near first barrier. Unwinding may occur. Whether or not unwinding occurs, maintain the vector sum of the new near first barrier stack. Wait for a larger release.

POST TREATMENT TESTING AND INQUIRY

Use the standard post treatment procedure for mobility testing and question asking detailed in the introduction to treatment methods section. Either treat this same area further, as indicated by this inquiry, or return to general assessment.

Stack and borrow example 3

ASSESSMENT

General assessment points to the head.

Local assessment, including local listening, manual thermal assessment, layer listening, and applied kinesiology questions, leads to a patch of stiff superficial fascia about 3 cm in diameter on the left occiput.

MOBILITY TESTING

Global active

- Ask the standing client to make a succession of several movements of the neck: flexion, extension, left side bending, right side bending, left rotation, and right rotation.

Global passive

- Ask the client to lie supine on the table.
- Sit comfortably at the head of the table.
- Place both hands under the back and sides of the head to test mobility in several directions, pausing at neutral between each direction.
- Left rotation, right rotation, left side bending, right side bending, flexion, extension, combined right side bending and flexion, combined left side bending, and extension.

Local passive

- Still seated at the head of the table, place fingertips on the portion of the occiput indicated by assessment methods.
- Attempt to glide the skin to a comfortable end-feel successively, medial, lateral, superior, and inferior.
- Similarly, test adjacent areas and on the right side of the occiput. By this means, both note the lack of skin movement in this area and define its edges.

TREATMENT

Continuing to sit at the head of the table, use your right hand under and to the right of the head to dynamically stabilize the head. Place finger pads of your left hand on the primary area of stiffness on the left occiput. Sink into the skin. Glide the skin to first barriers medial and lateral to determine which is near and which is far. Load the tissue to a far first barrier. Maintaining this load, mobility test the tissue to first barriers superior and inferior to locate the near and far first barriers. While maintaining the medial or lateral far first barrier load, now establish a superior–inferior dimension far first barrier load. Rotate the tissue clockwise and counterclockwise to first barriers. While maintaining the first two dimensions to far first barriers, load the tissue to a far first barrier in rotation. Select one of the three dimensions; transition it to a near first barrier. Then concurrently transition the other two first barriers to near first barrier. Maintain this near first barrier load. In the less likely event that an unwind ensues, maintain the vector sum of these three near first barrier loads during the unwind. Whether or not an unwind occurs, maintain this vector sum load until there is a larger, more general release.

POST TREATMENT TESTING AND INQUIRY

Use the standard post treatment procedure for mobility testing and question asking detailed in the introduction to treatment methods section. Either treat this same area further, as indicated by this inquiry, or return to general assessment.

Treatment method 10: standing adaptation of the sacro-occipital technique (SOT) type 4 correction: an application of the stack and borrow technique

Origin

Major Bertrand DeJarnette, DO, DC, 1889–1992, made many innovations, including the use of wedges under the pelvis in any of three different patterns known as sacro-occipital technique (SOT) corrections type 1, 2, and 3. His followers created ten more variants. Variant number 4 worked like this: If one ilium is rotated forward and the other backward around a transverse axis through the acetabula, have the client lie supine. Place a wedge under the posterior iliac spine of the posterior ilium. Place a second wedge under the other side of the pelvis under the greater trochanter. Wait until gravity settles the pelvis toward neutral.

One of the benefits of this type of correction is that if the body says it has had enough intervention, a type 4 correction will often give it enough stability to accept more intervention.

I have developed a standing adaptation of the SOT-4 correction which includes additional contacts on the sacrum.

Indications:

- a *no* response to the question "Is it beneficial to treat?" or
- a *yes* response to asking if it is safe and beneficial to apply this type 4 correction variant.

Pretest

1. General listen.
2. Look for the visual hallmarks of structural integration.
3. Have the client stand comfortably, with the feet in a natural position and the arms hanging free. Sit on a stool behind the client. Place your hands on the iliac crests to evaluate height. Then move the hands to the superior surfaces of the greater trochanters to evaluate anatomic leg length. Assuming the legs appear equal in length, the heights of the iliac crests can be taken at face value. If the greater trochanters are not at the same height, you must compare lines between the ASIS and PSIS on each side. Do the left and right lines have the same slope?
4. With one hand grasping each iliac crest, attempt to counter-rotate the ilia around a transverse axis through the acetabula. The high crest is expected to rotate anteriorly with greater ease, i.e., into aberration. The low crest is expected to rotate posteriorly with greater ease. Return to recheck iliac crest height if this is not the case. However, if the joints of the pelvis are very stiff, this mobility will not be observed.
5. If there is no mobility, the positional assessment is assumed to be correct; however, it may be necessary to treat the sacroiliac joint capsules before the type 4 correction can be performed.
6. Now place the thumbs in the sacroiliac joint sulcus first at the superior lateral angles and then at the inferior lateral angles. Note the least deep sulcus. This is the most posterior corner of the sacrum with respect to the diagonal axes. Which diagonal axis the sacrum is fixated on, and which way the front of the sacrum is facing, can be deduced from this:

Most posterior corner	Front of sacrum faces	On axis
Upper left	Left	Right
Lower left	Left	Left
Upper right	Right	Left
Lower right	Right	Right

Treatment

A complex stack and borrow technique is used:

1. Still seated behind the standing client, place the left hand on the left iliac crest and the right hand on the right iliac crest, with a thumb resting softly on the most posterior corner of the sacrum. Rotate the anterior crest further forward around a transverse acetabular axis somewhat past a first barrier. At the same time, posteriorly rotate the posterior crest in a similar fashion.

2. Maintaining this, gently push the client's pelvis slightly left and then slightly right to determine direction of ease. Maintain it just past a first barrier in ease.

3. Then gently push the client's pelvis slightly anterior and then posterior to determine biomechanical direction of ease. Maintain the pelvis just beyond a first barrier in direction of ease.

4. Maintaining all this, gently rotate the pelvis clockwise and counterclockwise around a set of vertical axes through the legs to determine ease and effort; maintain this just beyond a first barrier in direction of ease.

5. Maintaining all this, now use the thumb to push the most posterior corner of the sacrum anterior to a first barrier. Maintaining this sacral position, concurrently transition all other dimensions to a first barrier effort.

6. In this last maneuver, it will be found that little movement is possible as much of the slack generated by taking the several dimensions to ease has been used up by pushing the corner of the sacrum anterior. Nevertheless, maintain this atypical first barrier effort stack through a series of releases to a general release. Lines of tension from the pelvis through the feet to the ground will be noted during this. The process releases strain patterns in the lower limbs which have contributed to the pelvic malposition.

Post test

Same as pretest.

Treatment method 11: scrubbing the walls

Origin
Jeffrey Burch.

Concept
There are two elements to this concept, shape and load.

SHAPE
First barrier loads or stacks are traditionally made along either cardinal planes or physiologic axes. However, a first barrier will be encountered in any direction in which tissue is loaded from neutral. In other words, the six points found by mobility testing to first barriers in three axes are only six points on the surface of a volume which could be found by mobility testing in many directions. What then is the shape of this space? Looking at the first six points, we can connect them in our minds to form a rectangular shape or alternatively an approximation of a sphere that would just fit in such a rectangular solid. Reality is more variable and more complex. The shape of the space defined by first barrier loads in succession of many directions is an irregularly shaped volume, reminiscent of being inside a cave chamber. I call this irregular surface the first barrier horizon.

LOAD
For methods discussed up to now, therapeutic tissue loads, either single dimension or stacks, have been applied in a particular directional vector. The direction and force of that vector are then maintained as the tissue unwinds. That method is effective; however, as the tissue changes during the unwind, consistent loads of this type soon are no longer accurately perpendicular to the first barrier they approach. In fact, given the irregular shape of the first barrier force horizon, they may never have been perpendicular to that surface. The method described in this technique keeps the first barrier load constantly perpendicular to the first barrier's dynamic position as the tissue unwinds.

The initial load may be compression, torsion, shear, or stretch; however, some stretch loads have special characteristics which are described in the following section.

Image
Imagine you are inside a small cave in complete darkness. If you reach up with a hand you can feel the height of the ceiling and know its distance from the floor under your feet. If you reach out to the sides with each arm you can touch the walls, sensing the width of the cave. If you turn 90 degrees and again reach out with your arms you can feel a third dimension of the cave. Knowing these three dimensions gives a sense of the shape of the cave. However, the contour of the walls between the points touched with your hands remains unknown. Between the points of wall touched, the walls of the cave may bulge to the inside or enlarge to the outside in infinite possible variations.

Another assessment approach is to reach out to touch a wall of the cave and then follow it with your hand. Sweep over it at a moderate pace to feel the shape of the wall in detail.

Unlike a cave, the interior surface we approach with a first barrier load is not a solid wall, instead it is the distance we must travel from neutral in any direction to find a first barrier. We can call this a force horizon.

The properties of this force horizon include both elasticity and plasticity. If we push a little harder into it, we feel the spring of tissue elasticity. If we stay at the force barrier allowing unwind, the location and shape of the first barrier force horizon will progressively expand, expressing the force horizon's plasticity.

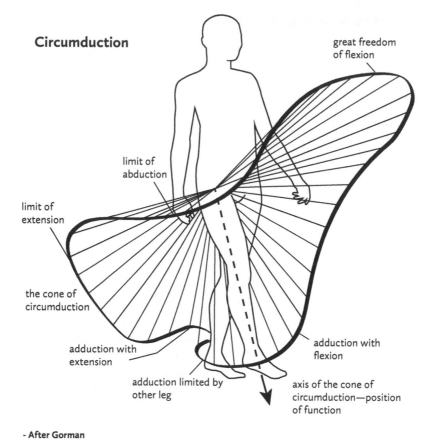

Circumduction

Important note—While the location and shape of the first barrier force horizon will change progressively with this method, achieving spherical shape or even symmetry are not goals. A reason for this is that physiologic limits of tissue impose important dimensional constraints. For example, the femero-acetabular joint is a ball and socket joint which allows movement in many axes; however, the nonuniform shape of the perimeter of the acetabulum, the contours of the head and neck of the femur, and the normal constraints of the ligamentous capsule of the hip joint and other associated soft tissue all interact to make the limits of normal healthy movement in the hip joint not perfectly circular.

Method

Pretest mobility in the usual ways both globally and locally.

Contact the primary tissue to move that tissue from its neutral resting place in any direction until a first barrier is encountered. Recognize the first barrier found in this way as one point on the first barrier force horizon which has a yet unknown irregular shape.

Once at the force horizon, maintain this pressure to stay at the force horizon while otherwise allowing a free unwind. You will find yourself gliding along the force horizon in paths directed by the client's tissue. Let yourself be surprised where your hand will be led. As you glide, releases will occur so that the shape of the force horizon will change, moving incrementally outward, enlarging the volume of the space bounded by the force horizon. As you glide, stay constantly alert to maintain pressure perpendicular to the surface of the irregularly shaped force horizon.

This is somewhat like a direction or ease, or direction of effort unwind. However, specific directionality of ease or effort is not maintained, rather a first barrier force horizon is hugged. In a physical room or cave, the walls, ceilings, and floors are continuous. Similarly, direction of ease and effort force horizons are continuous. In this technique, any part of this continuous surface is found by mobility testing to a first barrier. Once a single point on the first barrier force horizon has been found, the rest of the surface can be found by simply following the walls, while maintaining your force perpendicular to that part of the wall.

Following the walls also changes them. To follow the force horizon is to treat it. As treatment progresses, the volume of the space described by the force horizon will increase at a variable pace and in unequal increments. This increase in volume is not uniform in all dimensions. Some portions of the inside of the cave will yield sooner and/or further than other portions. Some portions will yield during the treatment, change will continue in the following weeks, yet other portions may remain to be worked on in future treatments.

Completion of treatment is recognized by a general softening of the area and cessation of movement.

Post treatment testing and inquiry

Use the standard post treatment procedure for mobility testing and question asking detailed in the introduction to treatment methods section. Either treat this same area further, as indicated by this inquiry, or return to general assessment.

Six factors varying among functional methods

TISSUE ENGAGEMENT

Tissue engagement is the same as for first barrier ease or first barrier effort methods. The handshake is initiated by the therapist loading tissue to a first barrier.

FORCE

Low. The therapist maintains a first barrier load into the force horizon.

SPEED

Slow. Tissue unwinding too fast is rare with this method but remain watchful for too rapid movement and slow the tissue down if this occurs. Similarly, repeated patterns are rare, but stay alert to this possibility.

CONSTRAINT

None. Unwinding is allowed in any direction so long as first barrier loading is maintained.

DIRECTIVENESS

Mild. A first barrier load at the first barrier force horizon is maintained, no other direction is given.

RELATIONSHIP TO EFFORT BARRIERS

First barrier load is always maintained.

Scrubbing the walls

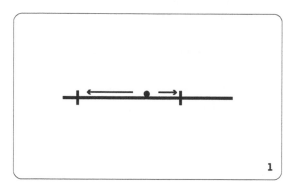

1

Begin by mobility testing tissue to a first barrier in two opposite directions, as you did for first barrier stacking techniques. The distance to the first barrier in the two directions will usually not be the same.

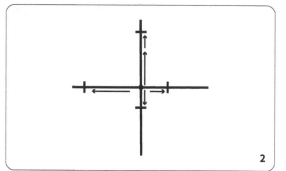

2

The distance to the first barrier can then be tested in another dimension at 90 degrees to the first. A new pair of points marking the location of the first barrier will be found.

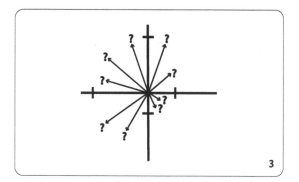

3

Where would you expect to find the first barrier if you test in several other directions other than at 90 degrees to the first dimensions tested?

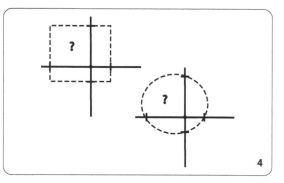

4

Would the first barriers all be on the perimeter of a rectangle defined by the first four points found? Or would the first barriers lie in an oval shape again including the first four points found?

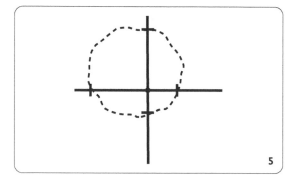

5

Neither of the above. If you mobility test the distance to a first barrier in many directions, the points found map an irregular curve. We call this irregular curve the first barrier force horizon.

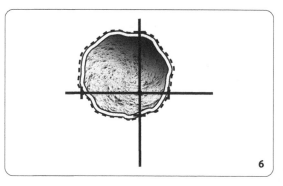

6

Multiple first barrier mobility tests in many directions using the third dimension will map a lumpy shallow bowl shape. We now have a three-dimensional first barrier force horizon.

Scrubbing the walls (*cont.*)

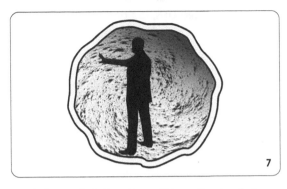

Unwinding can be initiated by mobility testing to a first barrier in any direction. It is as if you reach out in the dark to touch the wall of the cave.

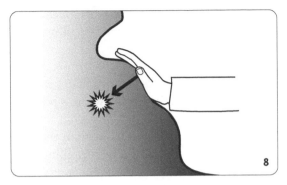

As the unwind proceeds, your contact will glide along the cave wall, changing direction as you encounter the hollows and bumps of the cave wall. Your hand will usually not move over the skin, but the felt sense of unwinding under the skin includes a gliding-like sensation.

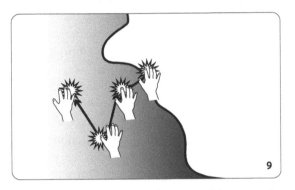

It is as if you are gently scrubbing the walls of the cave with your hand.

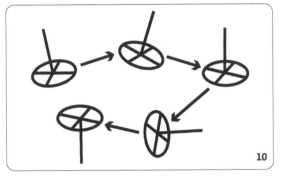

Your tasks are to a) maintain a first barrier pressure into the wall of the cave, and b) keep your hand perpendicular to each part of the cave wall you glide along.

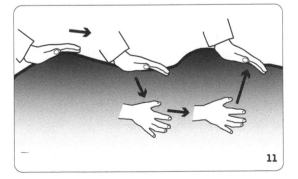

As the unwinding proceeds, the walls of the cave will soften and change shape, generally becoming smoother, and the volume of the cave expanding.

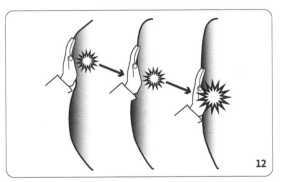

As with any unwinding, there will eventually be a larger release and softening, at which moment the unwind will stop. As usual, when the unwind ends, remove your hand and return to assessment.

Scrubbing the walls example 1

Caution—Do not do this on any client who is known to have osteoporosis or who has risk factors for osteoporosis but has not been tested for osteoporosis.

ASSESSMENT

General assessment leads to the right upper limb, confirmed by inhibition of the witness point at the right olecranon process.

Local assessment such as manual thermal assessment, local listening, layer listening, and applied kinesiology questioning pinpoints focal stiffness in the right humerus.

CLIENT INQUIRY

Ask the client:

- how they have been feeling in general, and
- of their awareness of their shoulders and arms.

MOBILITY TESTING

Global active

- Ask the client to walk; observe gait, particularly with respect to arm swing.
- Ask the client to circumduct the right shoulder.

Global passive

- Stand behind the client. Place your left hand on top of the right shoulder girdle to stabilize the clavicle and scapula. With your right hand, control the client's right elbow to circumduct the gleno-humeral joint while maintaining the elbow comfortably extended.

Focal passive

- Ask the client to lie supine on the table.
- With your two hands, contact the two ends of the humerus. Gently attempt to spiral bend it along its long axis.
- With fingertips, tap on the humerus in a succession of places from distal to proximal. Stiff areas of bone tend to have a duller, less bright resonance.
- Place fingers of your two hands next to each other, contacting the humerus just above the elbow. Gently make a slight focal bend of the bone. Shift your hands slightly superior along the humerus and repeat this test along the length of the bone. How does this data compare with the tap test?

TREATMENT

Place one hand supportively under the stiff portion of the humerus. With your other hand, contact the other side of the humerus; sink into bone to a first barrier. As an unwind begins, follow the unwind with your fingers, staying alert to the orientation and position of the first barrier horizon you are contacting. Stay perpendicular to this dynamically changing surface at a first barrier load. Regardless of the direction which the load takes, stay at first barrier force, perpendicular to the evolving first barrier force horizon. After seconds to minutes, the unwind will stop, usually with a larger release felt.

POST TREATMENT TESTING AND INQUIRY

Use the standard post treatment procedure for mobility testing and question asking detailed in the introduction to treatment methods section. Either treat this same area further, as indicated by this inquiry, or return to general assessment.

Scrubbing the walls example 2

ASSESSMENT

General assessment leads to the upper abdomen.

Local assessment such as manual thermal assessment, local listening, layer listening, and applied kinesiology questioning pinpoints the primary restriction as the round ligament of the liver.

The round ligament of the liver is derived from a portion of the umbilical vein. Its inferior end is fused into the scar tissue of the umbilicus. From there, it runs superiorly just posterior to the linea alba and exterior to the parietal peritoneum. At its superior end, it swings posterior to approach the liver where it is continuous with the ligamentum venosum lying within the groove on the inferior side of the liver which distinguishes the left and right lobes of the liver.

CLIENT INQUIRY

Ask the client:

- how they have been feeling in general, and
- of their awareness of their upper abdomen and mid back.

MOBILITY TESTING

Global active

- Ask the client to walk; observe gait, particularly with respect to mobility in the upper abdomen and lumbodorsal hinge area.
- Ask the client to extend their trunk. Observe the ability of the upper abdomen to lengthen.

Global passive

- Stand at the client's side. Place one hand at the lumbodorsal hinge as a fulcrum. Place your other hand on the client's upper sternum to apply a posterior load extending the client's trunk over the fulcrum at your posterior hand.

Local passive

- Ask the client to lie supine on the table. Sit at your client's right side.

- With the thumb and fingers of your right hand, contact the superior surface of the umbilicus.
- Place the heel of your left hand on the lower sternum. Bracket the midline just inferior to the sternum with your index and middle fingers. With your thumb and remaining fingers, contact the inferior surface of the costal arch, right and left of midline. In this way you have control of both ends of the round ligament of the liver. Provide a superior load dynamic stabilization with the left hand while you use your right hand to draw the umbilicus inferior, testing the span of the round ligament of the liver.

TREATMENT

Still seated or standing at the client's right side, shift your hands so your two thumbs are arranged vertically on the right edge of the linea alba, superior to the umbilicus, with the tips of the two thumbs touching each other. Arrange the tips of all your other fingers in a vertical row on the left side of the linea alba again, all superior to the umbilicus. With all your fingers, sink into the depth of the round ligament of the liver. Use these contacts to slowly bow the round ligament of the liver to a first barrier in any plane. An unwind will start. Follow the unwind, staying in contact with the round ligament of the liver. The direction of the bending load on the round ligament will change as the unwind proceeds and may shift to other types of loads, including compression, stretch, torsion, or shear. Regardless of the direction which the load takes, stay at first barrier force, perpendicular to the evolving first barrier force horizon. After seconds to minutes, the unwind will stop. Remove your hands.

POST TREATMENT TESTING AND INQUIRY

Use the standard post treatment procedure for mobility testing and question asking detailed in the introduction to treatment methods section. Either treat this same area further, as indicated by this inquiry, or return to general assessment.

Scrubbing the walls example 3

ASSESSMENT

General assessment leads to the right upper limb.

Local assessment such as manual thermal assessment, local listening, layer listening, and applied kinesiology questioning pinpoints the primary restriction as fibrosity in the intermuscular connective tissue between the long and short heads of the right biceps muscle in a focal area near mid shaft of the humerus.

This does not allow the two heads of the biceps to operate as independently of each other as they should.

CLIENT INQUIRY

Ask the client:

- how they have been feeling in general, and
- of their awareness of their shoulder and arm.

MOBILITY TESTING

Global active

- Ask the client to walk; observe gait, particularly with respect to mobility of the upper limbs.
- Ask the client to bring their hand to their shoulder, and then to return it to hanging at their side. Compare this between the left and right arms.

Global passive

- Stand behind the client shifted somewhat to the right. Place your left hand laterally on the top of the shoulder girdle to provide dynamic stabilization of the scapula and clavicle.
- Place your other right hand on the client's distal right forearm just above the elbow. Extend the right shoulder, allowing the elbow to naturally flex. Return the client's arm to hang naturally at their side.
- Shift your right hand a little distal on the arm to control the elbow so you can extend the arm while maintaining the elbow comfortably extended. Note the difference between extending the shoulder in these two ways.

Local passive

- Ask the client to lie supine on the table. Sit at your client's right side facing their right upper arm.
- Place your left hand under the middle of the right upper arm, wrapping your hand and fingers around the back side of the arm so you can control lateral movement of the short head of the biceps muscle with your fingertips and the heel of your hand.
- Place your right hand over the biceps muscle opposite your left hand, wrapping down around the long head of the biceps to control its medial–lateral position.
- Use these hand holds to test for medial–lateral counter movement between the long and short heads of the biceps muscle.

TREATMENT

Still seated at the client's right side and with your hands in the same position as for the passive focal, mobility test. Apply dynamic stabilization with your left hand on the posterior aspect of the arm as you apply a gentle load to the long head of the biceps in a frontal plane. This shear load is directed at and focused on the connective tissue between the long and short heads of the biceps muscle. This shear load may be initiated in any direction within the frontal plane.

An unwind will start. Follow the unwind staying in contact with the long and short heads of the biceps. The direction of the shear load on the intermuscular connective tissue will change as the unwind proceeds and may shift to other types of loads, including compression, stretch, torsion, or shear. Regardless of the direction which the load takes, stay at first barrier force, perpendicular to the evolving first barrier force horizon. After seconds to minutes, the unwind will stop. Remove your hands.

POST TREATMENT TESTING AND INQUIRY

Use the standard post treatment procedure for mobility testing and question asking detailed in the introduction to treatment methods section. Either treat this same area further, as indicated by this inquiry, or return to general assessment.

Treatment method 12: pendulum wall scrubbing

Origin
Jeffrey Burch.

Concept and image
This is a variant of wall scrubbing initiated as a stretch load from a dynamically stabilized point.

Pendulums usually hang down vertically in gravity from a fixed point above. In this technique, the load is created by the therapist rather than by the gravitational field of the earth and can thus be in any direction, not just vertical.

Pendulums usually swing in one plane, back and forth in a circular arc. As the pendulum loses energy to friction, the arc will grow progressively shorter until it stops.

A pendulum can be made to swing in a circular shape. If a circular pendulum path is initiated, the pendulum will gradually swing in smaller and smaller circles until it stops. In this situation, over time the pendulum describes the shape of an approximate spherical section, effectively a bowl.

In this technique, the tissue is unwinding so it neither follows a regular path nor loses energy to friction. It will describe an ever-changing approximation of a bowl shape of uneven contour. As a partial metaphor, picture a wooden bowl turned from green wood so that as it dries it warps. To complete the metaphor, the bowl would also have to exhibit plasticity like wet clay.

As for the previously described technique, the final goal for bowl shape is neither perfect spherical section nor symmetry, rather it is expansion and greater smoothness.

Method
Pretest mobility in the usual ways both globally and locally. This technique is usually used on a primary structure which is linear or at least has a longer axis.

Contact two ends of the primary structure with your two hands. Choose one end to establish a dynamic stabilization as the pivot of the pendulum. Use the other hand to begin to stretch the structure to be treated away from the dynamically stabilized pivot; load this to a first barrier, then as an unwind begins dynamically maintaining the first barrier stretch load from the pivot point. During the unwind, the direction will continuously change. The distance from the pivot will incrementally increase.

Completion of treatment is recognized by a general softening of the area and cessation of movement.

Post treatment testing and inquiry
Use the standard post treatment procedure for mobility testing and question asking detailed in the introduction to treatment methods section. Either treat this same area further, as indicated by this inquiry, or return to general assessment.

Six factor model: Pendulum wall scrubbing
TISSUE ENGAGEMENT
Tissue engagement is initiated by the therapist stretching tissue to a first barrier. Tissue engagement is the same as for first barrier ease or first barrier effort methods; however, no specific relationship to near or far first barriers is used.

FORCE
Low. The therapist maintains a first barrier load into the first barrier force horizon.

SPEED
Slow. Tissue unwinding too fast is rare with this method but remain watchful for too rapid movement and slow the tissue down if this occurs. Similarly, repeated patterns are rare but stay alert to this possibility.

CONSTRAINT
None. Unwinding is allowed in any direction so long as first barrier loading is maintained, and a

repeated pattern, or too fast movement, does not occur.

DIRECTIVENESS

Mild. A first barrier load into the first barrier force horizon is maintained; movement in all other directions is allowed.

RELATIONSHIP TO EFFORT BARRIERS

First barrier load is always maintained.

Pendulum wall scrubbing

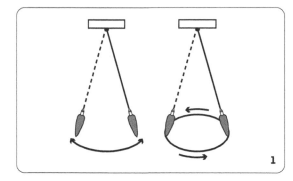

A pendulum is a weight suspended from a fixed point. The weight can swing back and forth in one plane describing an arc. A pendulum weight can also swing around in a circle.

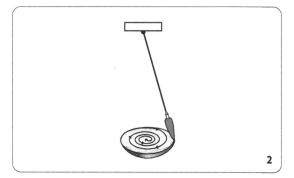

As a straight arc pendulum runs down, its arc will get shorter and shorter. As a circularly swinging pendulum runs down, it defines a shallow bowl which is a section of a sphere with the center of the sphere at the stable end of the pendulum.

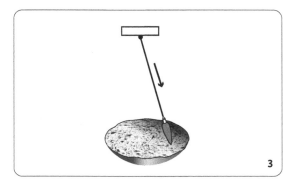

If a wall scrub technique is initiated with a gentle stretch rather than with pressure, the unwinding will describe part of a lumpy surfaced bowl sort of like a circular pendulum, but more irregular in path.

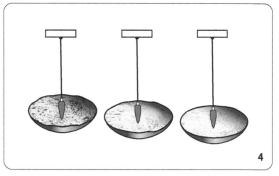

As this type of unwind proceeds, the string of the pendulum gradually gets longer; in effect it is being stretched. At the same time, the surface of the bowl becomes somewhat less lumpy.

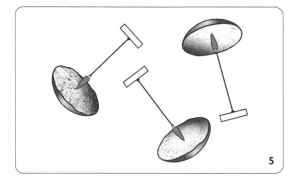

Real pendulums always hang vertically in gravity. Pendulum unwinding treatment technique can be done in any direction as long as there is a dynamic stabilizing hand at one end, and a mobile unwinding hand at the other end.

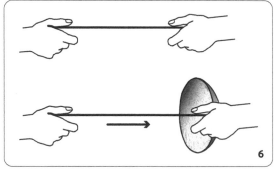

To initiate a pendulum unwind, use one hand to dynamically stabilize tissue at one point. Contact at the other end of the structure to be elongated with the other hand and use that hand to stretch away from the stabilized point to a first or early barrier. Follow the unwind with this second hand in the usual way.

Double ended pendulum wall scrubbing

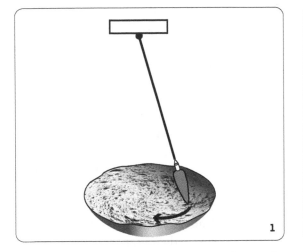

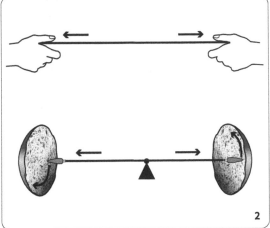

Pendulum wall scrubbing is performed with one dynamically stabilized point, and the other end of the gently stretched structure is free to unwind. The shape of the unwinding is the inner surface of a warped or lumpy bowl.

Instead of a fixed point at one end, it is possible to allow both ends of a gently stretched structure to unwind. In this situation, it is as if there is a pivot or fulcrum along the stretched structure instead of a fixed point at one end. Each of the two ends follow an irregular hollow curved surface unwinding path. The movement of the two ends mirror each other.

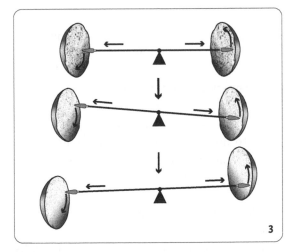

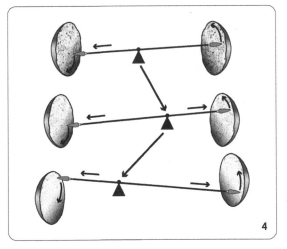

In addition to each end describing a convex unwinding path, there are two additional elements of unwinding. 1) The gently stretched line will tilt on the fulcrum along its length, and

2) The fulcrum will also seem to change position along the gently stretched line. This may either resemble the stretched line sliding over the fulcrum so the bowls at the ends move laterally, or the fulcrum sliding along the line so the distance to each end-unwind-bowls changes.

Pendulum wall scrubbing example 1

ASSESSMENT

General assessment leads to the right lower limb, confirmed by inhibition at the witness point at the right greater trochanter. The witness point at the lateral malleolus gives an equivocal answer suggesting the primary has some relationship to the foot or ankle but is not wholly located in it.

Local assessment such as manual thermal assessment, local listening, layer listening, and applied kinesiology questioning pinpoints stiffness in endomysium of the lateral head of the right gastrocnemius muscle.

CLIENT INQUIRY

Ask the client:

- how they have been feeling in general, and
- of their awareness of their knees, lower legs, and ankles.

MOBILITY TESTING

Global active

- Ask the client to walk; observe gait, particularly with respect to the knees and ankles.

Local active

- Ask the client to lie supine on the table with heels just off the end of the table. Ask the client to plantarflex and then dorsiflex each ankle, one at a time.

Local passive

- At the ankle, dynamically stabilize the distal lower leg with one hand and with the other hand control the calcaneus and talus to dorsiflex the ankle. Do this one leg at a time on each leg.
- Place a monitoring hand under the belly of the gastrocnemius muscle. With the other hand, control the talus and calcaneus to dorsiflex the ankle. Note which head of the gastrocnemius is more taut when in dorsiflexion. Do this one leg at a time on each leg.

TREATMENT

With the fingers of one hand, provide dynamic stabilization of the proximal tendon of the lateral head of the right gastrocnemius muscle and the distal femur to which it is attached. With your other hand, control the calcaneus. Use the calcaneus to slightly plantarflex the ankle. Then, again using the calcaneus as a handle, slowly dorsiflex the ankle, drawing the calcaneus inferior to a first barrier. As an unwind begins, use the calcaneal hand to follow the unwind while maintaining a first barrier stretch load. As you do this, maintain the dynamic stabilization of the proximal end of the lateral head of the distal femur to which it is attached. This will give a quality of an irregular pendulation movement of the calcaneus down from the pivot at the femoral end of the lateral gastrocnemius muscle. Proceed until a larger, more general release is felt and the unwinding stops. Remove your hands.

POST TREATMENT TESTING AND INQUIRY

Use the standard post treatment procedure for mobility testing and question asking detailed in the introduction to treatment methods section. Either treat this same area further, as indicated by this inquiry, or return to general assessment.

Pendulum wall scrubbing example 2

ASSESSMENT

General assessment leads to the head. Local listening and inhibition between the cranial vault, cranial base, and face leads to a co-dominance of the cranial base and the face.

Local assessment such as manual thermal assessment, local listening, layer listening, and applied kinesiology questioning pinpoints stiffness in the branch of the right facial nerve innervating the right cheek. The facial nerve is a cranial nerve which exits the cranial base through the styloid foramen in the basilar portion of the temporal bone. The facial branch spreads anterior from there into the cheek.

CLIENT INQUIRY
Ask the client:

- how they have been feeling in general, and
- of their awareness of any complaints.

MOBILITY TESTING
Global active

- Ask the client to walk; observe gait, particularly with respect to the head and neck.

Focal active

- Ask the standing client to move their head in left then right rotation, left then right side bending, flexion, and extension. Then ask the client to open their mouth to a comfortable degree; observe mandible tracking.
- Ask the client to move their mandible forward to a comfortable degree; observe tracking.
- Ask the client to move their mandible first left then right; observe ease and range of motion.

Focal passive

- Ask the client to lie supine on the table. With one hand, dynamically stabilize the maxillae; with the other hand, gently move the mandible swinging it left, then right. Compare excursion and ease of movement. Sitting at the head of the table, place your right hand under the client's occiput with your right thumb aligned along the mastoid process; place the fingers of your left hand on the right cheek and gently stretch soft tissue anterior, providing dynamic stabilization of the cranial base with your right hand. Repeat this last test on the other side for comparison.

TREATMENT
This treatment uses an assessment method called the source and target method. This is a double long lever process in which the nerve itself is not touched, rather the bone(s) from which the nerves emerge from the central nervous system are used as a handle at one end, and the tissue which the nerves supply are used as a handle on the other end.

Sitting at the head of the table, align your two hands as for the last mobility test above. Place your right hand under the client's occiput with your right thumb aligned along the mastoid process; place the fingers of your left hand on the right cheek and gently stretch soft tissue anterior, providing dynamic stabilization of the cranial base with your right hand. With your left hand, gently slack the tissue on the right cheek posteriorly to ensure the tension in the nerve is less than first barrier. Then allow the tissue on the right cheek to spring back anteriorly until a first barrier load is recognized; this may be either before or after the original equilibrium position of the tissue. With your right hand, maintain a dynamic stabilization of the cranial base, particularly the mastoid process. From this fixed point, maintain a first barrier stretch load on the right facial nerve as you allow an unwind. As the unwind proceeds, the perceived distance between your two hands from the mastoid to the cheek will incrementally shift, generally increasing. When the unwind stops and a generalized softening is felt, release your stretch load on the nerve and begin post treatment testing and inquiry.

POST TREATMENT TESTING AND INQUIRY

Use the standard post treatment procedure for mobility testing and question asking detailed in the introduction to treatment methods section. Either treat this same area further, as indicated by this inquiry, or return to general assessment.

Pendulum wall scrubbing example 3

ASSESSMENT

General assessment leads to the left upper limb, supported by inhibition of the witness point at the left olecranon process.

With local assessment, gliding inhibition points to a primary restriction in the hand. Manual thermal assessment, local listening, layer listening, and applied kinesiology questioning pinpoint stiffness in the third metacarpophalangeal joint of the left hand.

CLIENT INQUIRY

Ask the client:

- how they have been feeling in general, and
- of their awareness of any complaints.

MOBILITY TESTING

Global active

- Ask the client to walk; observe gait, particularly with respect to movement of the upper limbs.

Focal active

- Ask the standing client to move each shoulder in internal and external rotation, flexion, extension, and abduction.
- Ask the client to bring their fingertips to their shoulder and then to fully extend each elbow while allowing the shoulder to extend to neutral.
- Ask the client to circumduct each wrist.
- Ask the client to first close each hand into

a fist and then to fully extend the fingers of each hand.

Focal passive

- With the client supine on the table, sit or stand at the client's left side as is convenient for you to explore the client's hand.
- With one hand, dynamically stabilize the distal end of each metacarpal bone 2, 3, 4, and 5, and use the other hand to move the proximal phalanx on each of these to comfortable end-feel in flexion, extension, radial deviation, ulnar deviation, and long axis rotation.

TREATMENT

This treatment uses a double long lever process using the two bones of a joint as handles to treat the joint capsule spanning between the two bones. This contrasts with a shorter lever treatment where the joint capsule would be contacted through the overlying skin.

With the client supine on the table, sit or stand at the client's left side as is convenient for you to explore the client's hand. With one of your hands, provide dynamic stabilization of the distal end of the client's left third metacarpal bone. With your other hand, control the proximal end of the third proximal phalanx of the client's left hand. Gently make a long axis compaction of the metacarpophalangeal joint to make sure the tension in the joint capsule is less than first barrier. From this position, and continuing to dynamically stabilize the metacarpal bone, allow the proximal phalanx to slowly spring out distally, and possibly gently stretch it beyond the original neutral until a first barrier load is encountered. Continuing to maintain the dynamic stabilization of the metacarpal and the first barrier long axis load on this joint, allow an unwind to proceed. As the unwind proceeds, the perceived distance between your two hands will change incrementally, generally lengthening. When the unwind stops and a generalized softening is felt, release your load and contact on the two bones and begin post treatment testing and inquiry.

POST TREATMENT TESTING AND INQUIRY

Use the standard post treatment procedure for mobility testing and question asking detailed in the introduction to treatment methods section. Either treat this same area further, as indicated by this inquiry, or return to general assessment.

A variant of pendulum wall scrubbing is to allow both ends of the tensional line to move. In this situation there will also be a moving pivot along the line between the two ends.

TECHNIQUES IN WHICH THERAPEUTIC ENGAGEMENT IS MADE BY THE THERAPIST AND UNWINDING IS NOT USED

The techniques in this section have two common characteristics:

- therapeutic engagement is made by the therapist
- unwinding is not used.

In some of these techniques, the nature of the therapeutic engagement prevents unwinding; in other techniques, the therapist forbids unwinding in favor of other paths to changing tissue span.

Treatment method 13: recoil

Origin
Early osteopathic treatment method. Discoverer not known.

Concept
If tissue is first stabilized by the therapist's hands in a specifically loaded fashion, and then the stabilization is abruptly released, the resulting minor earthquake shakes things loose.

Pretreatment tests
It is often useful to point out test results to the client. Invite them to remember the pretest condition to compare with test results after the treatment.

Observe postural alignment in the person's body both locally and globally.

Test biomechanical ranges of motion in the area to be treated.

Recent perspectives
Classically, the initial loading for recoil was often applied at a force level near end-feel. More recently, I have discovered that loading just beyond a first barrier usually provides better results than end-feel loading. Hoover centralizing technique style less than first barrier loadings is also often effective. End-feel loaded recoil often feels harsh for the client.

Classically, the preparatory phase of recoil was always done in direction of near end-feel; however, I have found that sometimes far end-feel, or mixed near and far, is more effective. This also applies when barriers less than end-feel are used.

Method

1. Choose direction of ease, effort, or mixed.
2. As you mobility test dimensions of mobility, in each dimension load the tissue in the chosen direction to a little beyond a first barrier. Accumulate these directions of loading as you go. Loading beyond a first barrier prevents the tissue from beginning therapeutic release until all aspects of the treatment setup are complete.
3. Once the tissue is loaded beyond a first barrier in the available cardinal and/or physiologic dimensions, ask the person to take and release a full breath at a moderate pace. Observe tension under your hands throughout the cycle of breath. At some point in the breath cycle, the felt tension under your hands will be at a maximum. On the next breath cycle, wait for this tension maximum, and at that moment release your hands with utmost speed.

This procedure may be used up to three times

on the same tissue or body area on a given day. Beyond three applications, it is usually ineffective.

Secrets of speed:

- Note the direction of push each hand exerts to maintain the prerelease pressure loading. As the hands are quickly lifted from the body, allow them to move in the direction of the loading. This makes for a much quicker departure than reversing the muscular activity established in the setup phase.
- Supinate your hands as you release.

Post treatment tests

Test ranges of motion in the area treated.

Observe postural alignment in the person's body both locally and globally.

Six factor model: Recoil

TISSUE ENGAGEMENT

Tissue stacking a little beyond a first barrier.

FORCE

A little beyond first barrier during setup. None during release.

SPEED

Moderate during setup. As fast as possible during the release.

CONSTRAINT

High constraint is applied during the setup phase; tissue is loaded beyond a first barrier. No spontaneous movement is allowed during the setup phase.

No constraint is applied during the release phase. Any movement is allowed.

DIRECTIVENESS

None. No specific movement is required.

RELATIONSHIP TO EFFORT BARRIERS

A little beyond first barriers in the setup phase.

None in the release phase; contact is abruptly broken.

TREATMENT
METHOD 13

Recoil

TREATMENT
METHOD 13

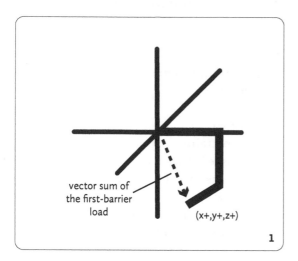

Mobility test the tissue and load it in three dimensions just beyond a first barrier. The load may be near barrier, far barrier, or mixed near and far barriers. Loading the tissue beyond a first barrier rather than to a first barrier prevents unwinding. The release happens in a different way with this technique.

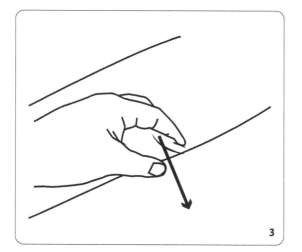

Observe the client's natural breath through a full cycle. At some phase of the breath cycle there will be an increase of tension under your hands. At the phase of the cycle where this increase of tension occurs, release the tissue as quickly as possible. The quicker the hands release the tissue, the more effective the recoil treatment.

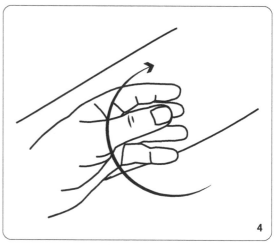

There are two secrets to speed which are to be used *together at the same time*. The first secret of speed is to move the hands in the direction you are already loading the tissue as you break contact. This makes a quicker release than if you reverse your effort.

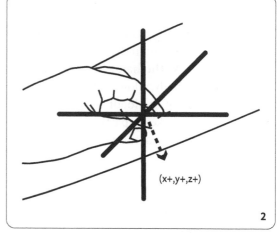

The second secret of speed is to turn your hand palm up as you release the tissue. This supination of the hand(s) also makes for a quicker release.

The two elements of speed, moving off the tissue in the direction it is already loaded shown in frame 3, and turning the hand palm up shown in frame 4, are both done at the same time. Together, these two directions of movement make for the quickest possible breaking of contact. The quicker the contact between the therapist's hand and the client's tissue is released, the more effective the recoil treatment.

Recoil example 1

Caution—Do not use this treatment method on clients known to have osteoporosis, or who have risk factors for osteoporosis but who have not recently been tested for osteoporosis.

ASSESSMENT

General assessment leads to the inferior part of the left thorax posterior–laterally.

Local assessment such as manual thermal assessment, local listening, layer listening, and applied kinesiology pinpoints this as the left tenth costotransverse joint.

CLIENT INQUIRY

Ask the client:

- how they have been feeling in general, and
- of their awareness of their mid and low back.

MOBILITY TESTING

Global active

- Ask the client to sit on a bench or stool, and in that position to move their trunk in:
  - flexion
  - extension
  - left side bending
  - right side bending
  - left rotation
  - right rotation.

Global passive

- Explain to the client the purpose and methods of the test you will do.
- With the client seated, stand or sit comfortably behind the client. With your two hands, contact and support the lower rib cage. Move the client successively:
  - left side bending
  - right side bending
  - left rotation
  - right rotation.

Passive focal

- With the client still seated, and sitting comfortably behind the client, use your right hand to contact the eleventh and twelfth thoracic vertebrae in a dynamic stabilization. With your left hand, contact the spinal end of the twelfth rib. Attempt to move the spinal end of the twelfth rib superior–laterally. Shift both of your hands one segment higher to mobility test the left eleventh costotransverse joint. Continue with the tenth, ninth, and eighth costotransverse joints. Similarly test the same joints on the other side.

TREATMENT

Choose near first barriers for this treatment. Return your hands to the left tenth rib and the ninth and tenth thoracic vertebrae in the same position as for mobility testing.

- Mobility test for the location of first barriers in a superior–inferior direction. Load the rib just beyond the near first barrier in the superior–inferior axis.
- Maintain this load as you mobility test the same joint in an anterior–posterior direction. Load this second dimension just beyond a first barrier in the near first barrier direction.
- Maintain these two directions of load as you mobility test the same joint for first barriers in a medial compaction–lateral stretch dimension. Load this third dimension just beyond a near first barrier.
- Maintain the vector sum of these three-dimensional loads as you observe the client's breath through a complete cycle. At some point in the cycle, you will feel

a maximum tension between your hands. As you continue to monitor breath through the next cycle, when you arrive at this tension maximum remove your hands as quickly as possible. To achieve maximum speed of departure, do these two things at the same time: 1) turn your hands palm up, and 2) depart in the same direction as the vector load you established in the tissue.

POST TREATMENT TESTING AND INQUIRY

Use the standard post treatment procedure for mobility testing and question asking detailed in the introduction to treatment methods section. Either treat this same area further, as indicated by this inquiry, or return to general assessment.

Recoil example 2

Caution—Do not use this treatment method on clients known to have osteoporosis, or who have risk factors for osteoporosis but who have not recently been tested for osteoporosis.

ASSESSMENT

General assessment leads to the right lateral part of the thorax.

Local assessment such as manual thermal assessment, local listening, layer listening, and yes–no questions pinpoints this as a fibrosity in superficial fascia in an irregularly shaped area of superficial fascia on the lateral aspect of the right side of the thorax overlying portions of ribs 7, 8, 9, and 10.

CLIENT INQUIRY

Ask the client:

- how they have been feeling in general, and
- of their awareness of their breath and thorax.

MOBILITY TESTING

Global active

- Ask the standing client to exhale fully and then inhale fully.
- Ask the client to sit on a bench or stool, and in that position to move their trunk in:
  - flexion
  - extension
  - left side bending
  - right side bending
  - left rotation
  - right rotation.

Global passive

- Explain to the client the purpose and methods of the test you will do.
- With the client seated, stand or sit comfortably behind the client. With your two hands, contact and support the lower rib cage. Move the client:
  - left side bending
  - right side bending
  - left rotation
  - right rotation.

Passive focal

- Ask the client to lie in a side-lying position with the right side up. Provide pillows under the head, in front of the torso, and if the client wishes, between the knees.
- With the fingers of one hand, contact skin inferior to the area of primacy on the lateral thorax. Move the skin over underlying tissue, anterior, posterior, superior, and inferior.
- Shift your fingers to the area of primacy and attempt the same glides.
- Do this same test in several adjacent areas to determine the margins of the region of fibrosed superficial fascia.

TREATMENT

- Choose far barrier load for this treatment.
- Depending on the size and shape of the irregular fibrosed area on the lateral chest wall, contact it with the hypothenar edge, eminence, or whole hand, sinking to the level of the superficial fascia. Match as well as you can the size and shape of the area to be treated.
- Drag the tissue anteriorly and posteriorly to find the first barrier. Load the tissue just beyond the first barrier in the far first barrier direction.
- Maintain this load as you drag the tissue superiorly and inferiorly to identify the first barriers in these directions. Additionally load the tissue to just beyond the far first barrier in this axis.
- Maintain these two axial loads just beyond a first barrier as you rotate this tissue clockwise and counterclockwise to find the first barrier in each direction. Load the tissue just beyond a first barrier in this third dimension.
- Maintain the vector sum of these three-dimensional loads as you observe the client's breath through a complete cycle. At some point in the cycle, you will feel a maximum tension between your hands. As you continue to monitor breath through the next cycle, when you arrive at this tension maximum remove your hands as quickly as possible. To achieve maximum speed of departure, do these two things at the same time: 1) turn your hands palm up, and 2) depart in the same direction as the vector load you established in the tissue.

POST TREATMENT TESTING AND INQUIRY

Use the standard post treatment procedure for mobility testing and question asking detailed in the introduction to treatment methods section.

Either treat this same area further, as indicated by this inquiry, or return to general assessment.

Recoil example 3

Caution—Do not use this treatment method on clients known to have osteoporosis, or who have risk factors for osteoporosis but who have not recently been tested for osteoporosis.

ASSESSMENT

General assessment leads to the right upper limb. This is supported by inhibition of the witness point at the right olecranon process.

Local assessment such as manual thermal assessment, gliding inhibition, local listening, layer listening, and applied kinesiology pinpoints this as strain in bone in the spine of the right scapula.

CLIENT INQUIRY

Ask the client:

- how they have been feeling in general, and
- of their awareness of their shoulders.

MOBILITY TESTING

Global active

- Ask the standing client to make shoulder movements with each arm one at a time, flexion, extension, abduction, internal and external rotation, and circumduction.

Global passive

- With the client standing, ask the client to allow you to move their shoulder in various directions without either assisting or resisting. Stand behind the client off center to the side of the shoulder to be investigated. Separately assess shoulder girdle and shoulder joint mobility.
- For the right shoulder girdle, stabilize the

thoracic axial skeleton by placing your left hand on top of the left shoulder girdle as close to the base of the neck as possible, and the tip of your left thumb against the left lateral aspect of the first thoracic vertebra. Use this contact to make a dynamic stabilization of the rib cage and thoracic spine as the right shoulder girdle is moved on it.

- Place your right hand on the top of the right shoulder girdle, more distally engaging the distal clavicle and more lateral part of the scapula and proximal humerus. Use this contact to move the right shoulder girdle on the dynamically stabilized trunk in protraction. Let the shoulder girdle settle back to neutral, then retract the right shoulder girdle.
- While maintaining the same left-handed thorax stabilization, shift your right hand to grasp the right deltoid muscle area over the proximal humerus. Use this upper arm contact to elevate the right shoulder girdle.
- Use a mirror image of these instructions to similarly mobility test the left shoulder girdle.

Focal passive

- With the client standing, seated, or in a side-lying position with the right side up,

use the fingers of both hands to broadly grasp the spine of the right scapula. Gently test the elasticity of the bone. Bow it in a frontal plane, then in a sagittal plane. Spiral twist it on a near transverse axis.

TREATMENT

Leave your hands in the same position, grasping the spine of the scapula as for the passive focal tests. Use the same dimensions as for the above end-feel mobility testing to test for first barriers. Load the tissue to a mixed near and far first barrier stack, just beyond first barrier.

Maintain the vector sum of these three-dimensional loads as you observe the client's breath through a complete cycle. At some point in the cycle, you will feel a maximum tension between your hands. As you continue to monitor breath through the next cycle, when you arrive at this tension maximum remove your hands as quickly as possible. To achieve maximum speed of departure, do these two things at the same time: 1) turn your hands palm up, and 2) depart in the same direction as the vector load you established in the tissue.

POST TREATMENT TESTING AND INQUIRY

Use the standard post treatment procedure for mobility testing and question asking detailed in the introduction to treatment methods section. Either treat this same area further, as indicated by this inquiry, or return to general assessment.

Treatment method 14: accordion technique, also known as alternating decompression

Origin
Jeffrey Burch.

Concept
If tissue is gently compressed from two ends, then the compression is relieved and at one end a pressure wave will propagate through the tissue toward the stabilized end creating tissue release.

1. Between two hands, make a linear compaction of tissue to a middle barrier. Call the two ends of the compaction A and B—naming is arbitrary.
2. At a measured pace, relieve the pressure on only one end of the compacted tissue, e.g., End A. If this is done at just the right pace, the tissue will begin to decompress at the end on which the pressure is being reduced, End A. This decompression will then ripple slowly across the tissue to the end, which is not being moved, End B.
3. Recompress the tissue from the end which was relieved (A). Once a middle barrier compression is established, relieve the pressure at the opposite end (B) at a similar measured pace so that a ripple of decompression proceeds from the end relieved (B) across the tissue toward End A.
4. Again, recompress the tissue from the end which was relieved (B). This time relieve the pressure from End A, so the ripple of decompression proceeds toward End B.
5. Continue to recompress, followed by pressure relief from alternating ends until either adequate tissue span change is achieved, or a first hint of edema is felt. Edema is recognized in this situation as fluid filling.

Six factor model: Accordion technique

TISSUE ENGAGEMENT
Tissue engagement is created entirely by the therapist's will and action. In this treatment method, unwinding phenomena are not only not utilized but suppressed.

FORCE
In the initial loading of tissue, compaction is to a comfortable end-feel. From there, load is slacked at a pace that allows for the domino effect release. This is done without respect to specific barriers.

SPEED
Speed of movement of the therapist's hands is moderate for the initial loading. Similarly, the pace of initial decompaction is moderate. As release occurs, the therapist's hands slow a little, adjusted to foster the release.

CONSTRAINT
Unwinding is unlikely to happen due to the high directive demand. If unwinding does occur, it is suppressed by actively modulated back force just sufficient to prevent movement. This is like the suppression of movement in Hoover technique.

DIRECTIVENESS
This technique is highly directive. The tissue is compacted to a comfortable end-feel, and then the relaxation from compaction is managed at a rate to produce a very particular kind of release.

RELATIONSHIP TO EFFORT BARRIERS
In the initial setup of each treatment chapter, treatment is at a comfortable end-feel. Load during the release phase of each chapter is modulated to produce a particular type of release, but without reference to any specific effort barrier.

Accordion technique

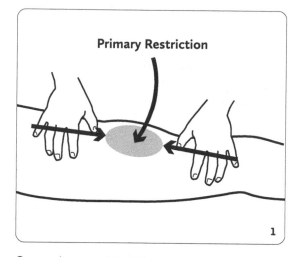

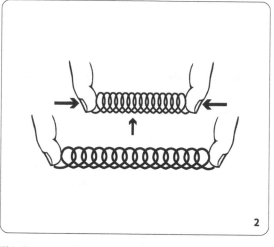

Once a primary restriction is located, the first step of the accordion treatment method is to compress the restriction between two hands or fingers at a moderate pace to a comfortable end-feel. As you compress the tissue you will feel its springy pushback into your hands.

This illustration shows the springy feel of the compressed tissue metaphorically as a coil spring.

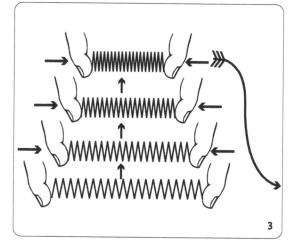

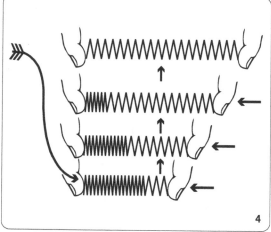

Here the metaphor is changed to an accordion spring. Compress the tissue in one smooth move at moderate pace to a comfortable end-feel. This illustration shows a succession of four degrees of compression as snapshots during the smooth continuous compression.

Once the tissue is compressed to a comfortable end-feel, begin to slowly release the compression from one end only, shown here as on the right end. Pressure from the stabilized end, in this instance the left end, is a dynamic stabilization, with pressure progressively slacked just enough to allow the tissue at the stabilized end to stay in the same location. If the pace of decompaction is correct, the spring will unfold in a wave, first at the end being moved during the decompaction and progressing to the other, stabilized end of the spring.

Accordion technique (*cont.*)

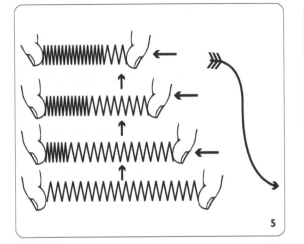

5

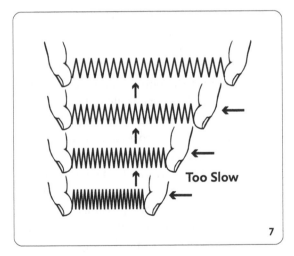

7

Once the compression on the tissue is fully released, stay in contact with the tissue and promptly begin to compact it again from only the same end just used to relieve the compression (in this instance the right end). Compact again at a moderate pace to a comfortable end-feel. During this compaction, the stable end stays in one place by a dynamic stabilization with the left end pressure increasing at a rate to match the increasing load from the right without moving the left end.

Similar to frame 4, decompact at a moderate rate from one end only, but this time from the opposite end from the last decompaction. In this instance, the decompaction is now from the left end as the right end is dynamically stabilized. If the pace of decompaction is correct, the spring will unfold first at the end being moved for the decompaction and progress to the other end of the spring in a regular way.

Pace of decompaction is critical to success. If the tissue is decompacted too slowly, the spring will unfold all along its length at the same time rather than as a wave starting at one end. This does not produce as full a tissue release as the wave of decompaction progressing from one end to the other.

If the pace of decompaction is too fast, the decompaction will happen in a haphazard irregular jumble. This produces less release in the tissue than when there is a wave of decompaction from one end to the other.

Continue to compact and decompact in this pattern from alternating ends.

TREATMENT METHOD 14

Accordion technique example 1

Caution—Do not do this on anyone who has or may have osteoporosis.

ASSESSMENT

General assessment leads to the right upper limb, confirmed by inhibition of the witness point at the right olecranon process.

Local assessment such as manual thermal assessment, local listening, layer listening, and applied kinesiology questioning pinpoints focal stiffness in the right humerus.

CLIENT INQUIRY

Ask the client:

- how they have been feeling in general, and
- of their awareness of their shoulders and arms.

MOBILITY TESTING

Global active

- Ask the client to walk; observe gait, particularly with respect to arm swing.
- Ask the client to circumduct the right shoulder.

Global passive

- Stand behind the client. Place your left hand on top of the right shoulder girdle to stabilize the clavicle and scapula. With your right hand, control the client's right elbow to circumduct the gleno-humeral joint while maintaining the elbow comfortably extended.

Focal passive

- Ask the client to lie supine on the table.
- With your two hands, contact the two ends of the humerus. Gently attempt to spiral bend it along its long axis.
- With fingertips, tap on the humerus in a succession of places from distal to proximal. Stiff areas of bone tend to have a duller, less bright resonance.
- Place fingers of your two hands next to each other, contacting the humerus just above the elbow. Gently make a slight focal bend of the bone. Shift your hands slightly superior along the humerus and repeat this test along the length of the bone. How does this data compare with the tap test?

TREATMENT

Place one hand supportively under the proximal end of the humerus. With your other hand, contact the distal end of the humerus. At a moderate pace, compact the bone between your two hands along its long axis to a comfortable end-feel. At a moderate pace, reduce the compacting force at only the distal end of the bone, while dynamically maintaining the position of the proximal end of the bone, until a release is felt in the bone near the distal end. Regulate the pace of decompaction to encourage propagation of a wave of release from the distal to the proximal end of the humerus. Then recompact the bone to end-feel from the distal end toward a dynamically stabilized proximal end. Next, start to reduce the compacting load but this time from the proximal end, at a pace to seek a release which begins at the proximal end and proceeds like a wave or set of falling dominoes toward the distal end. Continue to work back and forth distal to proximal, and proximal to distal in this fashion, until either a larger, more general release is felt or a hint of fluid filling suggesting the beginning of edema is felt.

POST TREATMENT TESTING AND INQUIRY

Use the standard post treatment procedure for mobility testing and question asking detailed in the introduction to treatment methods section. Either treat this same area further, as indicated by this inquiry, or return to general assessment.

Accordion technique example 2

ASSESSMENT

General assessment leads to the right upper limb, confirmed by inhibition of the witness point at the right olecranon process.

Local assessment such as manual thermal assessment, local listening, layer listening, and yes–no questioning pinpoints focal stiffness in the skin and superficial fascia overlying the right scapula.

CLIENT INQUIRY

Ask the client:

- how they have been feeling in general, and
- of their awareness of their shoulders and arms.

MOBILITY TESTING

Global active

- Ask the client to walk; observe gait, particularly with respect to arm swing.
- Ask the client to circumduct the right shoulder, then the left shoulder. Compare movement.
- Ask the client to first protract and then retract each shoulder. Compare movement.

Global passive

- Stand behind the client. Place your left hand on top of the right shoulder girdle to stabilize the clavicle and scapula. With your right hand, control the client's right elbow to circumduct the gleno-humeral joint while maintaining the elbow comfortably extended.

- Still standing behind the client, shift your position slightly to the left. Place your left hand on top of the left shoulder girdle as close to the base of the neck as possible, and with the tip of your left thumb against the left lateral aspect of the first thoracic vertebra. Place your right hand over the upper portion of the right deltoid area with thumb and fingers controlling the scapula and distal clavicle. Protract the shoulder girdle, let it rest to neutral, then retract the scapula. Repeat for the other upper limb. Compare ranges of motion.

Focal passive

- Ask the client to lie on the table right side up. Place a pillow under the client's head and another pillow in front of their thorax for the right arm to rest on.
- With your fingers, engage the skin over the posterior aspect of the scapula and attempt to glide it superior, inferior, lateral, and medial. Test adjacent areas to map the extent of the superficial fascia stiffness, which will usually be an irregularly shaped area.
- Using the fingers of two hands, engage skin on the posterior aspect to the scapula and gently stretch it medial to lateral, superior to inferior, and on 45-degree diagonals between these axes. Test several areas to map the skin stiffness which will typically be an irregular area overlapping but not identical to the superficial fascia stiffness.

TREATMENT

Place the fingers of two hands near edges of the stiff area of both skin and superficial fascia on the posterior aspect of the scapula. At a moderate pace, compact the skin and superficial fascia across their breadth between your two hands. As soon as end-feel is felt, begin to reduce the compacting load on the tissues at a moderate pace, moving *one hand only* until the beginning of release is felt in the skin and superficial fascia. Regulate the pace of further decompaction to encourage propagation of a wave of release across the planes of tissue from the end contacted by the hand you are moving toward the stable hand. Then recompact the skin and superficial fascia to end-feel from the end where the last release was initiated, toward the stabilized end. Next, start to reduce the compacting load but this time from the other end, the one previously stabilized. Pace this second episode of decompaction to allow a release which begins at the end and being decompacted and proceeding like a wave or set of falling dominoes toward the newly stabilized end. Continue to work back and forth in an alternating fashion between these two ends until either a larger, more general release is felt or a hint of fluid filling suggesting the beginning of edema is felt.

POST TREATMENT TESTING AND INQUIRY

Use the standard post treatment procedure for mobility testing and question asking detailed in the introduction to treatment methods section. Either treat this same area further, as indicated by this inquiry, or return to general assessment.

Accordion technique example 3

ASSESSMENT

General assessment leads to the left lower limb, confirmed by inhibition of the witness point at the left greater trochanter.

Local assessment such as manual thermal assessment, local listening, layer listening, and applied kinesiology questioning pinpoints focal stiffness in the distal left quadriceps muscles where they join.

CLIENT INQUIRY

Ask the client:

- how they have been feeling in general, and
- of their awareness of their legs.

MOBILITY TESTING

Global active

- Ask the client to walk; observe gait, particularly with respect to knee movement.
- Ask the client to squat down as far as they comfortably can and stand up again.

Global passive

- Ask the client to lie supine on the table. Using both of your hands, flex the client's left knee and hip at the same time at a moderate pace, and then return the leg to supine. Repeat with the other leg for comparison.

Focal passive

- With the client still supine on the table, stand at the client's left side.
- Place your left hand under the condyles of the distal left femur for a dynamic stabilization.
- With your right hand, grasp the distal end of the left quadriceps. At a moderate pace, attempt to move the distal quadriceps medially over the distal femur, let them settle to neutral, then move them laterally. For comparison, try the same thing a handwidth superior on the thigh, and on the other leg.
- Place your left hand on the left patella and the distal most portion of the left quadriceps muscle. Place your right hand adjacent to your left hand immediately superior to it on the left quadriceps. Using your left hand, drag that portion of the quadriceps toward you, while with your right hand take the next most superior hand full of quadriceps medial, creating a shearing motion between the two hands. Repeat this on the other leg for comparison.

TREATMENT

Place your left hand on the lateral aspect of the most distal portion of the left quadriceps muscle. Similarly, place your right hand on the medial aspect of the most distal portion of the left quadriceps muscle opposite your left hand. Compact between your two hands to a comfortable end-feel. Maintain your right hand where it is and begin to reduce the pressure with your left hand at a pace that allows tissue near your left hand to release, and for the release to propagate across the width of the distal quadriceps toward your right hand in a wavelike or falling domino fashion. Recompact the distal quadriceps with your left hand toward the stable right hand. Then begin to slack the compression of your right hand until a wave of release starts at the medial side of the quadriceps and propagates toward the stable lateral aspect supported by your left hand. Compact again with your right hand from the medial aspect of the quadriceps. Continue to play the accordion back and forth from side to side until a larger, more general release is felt or until the first hint of fluid filling.

POST TREATMENT TESTING AND INQUIRY

Use the standard post treatment procedure for mobility testing and question asking detailed in the introduction to treatment methods section. Either treat this same area further, as indicated by this inquiry, or return to general assessment.

TREATMENT
METHOD 14

Treatment method 15: centralizing (Hoover) technique

Origin
Harold V. Hoover DO, c. 1950.

Concept
In some techniques, tissue is loaded to a first barrier. In other techniques, a load greater than first barrier is applied. In centralizing technique, tissue is stabilized to a specific position rather than to a specific barrier.

Pretest
Observe alignment in the person's body both locally and globally. Test range of motion in the area to be treated. It is vital to know the starting place both in the big picture and locally.

Therapeutic method
Test each dimension separately and note the location of the first barriers. Then stack the tissue to the geographic center between the near and far first barriers in each dimension. One might think stacking tissue to a geographic center would return the tissue to the original position, but this is not the case. As an example, excursion to a first barrier may be 6 mm superior and 2 mm inferior. Within this 8-mm range between opposite first barriers, the geographic center is 2 mm superior from the original equilibrium point. Force required for stabilization is low since this is a sub first barrier technique; however, absolute stillness must be maintained.

Completion and repetition
Once the geographic center has been found, stabilize tissue at this point until a release is felt; this will be felt as a generalized spreading and softening of tissue. Often, but not always, this will be a large release. Once a release has occurred, the new resting equilibrium point will have shifted, and the location of the barriers will have changed. These may be retested to establish a new centralizing stack. A single treatment may produce satisfactory mobility. Two or more cycles of treatment in the same area may be required to produce satisfactory mobility. It is important to be sensitive to any hint of edema arising and when it is present to stop, avoiding overtreatment.

Post test
Observe alignment and test range of motion. Point out change to client.

Application
This method may be applied to most structures. Hoover technique is a big hammer. It will free up almost anything. Occasionally someone becomes enamored of Hoover technique and makes it a mainstay of their practice. This is like hitting everything with a sledgehammer whether it is a railroad spike, framing nail, finish nail, or tack. Most tissues that are currently the primary restriction can be released with other less powerful techniques. Still, it is useful to have a big hammer in the tool kit, as occasionally it is the tool of choice.

Contraindications
Never apply this method to the pancreas, spleen, eyeball, or other fragile tissue.

Centralizing technique—Harold V. Hoover DO's original functional treatment method

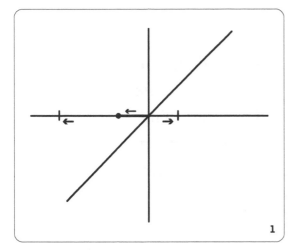

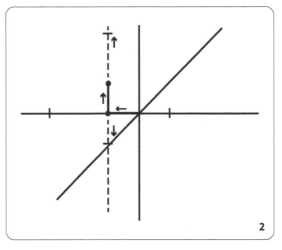

In a first dimension, mobility test to locate near and far first barriers. Then load the tissue to a geographic center between these two first barriers. This will be a very light force, less than first barrier. Maintain that load.

As you maintain the first directional load, mobility test to near and far first barriers in a second dimension. Again, load the tissue to the geographic center between these new first barriers, while maintaining the first dimension load.

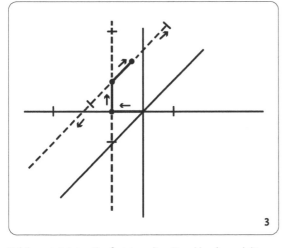

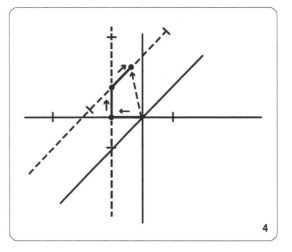

While maintaining the first two directional loads, mobility test the tissue in a third dimension. Again, load the tissue to the geographic center between this third set of first barriers while maintaining the first two directional loads.

The final load will be the vector sum of the three-dimensional loads. Maintain the tissue at this spot with minimum force to prevent movement. This is a dynamic stabilization, which means that as the tissue tries to move, match its attempted movement with a precise gentle counterforce to prevent movement.

Do not allow unwinding. Do not grip hard; use the minimum force necessary to securely maintain this location.

Centralizing technique—Harold V. Hoover DO's original functional treatment method (*cont.*)

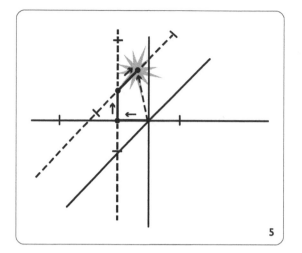

5

General Listening

Manual Thermal Evaluation

Local Listening

Layer Listening

Mobility Testing

Etcetera

6

In seconds to minutes, there will be a broad release in the tissue similar to that at the end of an unwind. As soon as this occurs, release the tissue. Post mobility test this area to assess the effect of your treatment. If it is not sufficiently treated and there is no hint of edema, treat again. If it is not sufficiently treated but there is any hint of edema, make a note to return another day and return to general assessment. If it is sufficiently treated, return to general assessment.

Return to general assessment to find the next primary restriction.

TREATMENT
METHOD 15

Six factor model: Harold Hoover DO's centralizing technique

TISSUE ENGAGEMENT

Tissue engagement is created entirely by the therapist's volition and action. In this treatment method, unwinding phenomena are not only not utilized but suppressed.

FORCE

In the exploratory phase, first barriers are found but not exceeded. In the setup phase, the force applied is distinctly less than first barrier. At the release, application of force dissolves and contact is promptly broken by the therapist.

SPEED

Speed of movement of the therapist's hands in the exploratory and setup phases is slow. Once the therapeutic setup is established, there is no movement of the therapist's hands and unwinding of the client's tissues is forbidden. As the tissues release, the therapist's hands are removed at a moderate pace.

CONSTRAINT

Throughout this technique, tissue unwinding is opposed and forbidden by the therapist. Once the setup phase is established, constraint is high in the sense that no tissue movement is permitted; however, the force required to maintain this constraint is low. The release at the end is fully allowed, signaling the prompt removal of the therapist's hands.

DIRECTIVENESS

In the exploratory phase, the tissue is moved in the several cardinal or physiologic directions by the will and action of the therapist. In the setup phase, the tissue is moved by the therapist to a very particular location and loading. Once this loading is established, there is no further direction given to the tissue.

RELATIONSHIP TO EFFORT BARRIERS

In the exploratory phase, first barriers are found in three or more dimensions; however, loading to those first barriers is only transient. In the setup phase, forces applied are distinctly less than first barrier. As the setup phase is maintained, precise forces, unrelated to but generally less than first barrier, are applied as needed to counter and prevent any attempt of the tissue to unwind. At the moment of release, the resistance against which the therapist has applied load dissolves, followed promptly by the therapist breaking contact.

Centralizing (Hoover) technique example 1

ASSESSMENT

General assessment points to the left lower limb. This general assessment is supported by an inhibitory contact at the left greater trochanter and refined to the foot or ankle by an inhibitory contact at the left lateral malleolus.

Local assessment including manual thermal assessment, local listening and inhibition, layer listening, and applied kinesiology questioning refines this to the left first tarso-metatarsal joint.

CLIENT INQUIRY

Ask the client:

- how they are feeling in general, and
- in their feet.

MOBILITY ASSESSMENT

Global active

- Ask the client to walk barefoot.
- Observe gait, particularly with respect to the feet and ankles.

Local active

- Ask the client to lie supine on the table with feet just off the end of the table. In this position, ask the client to:

- dorsiflex and plantarflex each ankle
- circumduct each foot.

Passive

- Explain to the client the method and purpose of your test.
- With the client supine on the table, heels just off the end of the table, use one of your hands to dynamically stabilize the first cuneiform bone; with your other hand, contact the adjacent proximal end of the first metatarsal bone. Test flexion and extension of the first metatarsal on the cuneiform.
- Make a similar set of local active and passive tests on the other tarso-metatarsal joints of this foot and of the other foot.

TREATMENT

With your hands still in the same position on the first cuneiform and first metatarsal bones, make slow movements of the first metatarsal on the cuneiform looking for pairs of opposite first barriers.

- Flexion–extension
- Adduction–abduction
- Long axis rotation, internal rotation–external rotation.

For each axis pair of movements such as flexion and extension, note the distance traveled in each direction to the first barrier. Then move the first metatarsal to the geographic midpoint between these two first barrier distances. Maintain this position for the first dimension as you test the second dimension. Add the midpoint for the second dimension. Test the third dimension and add its midpoint to the stack.

The force used to maintain this stack will be distinctly less than first barrier. Do *not* allow unwinding to occur. In addition to your centralizing stack, add dynamic counter-loads to

prevent any attempted unwinding or any other movement. Eventually a generalized sense of release will be felt, which is like the larger, more general release at the end of unwinding.

POST TREATMENT TESTING AND INQUIRY

Use the standard post treatment procedure for mobility testing and question asking detailed in the introduction to treatment methods section. Either treat this same area further, as indicated by this inquiry, or return to general assessment.

Centralizing (Hoover) technique example 2

ASSESSMENT

General assessment points to the right upper limb. This general assessment is supported by an inhibitory contact at the right olecranon process.

Local assessment including manual thermal assessment, local listening and inhibition, layer listening, and applied kinesiology questioning refines this to the right acromioclavicular joint.

CLIENT INQUIRY

Ask the client:

- how they are feeling in general, and
- in their shoulders.

MOBILITY ASSESSMENT

Global active

- Ask the client to walk.
- Observe arm swing during gait.

Local active

- Ask the client to circumduct each shoulder.
- Ask the client to sequentially move the right shoulder in:
  - protraction
  - retraction
  - elevation.

Global passive

- Explain to the client the method and purpose of your test.
- Stand behind the client a little right of center.
- Place your left hand on top of the right shoulder girdle to dynamically stabilize the scapula and clavicle. With your right hand, control the right elbow to make a circumduction of the right gleno-humeral joint while maintaining the elbow in a comfortable extension.
- Move your left hand to the top of the left shoulder girdle as close to the base of the neck as possible. Place the tip of your left thumb against the lateral surface of the spinous process of T1 to create a dynamic stabilization of the axial trunk.
- Place your right hand over the proximal humerus and glenoid region of the scapula. Successively move the shoulder girdle in protraction, retraction, and elevation.
- Make a similar set of global active and passive tests on the other shoulder for comparison.

Local passive

- Ask the client to lie supine.
- Stand at the head of the table a little to the client's right.
- With your left hand, grasp the distal end of the right clavicle to dynamically stabilize it.
- With your right hand, use the thumb and forefinger to grasp the acromion process of the scapula while the other fingers and palm of your hand control more distal portions of the scapula.
- With your right hand, move the scapula on the clavicle at the acromioclavicular joint, moving the scapula successively anterior, posterior, superior, inferior, protract, and retract.
- Similarly test the mobility of the left acromioclavicular joint.

TREATMENT

Ask the client to continue to lie supine on the table. Stand at the right side of the client facing the client's right shoulder. Locate the right acromioclavicular joint. With the fingertips of your right hand, grasp the distal end of the clavicle. With the palm of your left hand, support the scapula, and with the fingertips of the left hand, grasp the acromion process. Using these two contacts, gently mobility test the acromioclavicular joint to first barriers in anterior–posterior glide. Note the distance traveled to the first barrier in each direction; one distance will be longer than the other. Move the bone ends to the geographic midpoint between these two first barriers. Maintain that anterior–posterior position of the two bones. While maintaining this position, mobility test between the two bones in a superior–inferior direction to first barrier, noting the distance traveled in each direction. Position the two bones at the midpoint between these two first barriers. You now have two dimensions stacked.

For a third dimension, compact and decompact the acromioclavicular joint to first barriers. Position the two bones at the geographic center between these two first barriers. You now have three dimensions held at midpoints between first barriers. The force to hold the bones here is low, less than a first barrier load. The tissue will attempt to unwind. Exert just enough back force to prevent each direction of unwind. This is a low force dynamic stabilization, using the minimum force to prevent each movement. Within seconds to a few minutes, a substantial release will be felt like the release usually felt at the end of an unwind. Break contact.

POST TREATMENT TESTING AND INQUIRY

Use the standard post treatment procedure for mobility testing and question asking detailed in the introduction to treatment methods section. Either treat this same area further, as indicated by this inquiry, or return to general assessment.

Centralizing (Hoover) technique example 3

ASSESSMENT

General assessment points to the anterior central portion of the inferior abdomen.

Local assessment including manual thermal assessment, local listening and inhibition, layer listening, and applied kinesiology questioning refines this to the glide plane of the posterior surface of the urinary bladder.

CLIENT INQUIRY

Ask the client:

- how they are feeling in general
- in their abdomen and pelvis, and
- how well urinary function is working for them.

MOBILITY ASSESSMENT

Global active

- Ask the client to walk barefoot.
- Observe gait, particularly with respect to movement associated with the pelvis and lower abdomen.

Local active

- Ask the seated client to rotate the trunk successively right then left.

Local passive

- Explain to the client the method and purpose of your tests. Use anatomic models and/or illustrations.
- Ask the client to lie supine on the table;

place a pillow under the client's knees to create a mild relaxed flexion of the hips.

- Ask the client to touch the superior surface of their pubic symphysis.
- Stand at the client's right side.
- Palpate the right anterior superior spine of the iliac crest. Palpating, follow the superior surface of the pelvic rim to the superior surface of the pubic symphysis.
- With the tips of the thumb and forefinger of the right hand, sink into the abdomen in the first finger width superior to the pubic symphysis area with about 5 cm between the thumb and finger. Gently grasp the anterior–superior portion of the bladder.
- Place the thumb and forefinger of your left hand immediately superior to those of your right hand and again sink in to engage tissue posterior–superior to the urinary bladder. Depending on whether a uterus is present, this contact will be either on the uterus or the rectum.
- With these fingers, gently sink into the client's abdomen watching the client's response. Ask if the client is comfortable with this pressure. Reduce your pressure but maintain contact with these landmarks.
- With the fingers of both hands at these landmarks, gently test the glide plane posterior to the bladder by dragging the bladder left and the tissue posterior to it right, then reverse directions.

TREATMENT

With the fingers of both hands at these same landmarks on the bladder and the tissue posterior to it, gently test the glide plane posterior to the bladder by dragging the bladder left and the tissue posterior to it right, then reverse directions. Note the distance to the first barrier in each direction. Position the bladder at the midpoint between these two first barriers. Maintain this position. Next, similarly test superior–inferior glide between the bladder and the tissue behind it to first barriers. Position the bladder at the midpoint between these first barriers. You now have a two-dimensional stack. Maintaining this two-dimensional stack, rotate the bladder first clockwise, while stabilizing the tissue behind it, and then counterclockwise, again noting first barriers. Position the bladder at the midpoint between these two first barrier distances. You now have a three-dimensional first barrier stack. Maintain these two structures at this position with a minimum effort dynamic load. Prevent each attempt to unwind with a minimum force dynamic stabilization. After seconds to a few minutes, a release will be felt like the release at the end of an unwinding.

POST TREATMENT TESTING AND INQUIRY

Use the standard post treatment procedure for mobility testing and question asking detailed in the introduction to treatment methods section. Either treat this same area further, as indicated by this inquiry, or return to general assessment.

TREATMENT
METHOD 15

Treatment method 16: induction of a bodily rhythm

Origin

Early functional technique, following the work of H. V. Hoover DO. Original discoverer not known. Originally used for the craniosacral rhythm (CSR). Applied to internal organ motility by Jean-Pierre Barral DO. Applied to pulmonary respiration and cardiac pulse by Jeffrey Burch.

Concept

There are several rhythmic processes in our bodies, including heartbeat, breath, craniosacral rhythm (CSR),[1] and organ motility.[2] While all these rhythms continue throughout life with only rare pauses, they are never synchronized with each other.

Each rhythm varies from time to time in several dimensions. One of these dimensions is balance between movement toward the center of the body versus movement away from the center of the body. It is desirable for ease in expansion to equal ease in contraction to be full and equal. Often one or more of these rhythmic movements is not balanced. For example, the CSR may expand easily but contract effortfully, or the opposite. Similarly, pulmonary exhales may happen easily, while inhales are effortful, or the opposite.

Sometimes bringing a rhythm to balance requires release of specific fibrosities, limiting movement of the system. Sometimes balance can be achieved by working with the rhythm directly.

In mathematics, induction is a form of proof in which a series of similar events such as falling dominoes can be described by the first event in the series.

Assessment

Follow the rhythm through two or three full cycles, assessing for any difference between the ease of movement in the two phases of the cycle. For breath, this can be done visually. The CSR and the visceral motility must be felt with the hand. Specifically:

- *Breath*—Watch the person's natural breathing. Do not tell them what you are doing as they may take active control of their breath. One way to do it is to explain something of mild interest not related to breath to them, watching their breath as you speak. Resting breath rate for adults is typically 3–5 seconds per cycle. Does breath move with equal ease through inhale and through exhale?

- *CSR*—This rhythm can be felt anywhere on the body; with expansion, limbs roll subtly out, the torso widens, the frontal bone rocks anterior–inferior, and the occiput swings posterior. It usually takes 10–14 seconds to complete a cycle. To feel this small, low force cyclical movement, the hand and whole body of the therapist must be very relaxed and soft. Do the expansive movement and contracting movement happen with equal ease or does one direction happen more easily than the other?

- *Organ motility*—Similar to assessing the CSR, rest the hand softly over the organ in question; feel for the movement rocking away from the midline of the body

---

1   The CSR first described by William Garner Sutherland DO is a rhythmic contraction and expansion of not just the head, but the whole body. The period of expansion and contraction is typically 10–14 seconds. All parts of the body should expand together and contract together with equal ease. This oscillation is also called the primary respiratory mechanism and has been shown to correlate well with blood pressure fluctuations described by Mayer, Traube, and Hering.

2   In this context organ motility does not refer to the slow contractions of digestive organs, which move digesting food along, but rather to the 7.8 seconds per cycle rocking motion made by each internal organ. All organs should move away from midline together at the same time, and then back to midline together at the same time.

and then back toward the midline of the body. Each organ has its own pattern of movement, and all of them should move together. See the recommended reading for books of Jean-Pierre Barral for details or each organ's movements.

- *Heartbeat*—Feel the pulse in the usual way at a superficial artery such as the radial artery. Note the rhythmic expansion and relaxation of the artery. How similar are these two phases of movement? Also note that with the expansion of the artery there is also a subtle distal glide of the artery, and as the heart relaxes and fills, the arteries subtly glide toward the heart.

Treatment

BREATH

If the exhale is less effortful than the inhale, rest the hands on the lower rib cage; passively follow the breath to the end of its exhale. At the moment the breath would begin to expand, use your hands to gently move the ribs a little farther into the exhale just for a second or two, then release. Then watch the breath: within three cycles does it settle into a balanced rhythm? If not, repeat the treatment, and again observe the result. This may be repeated a third time, but not more in the same treatment session. If this method does not correct the breath balance, then there are mechanical restrictions to be found and released.

If the breath is easier with the inhale follow the same procedure, except have the hands under the costal arches, and at the end of the inhale gently lift the ribs a little farther in the directions of inhale for just a second or two.

CSR

With a very soft and relaxed hand or hands contact any safe part of the body. Feel for a 10–14-second cycle rhythmic movement. On expansion, the limbs will subtly roll out, the torso will expand, the frontal bone will roll forward, and the occiput will roll back. Is this rhythm balanced between expansion and contraction? If not, passively follow the movement to the end of its easy direction. At the moment when it would like to reverse directions, gently take the tissue a little further in the direction of preference for just a second. Then release the tissue and observe its movement. Does it settle into balance? If not, repeat up to two more times.

ORGAN "MOTILITY"

Read Jean-Pierre Barral DO's books (listed in the recommended reading) to learn the 7.8-second oscillating movement pattern for each organ. Place your relaxed hand over the organ to be assessed. Is the motility balanced between movement away from the midline and toward the midline? If not, passively follow the movement to the end of its easy direction. At the moment when it would like to reverse directions, gently take the organ a little further in the direction of preference for just a second. Then release the tissue and observe its movement. Does it settle into balance? If not, repeat up to two more times.

HEARTBEAT

Gently contact a safe artery to feel the pulse. The radial artery at the wrist is often used. Do not use the carotid arteries or the aorta. Observe the pulse. With each heartbeat, the artery is stretched fuller with blood, then as the heart relaxes the stretched artery wall acts like a spring pushing the blood along, as it is able to contact. Are the expansion and relaxation of the artery equally easy? If not, apply the same "induction" method as for the other rhythms.

Post treatment testing

Repeat all mobility tests and postural examinations used as pretests. Compare results. Discuss with the client.

Induction of a bodily rhythm

For rhythmic body processes, including the craniosacral rhythm, Barral's organ motility, breath, and arterial pulse, the expanding phase and the contracting phase should feel equally easy. Often one will feel less smooth or easy than the other. Restoring balance is easy.

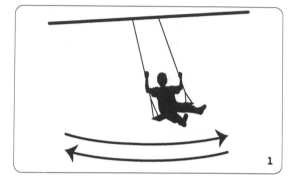

First assess the rhythmic process by feeling the rhythm through two cycles. Is it equally easy in both directions?

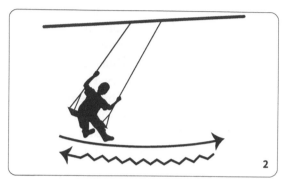

Or is it less easy or smooth in one direction than the other?

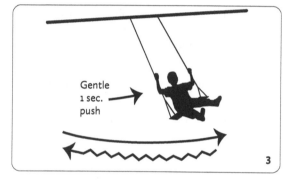

If one direction is easier than the other, follow the rhythm to the end of the easy direction, then give it a brief gentle push farther in the easy direction, like gently pushing a swing.

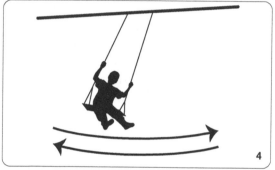

Monitor the pulse again through two cycles. It may be balanced now or not. If it is balanced, this treatment episode is done. Return to assessment.

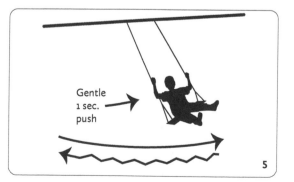

If the rhythmic process is not yet balanced, once again follow the process to the end of its easier range. At the end of the easy direction, push the tissue gently and briefly farther in the easy direction.

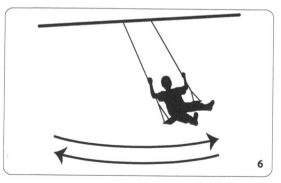

Reassess the rhythm observing it through two cycles. If it is balanced, you are done. If it is not balanced, push the swing a third time as in frame 3 above, then reassess.

Six factor model: Induction of a bodily rhythm

TISSUE ENGAGEMENT

Tissue engagement is made by the therapist and is quick and brief.

FORCE

Moderate. Load is in the range of middle barrier, about one-third of the way toward end-feel, but not calibrated to a particular barrier.

SPEED

Quick.

CONSTRAINT

None.

DIRECTIVENESS

Mixed. The corrective load is highly directional but very brief. The further movement of tissue after the quick motion is not directed.

RELATIONSHIP TO EFFORT BARRIERS

While the brief load is in the range of one-third of the way toward end-feel, no specific barrier is sought or addressed.

Note—The term induction is sometimes used to describe other therapeutic methods including near barrier treatments, also known as direction of ease treatments or indirect treatments.

Induction of a bodily rhythm example 1

GENERAL ASSESSMENT

General listening leads to the left upper abdomen. Localization with local listening, manual thermal assessment, layer listening, and applied kinesiology points to the liver. Assessment of the motility of the liver shows a marked inspir preference. Applied kinesiology questioning indicates induction of liver motility is the treatment of choice.

MOTILITY OBSERVATION

The visceral motility of the liver follows normal lines of movement, that is inspir is a combined superior–lateral–posterior roll and expir is the opposite. However, the expir movement is markedly fuller and easier than the inspir movement.

TREATMENT

Follow the motility of the liver to the end of its easier direction of movement, in this case expir. As soon as the motility tries to turn around into inspir, gently push the liver slightly farther in the expir direction for just a second. This process called induction is described more fully in the preceding pages.

POST TREATMENT TESTING AND INQUIRY

Immediately after the induction, follow the motility through two cycles to observe the degree of correction. If it is not fully corrected, induce it again. Again, observe two cycles of motility. If it is still not fully corrected, induce a third time. One to three inductions will usually correct motility; return to check it another day.

Return to global assessment to find the next primary.

Induction of a bodily rhythm example 2

GENERAL ASSESSMENT

General listening points to something in the head; however, attempts to further localize this give weak and mixed results. The CSR as expressed at the greater wings of the sphenoid and the occiput shows a persistent contraction (extension) preference. Applied kinesiology questioning indicated that induction of the CSR at the head is the most fruitful treatment at this moment.

CLIENT INQUIRY

- Ask the client how they feel.
- Invite the client to move around the room and to report any awareness in movement.

TREATMENT
METHOD 16

CSR ASSESSMENT

Ask the client to lie supine on the table with the head about 6 inches (15 cm) down from the end of the table. Adjust the table to a comfortable height so that you can sit at the head of the table facing the client with your forearms resting on the table and your hands on the client's head. With the pads of your thumbs, locate the lateral margins of the orbits. Place the pads of your thumbs very softly just posterior to the lateral margins of the orbits where they will lie over the greater wings of the sphenoid. Let your contact be gentle as if you are handling butterfly wings. Wrap the rest of your hand gently and comfortably down around the sides of the head so at least your fifth fingers contact the occiput. Note a rhythmic motion with an 8–12-second cycle in which the top of the head opens like a clam shell with the greater wings of the sphenoid swinging anterior and inferior while the occiput swings posterior and interior, followed by opposite motions of both. Let your hands and whole body be relaxed so you can feel this small slow movement.

The expansion and contraction phases of the movement should be equal in ease and smoothness. In the present case, the closing of the top of the head feels easier and smoother.

TREATMENT AND POST TREATMENT OBSERVATION

Follow the CSR to the end of its direction of ease, in this case contraction, also known as extension. As the CSR would begin to turn around into expansion, gently push it further into contraction for just a second. Then, with your hands still in place, return to monitoring, following the cranial movement through two cycles. If it is fully corrected, the induction of the CSR is complete. If the CSR is not yet fully balanced, induce it a second time, then monitor it through two more cycles. If necessary, induce the CSR a third time. If it is not yet fully balanced, move on to other treatment, and return to assess the CSR another day.

POST TREATMENT CLIENT INQUIRY

- Ask the client how they feel.
- Invite the client to move around the room and to report any awareness in movement.

RETURN TO GENERAL ASSESSMENT

Locate the next primary area or issue to treat.

Induction of a bodily rhythm example 3

GENERAL ASSESSMENT

General listening points to something broad in the thorax; however, attempts to further localize this give weak and mixed results. The pulmonary respiratory cycle as expressed in the thorax shows persistent greater ease on inhale. Yes–no questioning indicated that induction of the pulmonary respiration at the thorax is the most fruitful treatment at this moment. Note that pulmonary respiration is observable in all parts of the body. Induction of the pulmonary respiration could potentially be done at any location on the body.

BREATH RHYTHM ASSESSMENT

Ask the client to stand. As you observe other aspects of alignment, observe the client's breath. Do this before you ask the client about their awareness of their breath. Bringing their attention to breath may alter the pattern.

- How deep or shallow is breath?
- Is there a difference in ease or smoothness between inhale and exhale?

CLIENT INQUIRY

Ask the client:

- how they feel in general
- about their awareness of breath, and
- about their exercise stamina.

TREATMENT AND CONTINUING OBSERVATION

Stand behind the client. Place your relaxed hands broadly on the lateral aspects of the lower thorax. Observe breath through two cycles. Feel the difference between the ease and smoothness of inhale and exhale. Do not ask the client to actively control their breath.

On the next inhale (phase of ease), follow breath to the end of inhale, then for just a second gently push the rib cage up and out into further inhale.

Remove your hands. Watch breath through two more cycles. Is it normalized? One application will usually balance the cycle. If necessary, induce up to twice more, a total of three applications of this treatment.

POST TREATMENT CLIENT INQUIRY

- Ask the client what they feel. The client often will not have a lot to say.
- Ask again at the beginning of the next visit, after the client has had some days or weeks in which to experience change.

RETURN TO GENERAL ASSESSMENT

Locate the next primary area or issue to treat.

Induction of a bodily rhythm example 4

CONCEPT

This example shows a related treatment used to coordinate the motility of two internal organs. While this is not the "pushing the swing" process described in the earlier examples, it is an induction in the mathematical sense that a new first event is created which will be followed by a long succession of similarly coordinated events.

ASSESSMENT

General assessment points to a primary dysfunction broadly in the subcostal region.

Local assessment methods provide mixed and inconclusive results pointing to both liver and stomach. Liver motility and stomach motility are each observed to be balanced in terms of inspir and expir; however, the motility of the liver and the motility of the stomach are about 90 degrees out of phase with each other.

Liver motility is described in example 1 in this section. Stomach motility is a mirror image of liver motility with the stomach inspir also a superior–lateral–posterior roll.

CLIENT INQUIRY

Ask the client:

- how they have been feeling in general and
- how their digestion has felt lately.

TREATMENT AND POST TREATMENT OBSERVATION

Ask the client to lie supine on a table. Sit or stand comfortably at the client's left side. Place your left hand over the client's liver and your right hand over the client's stomach. Concurrently observe the motility of the two organs through two cycles. Then when one of the organs has reached the end of its inspir phase, exert just enough force with the hand on that organ to block its return into expir. Wait until the other organ has reached the end of its inspir, and at that moment release the organ whose movement had been blocked. The two organs will now move into expir. Monitor movement through two cycles. This usually takes only one application of treatment. If necessary, treat the same way up to three times.

POST TREATMENT CLIENT INQUIRY

Invite the client to stand and move around the room. Ask how they feel. The results may not be immediately perceptible to the client. In the days to come they are likely to notice a greater sense of wellbeing.

Treatment method 17: reconstructed A. T. Still technique

Origin

Reconstructed by Richard L. Van Buskirk DO from silent film footage of Andrew Taylor Still MD and notes by Still's early students.

Andrew Taylor Still, the creator of osteopathy, used many different techniques in his practice; however, he did not teach technique. He taught anatomy in great detail and had his students make up their own techniques from that.

During the 1990s, Richard L. Van Buskirk DO was able to reconstruct one of Still's techniques from the only film footage of Still working, a ten-second clip of his working on a shoulder, and from notes from his early students. This technique is applicable to a wide range of tissue types.

1. Pretest tissue mobility locally and globally in the usual ways, relevant to that area.
2. Begin to compress[3] the tissue at a moderate pace. If it is a joint, compress along the central or long axis of the joint. Compress toward end-feel and maintain this compression throughout steps 3 and 4; release the compression during step 5.
3. As the tissue is compressed, notice any natural tendency the tissue has to pull in a particular direction. Gently encourage the tissue to go further in this direction or succession of directions. Load the tissue to near end-feel in these directions, all the while maintaining the compression.
4. While fully maintaining the compression, reverse the direction the tissue was loaded following the pull in it. Make the reversal at a moderate pace allowing time for tissue to release. Load in this opposite direction to near end-feel.
5. As soon as you arrive at end-feel in step 4, begin to slack the compaction at a moderate pace, and concurrent with slacking the compression, move the joint or other tissue in a circumduction, timing the decompaction to coincide with one full circle of circumduction.
6. Repeat the mobility tests used in step 1 to evaluate how much change was made.

Note—Steps 2–6 may be repeated several times. However, this is a shotgun technique that will clear many, but often not all, portions of a restriction. After three or so applications it is often useful to make more discriminate mobility testing of the area and either refocus this technique on remaining focal restrictions or shift to another technique for those areas. As usual, be alert to the first signs of edema as a signal to stop treating this area for this day.

For a fuller description of this technique with a history of its reconstruction and many examples, see: Van Buskirk, Richard L. (2006) *The Still Technique Manual*. Indianapolis, IN: American Academy of Osteopathy.

---

3   Distraction may be used in place of compression; all other elements of the technique remain the same—just replace the word compression with distraction throughout.

Reconstructed A. T. Still technique

Andrew Taylor Still MD, the discoverer of osteopathy, used many different techniques in his practice. In teaching, he taught extensive anatomy and principles of technique. Still expected his students to make up their own treatment techniques. None of Still's original techniques were recorded. In the 1990s, Richard L. Van Buskirk DO reconstructed one of Still's techniques from a silent, grainy ten-second film of Still treating, and from notes of early students. This technique is applicable to a wide range of tissue types.

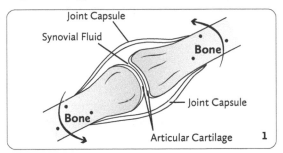

Pretest the mobility of the tissue to be treated both locally and globally in the usual ways, as relevant to that tissue.

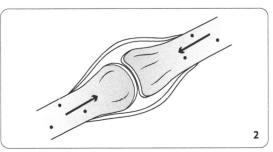

Begin to compress the tissue at a moderate pace. If it is a joint, compress along the central or long axis of the joint. Compress to end-feel and maintain this compaction throughout steps 3 and 4. Release the compression during step 5.

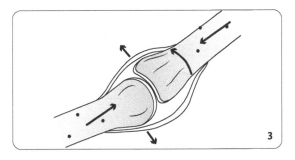

As the tissue is compressed, notice any natural tendency the tissue has to pull in a particular direction. At a moderate pace, encourage the tissue to go further in this direction or succession of directions. Load the tissue to near end-feel in these directions, all the while maintaining the compression.

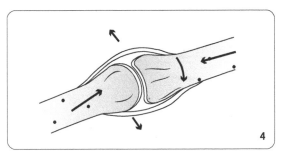

While fully maintaining the compression, reverse the direction the tissue was loaded exaggerating the natural pull in it. Make the reversal at a moderate pace allowing time for tissue to release. Load in this opposite direction to near end-feel.

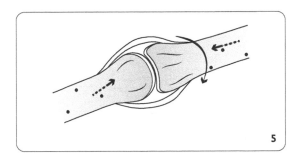

As soon as you arrive at end-feel in step 4, begin to slack the compaction at a moderate pace, and concurrent with slacking the compression move the joint or other tissue in a circumduction, timing the decompaction to coincide with one full circle of circumduction.

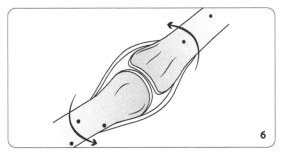

Repeat the mobility tests used in step 1 to evaluate how much change was made.

TREATMENT
METHOD 17

Stretch actuated variant of Van Buskirk's reconstructed A. T. Still technique

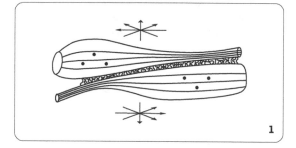

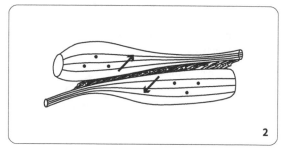

Shown here are two muscles and the intermuscular septum between them. Intermuscular septa are elastic connective tissue broadly attached to both muscles. The elasticity of the intermuscular septum allows the two muscles to move relative to one another without rubbing each other; however, it can lose its elasticity. Assess the elasticity of the intermuscular septum by moving the two muscles in several opposite directions.

If the available counter movement between the two muscles is insufficient in any directions, treat by choosing a relatively mobile direction in which to oppositely load the two muscles, thereby stretching the intermuscular septum. If improvement is insufficient with a first application of this treatment, then in the second treatment episode treat in a less mobile direction.

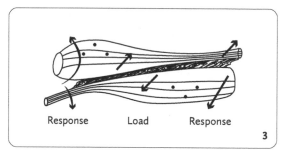

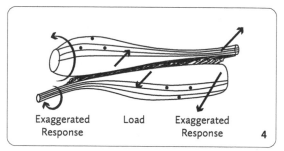

The intermuscular septum will respond to your stretch by moving the muscles in some direction. This movement(s) can be any combination of rotation and shear. Maintain your stretch load.

While maintaining your stretch load, exaggerate the natural counter movement(s) of the two muscles to end-feel.

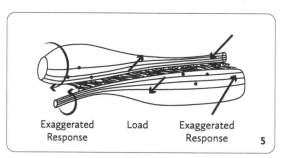

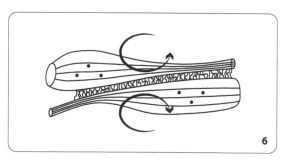

While continuing to maintain your stretch load, slowly reverse the response load taking the two muscles in the opposite direction to their natural movement to end-feel. Make this transition from natural direction of movement to its opposite at a moderate pace respecting the rate at which the tissue can change.

After the tissue has reached end-feel in the direction opposite to the natural pull of the tissue, release your stretch load at a moderate pace while making a circumduction of the two muscles relative to each other. Then briefly release your grip before post mobility testing the elasticity of the intermuscular septum to decide whether or not to treat it further.

Six factor model: Reconstructed A. T. Still technique

FORCE

The force applied in this technique varies from moderate to high.

- In step 2, the compaction is made at a moderated pace increasing through the range of compression up to near end-feel.
- In step 3, force used following the tissues listening like pull is initially moderate and increases at the end to near end-feel. The compaction of the tissue in this step continues near end-feel throughout.
- In step 4, force initially backs off from near end-feel to moderate, then at the other end of the range of movement approaches end-feel again. The compaction of the tissue in this step continues near end-feel throughout.
- In step 5, the compaction into the tissue is slacked at a moderate pace ending at zero force. Concurrent with the slacking of the compaction a circumduction is performed; force for this starts moderate as needed to work through the load of the compaction, and then lightens to near zero at the end.

SPEED

Speed is moderate throughout. During all phases of the treatment, stay alert to the release happening in the tissue. Too fast movement would not allow the tissue to change. Too slow movement could allow unwinding to occur, which is undesirable.

CONSTRAINT

In this technique, the levels of directiveness, speed, and force levels are high enough that there just is not much possibility of client tissue directed activity. The only client tissue directed activity is the tissue pull noted and utilized in step 3. Unwinding is specifically forbidden; however, preventing unwinding does not require watchfulness as in Hoover technique since the higher force levels used forestall unwinding.

DIRECTIVENESS

This is a highly directive technique throughout. In all steps, the therapist directs tissue movement.

TISSUE ENGAGEMENT

Tissue engagement is made by the therapist in most phases of this method; however, in step 2, the client's tissue pulls the therapist's hand in a particular direction.

RELATIONSHIP TO EFFORT BARRIERS

Effort barriers are not directly considered in this technique. Forces used vary from moderate through end-feel.

Reconstructed A. T. Still technique example 1

ASSESSMENT

General assessment leads to the right upper limb; assessment is supported by the witness point at the right olecranon process.

Local assessment, including gliding inhibition, manual thermal assessment, local listening, layer listening, and yes–no question asking, pinpoints this as the gleno-humeral joint capsule.

CLIENT INQUIRY

Ask about the client's awareness of their body:

- in general, and
- in their right arm and shoulder.

MOBILITY TESTING

Global active

- Observe the client walking, noting particularly arm and shoulder movement with gait.
- Ask the client to stand and then make a circumduction of first the right arm and then the left.

- Ask the client to forward flex the arm at the shoulder, return it to neutral, then extend it at the shoulder.
- Ask the client to abduct the arm, then return it to a neutral hanging position.
- Ask the client to internally rotate the arm at the shoulder joint, return it to neutral, then externally rotate it.
- Repeat all this with the other arm for comparison.

Global passive

- With the client standing, stand behind the client, slightly right of center. Place your left hand on top of the client's right shoulder girdle to stabilize the scapula and clavicle. With your right hand, grasp the right elbow and extend the arm back while maintaining the elbow comfortably extended. Return the arm to neutral, then similarly flex the arm at the shoulder. Return the arm to neutral, then abduct the arm. Return the arm to neutral, then internally rotate it at the shoulder, return it to neutral, then externally rotate it. Return the arm to neutral, then slightly flex the arm at the shoulder and adduct it in front of the torso to a comfortable end range. Hug this end-feel as you circumduct the arm; note where the arm deviates from a smooth curved path in its circumduction.
- Shift your right hand distal to control the elbow, so you can again extend the shoulder while maintaining the elbow in full extension. Note how the shoulder movement appears different from the previous test.
- Make the same passive tests on the other arm for comparison.

Focal passive

- Ask the client to lie supine on the table. Sit at the client's right side facing the shoulder. Place your left hand on the distal clavicle and scapula to provide a dynamic stabilization. With your right hand, grasp the proximal end of the humerus. At a moderately slow pace, glide the head of the humerus in a succession of directions in the glenoid fossa, returning it to neutral after each direction, before testing the next directions:
  - anterior
  - posterior
  - superior
  - inferior.
- Make all the same assessments on the other arm for comparison.

TREATMENT

Using the same hand holds as for the focal passive assessment mobility test:

- Maintain a dynamic stabilization of the shoulder girdle with your left hand.
- At a moderately fast pace, compact the head of the humerus into the glenoid fossa to a comfortable end-feel. *Maintain this compaction through all of the following steps until the last step. Maintaining this compaction is critical to success of this technique.*
- As you make this compaction, the head of the humerus will glide and/or rotate in some direction. Promptly load the head of the humerus to increase this natural glide and/or rotation to a comfortable end-feel.
- Be alert to the possibility of a succession of more than one leg of glide or rotation. Often there will be only one leg of displacement, but occasionally up

to three legs. A larger number of legs is conceivable.

- Once you have loaded the head of the humerus to end-feel in the single or several directions of natural glide, *maintain the compaction*, as you reverse this glide direction or succession of glide directions to load the tissue to end-feel in the opposite direction.
- As soon as you arrive at the end-feel in this reversed direction(s), begin to allow the humerus to decompact out of the glenoid fossa at a moderate pace. During the decompaction, make a moderately paced circumduction of the humerus on the scapula.
- Release all contacts. Remove your hands. Proceed to post treatment testing.

POST TREATMENT TESTING AND INQUIRY

Use the standard post treatment procedure for mobility testing and question asking detailed in the introduction to treatment methods section. Either treat this same area further, as indicated by this inquiry, or return to general assessment.

Reconstructed A. T. Still technique example 2

Caution—Do not do this on a person known to have osteoporosis or a person who has risk factors for osteoporosis but who has not been recently tested for osteoporosis.

ASSESSMENT

General assessment leads to the left lower limb. This is confirmed by the witness point at the left greater trochanter and refined to the left foot or ankle by the witness point at the left lateral malleolus.

Local assessment, including manual thermal assessment, local listening and inhibition, layer listening, and applied kinesiology questioning, narrows this to bone in the left calcaneus.

CLIENT INQUIRY

Ask about the client's awareness of their body:

- in general, and
- in their left foot and ankle.

MOBILITY TESTING

Global active

- Observe the client walking, noting particularly foot and ankle movement with gait.
- Ask the client to lie supine on the table with heels just off the end, then:
  - plantarflex the foot
  - dorsiflex the foot
  - circumduct the foot.

Global passive

- With the client supine on the table with heels off the end as for the previous test.
- Dynamically stabilize the distal lower leg with one hand. With the other hand, contact the metatarsals to first dorsiflex and then plantarflex the foot. This looks not only at ankle movement but elements of movement within the foot.
- With one hand, grasp the calcaneus; with the other hand, grasp the metatarsal heads. Mobility test the several joints of the foot collectively with a spiral movement through the foot on an anterior–posterior axis, first clockwise, then counterclockwise. Unlike many tests, this does not involve a dynamic stabilization of one part, and movement of the other part, but rather counter movement of two parts.

Focal passive

- With one hand, grasp the calcaneus; with the other hand, the talus. Test small gliding movements between these two bones A–P, medial–lateral, and rotary.

- With two hands grasp the calcaneus, one hand more posterior, one more anterior. Test the flexibility of this bone, bending it slightly:
  - bowed in a transverse plane
  - bowed in a sagittal plane
  - spiraled around an a–p axis.

TREATMENT

Using the same hand holds as for the focal passive assessment mobility test:

- Compact the bone in an A–P direction at a moderate pace to a comfortable end-feel. Maintain this compaction throughout this treatment until the last step. Maintaining this compaction is critical to the success of this treatment.
- Note the tendency of the bone to internally bend or rotate in response to this compacting load.
- Promptly load the tissue to a comfortable end-feel. Be alert to the possibility of more than one leg of bend or rotation. If there is more than one leg of bend and/or rotation, follow the tissue to a comfortable end range in each leg of movement.
- As soon as end-feel is reached, continue to maintain the original compaction, as you reverse the direction of the secondary compactions to the opposite end-feel.
- As soon as you arrive at this end-feel in the reverse direction, start to allow decompaction of the original load at a moderate pace, and circumduct within the bone as you decompact.

POST TREATMENT TESTING AND INQUIRY

Use the standard post treatment procedure for mobility testing and question asking detailed in the introduction to treatment methods section. Either treat this same area further, as indicated by this inquiry, or return to general assessment.

Reconstructed A. T. Still technique example 3
ASSESSMENT

General assessment leads to the right lower limb. This is supported by the witness point at the greater trochanter. The witness point at the lateral malleolus rules out the foot and ankle.

Local assessment including gliding inhibition, manual thermal assessment, local listening and inhibition, layer listening, and yes–no questioning narrows this to the medial portion of the patellar retinaculum. The patellar retinaculum is the portion of the knee joint capsule attached laterally and medially to the kneecap and running from there back to attach to the humerus and tibia and continuing into the capsule of the femero-tibial joint.

CLIENT INQUIRY

Ask about the client's awareness of their body:

- in general, and
- in their right leg, particularly the knee.

MOBILITY TESTING
Global active

- Observe the client walking, noting particularly knee movement in gait.

Global passive

- Explain to the client the process and reasons for testing.

- Ask the client to lie supine on the table. For each knee, test the range of motion of the knee noting range, ease, and smoothness of movement.

Focal passive

- With the client still supine on the table, stand at the side of the table for the knee to be tested. With both thumbs and forefingers, contact the lateral and medial aspects of the patella so that you can move it. With your other fingers and hypothenar edges of your hand, provide dynamic stabilization of the distal femur and proximal tibia. Slowly glide the patella to a soft comfortable end-feel:
  - medial
  - lateral
  - superior
  - inferior
  - diagonals between the above cardinal directions.
- Stay alert to signs of distress from the client. For some few clients, some of these movements may be uncomfortable, anxiety provoking, or both. Do not persist with testing which is distressing.
- For all these directions, note both range and ease of movement.
- Do all the above tests for the other knee for comparison.

General and local assessment led to dysfunction in a medial portion of the right patellar retinaculum. This could be either fibrosity or less commonly laxity. Either one will contribute to poor patellar tracking. Both conditions can be present in different portions of the same patellar retinaculum. Fibrosity will appear in mobility testing as reduced range and/or resistance to movement. Laxity will appear as excessive movement. The following treatment is for fibrosity.

TREATMENT

Using the same hand holds as for the focal passive assessment mobility test, begin to stretch the stiff portion of patellar retinaculum. *Maintain this stretch load throughout the following treatment until the last step. Maintaining this stretch load is essential to success of the treatment.*

As you start to stretch that portion of the patellar retinaculum, notice any tissue pull or deviation movement in any direction other than the direction of your stretch load. While maintaining the original stretch load to a comfortable extent, load the tissue in the direction of the observed tissue pull to a comfortable end range. Stay alert to the possibility of a second or third direction of pull; load each direction to end-feel. Once you have arrived at end-feel in these directions of pull, *maintain the original stretch load* as you reverse the direction of the pulls to the opposite end-feel. As soon as you arrive at this opposite end range, begin at a moderate pace to release your original stretch. During the time you are releasing the stretch, make a circumduction of the patella in the plane of original stretch.

POST TREATMENT TESTING AND INQUIRY

Use the standard post treatment procedure for mobility testing and question asking detailed in the introduction to treatment methods section. Either treat this same area further, as indicated by this inquiry, or return to general assessment.

Treatment method 18: listen and follow

Origin
Jean-Pierre Barral DO.

Concept
If we know how to listen, the body will show us a good way to treat it.

Pretest
Determine an area of primacy using the general assessment methods. Refine the definition of this area with local assessment methods. Once the area of primacy is identified and specified, mobility test that tissue. The mobility tests to be used will be determined by the nature and location of the tissue found. Point out the results of mobility testing to the client.

Treatment method
As you contact the tissue at the primary site with local listening, the tissue will pull your hand in a particular direction, and at a particular speed. The "listening" movement may be linear or curved. If it is curved, the amount of curve may vary from slightly curved through any amount of curve, up to a spin in place. As soon as the tissue stops moving at the end of this "listening" pull, load the tissue in the direction in which it has moved. The initial therapeutic load will be at first barrier. Soon, tissue will usually be felt to begin to release. There may be a succession of releases or various sizes, or a single larger release. If the tissue does not adequately release, gradually increase force up to mid-range until an amount of force is found which will produce tissue release.

Post test
Immediately after treatment, repeat the same mobility tests used as pretests. Note the changes in range of motion and elasticity. Point out the changes to the client.

Six factor model: Listen and follow
TISSUE ENGAGEMENT
Tissue engagement is made by the client's tissue. The therapist contacts the client's body at an area identified as primary. The client's tissue moves the therapist's hand in a particular direction.

FORCE
Variable, first barrier to moderate.

SPEED
During the initial "listening" tissue movement, follow the speed of tissue movement. Neither retard nor accelerate it.

Once the end of the listening directional pull is reached, maintain a gentle load in the exact direction of the listening movement. During this second phase, movement will be quite slow or absent. As tissue releases, follow the releasing tissue gently in the same direction to maintain the same load.

CONSTRAINT
No constraint. As the tissue releases, any movement is allowed; however, this will usually be in the direction of load, due to the high level of directiveness.

DIRECTIVENESS
High. The direction of movement is taken from the body's initial movement; however, once the initial movement has ceased, the therapist keeps a gentle load on the tissue in this same direction.

RELATIONSHIP TO EFFORT BARRIERS
Variable. Often, treatment is accomplished at a first barrier load; however, if the tissue does not change readily at this effort level, somewhat higher force may be tried.

Listen and follow

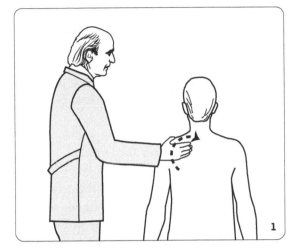

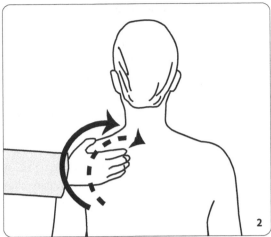

Contact the area identified as the current primary. Notice the local listening tissue pull in this area.

Move your hand just enough to follow the local listening tissue pull.

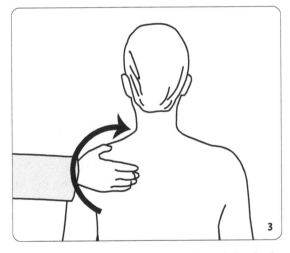

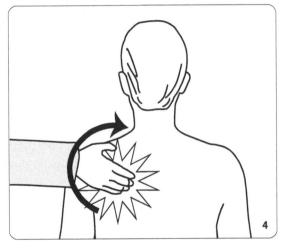

When the local listening pull has reached its end, then load the tissue further in the direction of the local listening. Start with a first barrier load. As tissue begins to release, continue to load the tissue at a first barrier force level, in the direction in which the listening traveled. There may be several increments of release. Occasionally, a first barrier load will not produce sufficient release, in which case gradually increase force up to a middle barrier force level.

When the tissue is sufficiently released, break contact. Post treatment mobility test the tissue. Describe and demonstrate the change to the client. Return to assessment to find the next primary.

Listen and follow example 1

ASSESSMENT

General assessment leads to the left side of the occiput.

With local assessment, local listening supports that there is an actively changing lesion in this area. The pull of this local listening is linear, suggesting that the active lesion is near the surface. Layer listening pinpoints this as in the superficial fascia. Manual thermal assessment further supports the existence of an active lesion in this area and suggests an area covering most of the left occiput. Mobility testing confirms that the skin will not slide over underlying tissues in this area.

CLIENT INQUIRY

The client is asked about their awareness of their neck mobility. The client indicates that they are aware that their neck does not move as freely as in earlier years, but there is no associated discomfort. The client reiterates that their main complaint is at their right hip.

MOBILITY TESTING

Global mobility testing of the neck shows that it is limited in both right rotation and in right side bending.

Focal mobility testing of the left and right atlantooccipital joints and C1–C2 articulations show that each has good mobility.

An ultraslow mobility test is performed by placing the neck in its easier direction of movement, left rotation with left side bending, then moving slowly back toward neutral. This shows the lack of skin glide over the occiput as the first limiting factor for neck mobility. This is typical that when skin cannot glide or stretch on the head it limits neck mobility. Neck mobility requires superficial tissue slack from the head.

TREATMENT

A broad contact is made with several finger pads on the tissue overlying the primary area on the left occiput. The direction of local listening pull is noted, in this instance inferomedial. A first barrier load is applied and maintained in this inferomedial direction. Several increments of release are felt as this vector is maintained. Then recheck both the mobility of the skin on the occiput and the range of motion in the neck. Treat further if indicated unless a slight edema has appeared in the area treated.

POST TREATMENT TESTING AND INQUIRY

Use the standard post treatment procedure for mobility testing and question asking detailed in the introduction to treatment methods section. Either treat this same area further, as indicated by this inquiry, or return to general assessment.

Listen and follow example 2

GENERAL ASSESSMENT

General assessment leads to the right lower limb. This is confirmed by a contact on the witness point at the right greater trochanter. Then contact at the right lateral malleolus narrows the search area by ruling in the right foot and ankle.

GLOBAL ASSESSMENT

The client is asked to walk, and gait is observed. Slightly less push off is seen with the right foot.

In local assessment, the client is asked to lie supine on the table with heels just off the end of the table. A manual thermal sweep of the right foot and ankle shows active lesions on the superior half of the posterior aspect of the heel, and near the first metatarsophalangeal joint. Local listening and inhibition between these two areas rules in the posterior heel. Local listening narrows this to the area where the distal end of the Achilles tendon overlies the superior third of the posterior aspect of the calcaneus. The local listening pull has a moderate amount of curve, suggesting intermediate depth. Layer listening refines this to just deep to the Achilles tendon. The Achilles bursa is suspected. The Achilles tendon attaches to the calcaneus about one-third of the way down from the top of the calcaneus. With the tendon running over bone in this area, there is friction potential. A small bursa here between tendon and bone mitigates this. It is an area of high mechanical stress, and this bursa frequently becomes adhered. This area is mobility tested by grasping the calcaneus with the fingers of one hand and grasping the overlying portion of the Achilles tendon with the other hand and attempting medial-lateral gliding motions between them. Nearly no glide is observable.

Both ankles are passively mobility tested. The right ankle is found to have somewhat less dorsiflexion than the left.

TREATMENT

A slightly long lever approach is taken. The calcaneus is held with the fingers of one hand and the distal Achilles tendon is held with the finger pads of the other hand. This double long lever approach is used to affect the bursa between the tendon and the bone. A local listening pull is observed which is medial glide with a moderate clockwise curve viewed from the back of the foot. This listening pull is followed and then exaggerated to a first barrier. This vector is maintained through a succession of releases. Recheck mobility within the Achilles bursa. Treat further, if indicated, unless a slight edema has appeared.

POST TREATMENT TESTING AND INQUIRY

Use the standard post treatment procedure for mobility testing and question asking detailed in the introduction to treatment methods section. Either treat this same area further, as indicated by this inquiry, or return to general assessment.

Listen and follow example 3

ASSESSMENT

General assessment leads to the right upper neck, posterolateral.

Manual thermal assessment in this area shows a 1 cm circular shaped area. Local listening suggests a moderate depth within the tissue. Layer listening suggests a lesion within vertebral mechanics, not as deep as the neural canal.

MOBILITY TESTING

The client is placed supine on the table. Global testing of neck mobility shows right side bending range a little greater than left, and neck rotation is about 50 percent of normal both left and right. Mobility testing of each atlantooccipital articulation shows good mobility both left and right. Testing rotation between C1 and C2 shows very little mobility. Testing side bending between C1 and C2 shows that the left C1–C2 joint can open, but not the right. The primary lesion is identified as the right C1–C2 facet joint.

TREATMENT

With the client supine, cradle the occiput with the left hand. With the fingers of the right hand, use the pads of the thumb and fourth finger to grasp the right transverse process of C1, and the tips of the second and third fingers to grasp the C2 right transverse process. Use these contacts to local listen into this area. Follow the local listening to its end. Then add a further first barrier load in this direction. Maintain that vector as the tissue releases. After several releases are felt, soften or break contact and return to mobility testing.

POST TREATMENT TESTING AND INQUIRY

Use the standard post treatment procedure for mobility testing and question asking detailed in the introduction to treatment methods section. Either treat this same area further, as indicated by this inquiry, or return to general assessment.

Treatment method 19: load and tap

Origin
Jeffrey Burch.

Concept
A structure which is stiff, distorted, or adhered to another structure may be corrected by loading the tissue toward correction, and while loaded, delivering a single tap of medium velocity and medium amplitude.

Pretreatment tests
It is often useful to point out test results to the client. Invite the client to remember the pretest condition to compare with test results after the treatment.

- Observe postural alignment in the person's body both locally and globally.
- Test biomechanical ranges of motion in the area to be treated.
- Discern directions in which tissue could be loaded to bring it toward a corrected state. This may be moderate bending of a kinked structure toward straight, or a moderate shear load through an adhesion.

Method
Load the tissue toward correction to barrier about three-quarters of the way toward a corrected state. With another hand, deliver a quick tap. The tap should be of medium velocity and medium amplitude. This tap must not be confused with a thrust.

Tissue distortion may be of several types. Here are examples:

- If a tissue is stiff the tissue will usually be stiff unevenly in different directions. Test the flexibility of the tissue in several directions. Load the tissue in the direction it least easily bends to a barrier, about three-quarters of the way toward end-feel. Deliver a quick tap to the tissue.
- Sometimes when tissue is stiff it is also bent or twisted. If an inflection point of this bend is discerned focus your bending load on the inflection and deliver the tap there.
- If two structures which should have a lubricated glide plane between them are adhered together, establish a shear force through the adhesion at a force level about three-quarters of the way toward end-feel. Deliver the corrective tap to the adhered area. If the area of adhesion is small, the tap may be delivered to its center. If the area of adhesion is larger, it will often be more productive to deliver the tap at an edge of the adhesion. To select which edge to use, local listening and inhibition may show the area most prone to change. Alternatively, select a portion of the adhesion which is demonstrably less firmly bound.

Post treatment tests

- Test ranges of motion in the area treated.
- Observe postural alignment in the person's body both locally and globally.
- Discuss results with the client.

*Caution—Do **not** use this method on any structure which is inherently or situationally fragile to an extent that such a tap has any potential to injure. Examples of structures never to use this method on are eyes, pancreas, blood vessels, and nerves. For these last, all areas of the body have blood supply and innervation, thus any tap in addition to addressing its target tissue will also be incidentally toward some small nerves and blood vessels. This is different than setting up this type of treatment to directly impact a nerve or blood vessel.*

TREATMENT
METHOD 19

Any structure may be situationally damaged, so it is more fragile than usual. Examples of such situationally weakened tissues include:

- a bone known or suspected to be cracked
- a bruised area
- any tissue damaged by an infectious process and not yet healed.

Err on the side of caution.

Six factor model: Load and tap

TISSUE ENGAGEMENT

Tissue engagement is made by the therapist. The tissue is loaded to about three quarters of the way to end-feel. This may be a bend load, or a shear load as appropriate to the situation.

FORCE

During set up, about three-quarters of the way toward end-feel. For the release phase, a medium velocity, medium amplitude tap.

Note: A tap is not a thrust.

SPEED

- Moderately slow to establish the setup.
- Fairly fast for the release tap.

CONSTRAINT

- High constraint is applied during the setup phase; tissue is loaded beyond a first barrier. No spontaneous movement is allowed during the setup phase.
- The constraint during the release phase is that the tissue may not move counter to the setup load. Any other movement is allowed.

DIRECTIVENESS

- Setup phase: Highly directive. The tissue is loaded moderately strongly in a particular direction.
- Release phase: Mixed. The tissue will move in the direction of the preload. No other direction is given.

RELATIONSHIP TO EFFORT BARRIERS

- Setup phase: About three-quarters of the way to end-feel.
- Release phase: a) At the moment of tap, the load on the tissue from the preload is still three-quarters of the way to end-feel; however, this rapidly diminishes as the tissue releases. b) The intensity of the tap is not related to specific barrier loads.

Load and tap

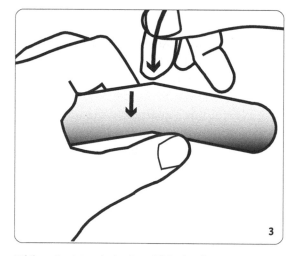

A body structure which is stiffened around a bent area in it.

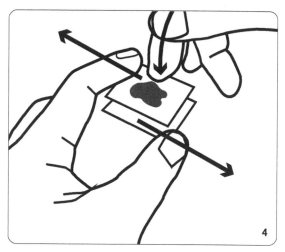

Mobility test the flexibility of the structure in several directions. Then load the structure toward correction of the bend, about three-quarters of the way toward end-feel.

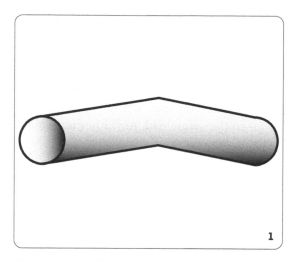

While maintaining the load established in the previous step, deliver a medium velocity, medium amplitude tap to the apex of the bend in the structure.

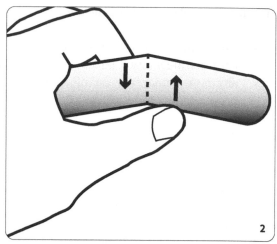

If the problem is an adhesion rather than a contracture, apply a moderate shear load through the adhesion and while maintaining this shear load tap the adhesion.

Load and tap example 1

ASSESSMENT

General assessment points to the area of the right deltoid muscle.

Manual thermal assessment shows a tongue shaped area posterolateral and more superior within the deltoid area. The base of the tongue shape is superior. Local listening has a moderate amount of curve suggesting the structure is at moderate depth. Layer listening refines this to just deep to the deltoid muscle. An adhesion of the subdeltoid bursa is hypothesized. Yes–no questioning supports this.

MOBILITY TESTING

As a global mobility test, perform a circumduction mobility test of the client's right shoulder. With the client standing, stand behind and slightly to the right of the client. With the left hand, stabilize the client's right scapula and clavicle. With the right hand, grasp the client's elbow to control both humerus and ulna. Move the shoulder to an end of range of motion. Proceed at a moderate pace through a circumduction, hugging the end of range of motion, throughout the range. Note any deviations from a smooth circle in the motion of the shoulder.

With the client supine and standing at the client's right side, the left hand is placed in the axilla supporting the upper arm. The right hand grasps the deltoid muscle and attempts to glide it anterior and posterior. Little mobility is observed confirming the presence of an adhesion in the subdeltoid bursa. The subdeltoid bursa is a flat extension of the shoulder joint capsule extending deep to the deltoid muscle. The continuity of the bursa with the joint capsule accounts for the tongue shape of the manual thermal projection.

TREATMENT

With the client supine on the table, stand at the client's right side facing their head. With the thumb and fingers of the right hand, grasp the deltoid muscle and apply a posteriorly directed shear load to the muscle directed at the depth of the subdeltoid bursa. Initiating at the therapist's left shoulder, make a whip motion to deliver a moderately strong tap with the left middle finger to the lateral aspect of the client's right deltoid muscle. Again, mobility test the glide of the subdeltoid bursa, and assess for the presence of slight edema.

POST TREATMENT TESTING AND INQUIRY

Use the standard post treatment procedure for mobility testing and question asking detailed in the introduction to treatment methods section. Either treat this same area further, as indicated by this inquiry, or return to general assessment.

Load and tap example 2

ASSESSMENT

General assessment is a lean to the right in the upper thorax. An inhibitory contact at the middle scalene muscle rules out the pleura. An inhibitory contact at the right olecranon process rules in the right upper limb. A manual thermal sweep of the right shoulder girdle, arm, and hand shows three thermal projections over the acromioclavicular joint, a linear area about 4 cm long just proximal to the radial side of the wrist, and an irregular shaped area about 3 cm in diameter at the mid-ulnar side of the forearm. Pairwise comparison of these three areas using local listening with inhibition suggests the wrist area is the most primary. Local listening is a nearly circular rotation. Layer listening suggests that the lesion is in bone.

CLIENT INQUIRY

Client inquiry confirms no history or risk factors for osteoporosis, and no recent injury to the wrist.

MOBILITY TESTING

With the client supine each wrist is mobility tested showing mild limitation in both extension and supination of the right wrist. The flexibility of the whole of both radiuses is tested by grasping both ends of the bone and gently torsioning it along its length. The right radius is found to be somewhat less elastic. The flexibility of the right radius is tested incrementally along its length by making gentle focal bends with both hands. The distal 5 cm of the radius is found to be stiffer than the rest of the bone.

TREATMENT

Standing at the client's right side, use the first three fingers of the right hand to apply a moderate bending load to the stiff distal portion of the right radius. While maintaining this load, initiate a whiplike motion of the left arm, starting at the shoulder, to deliver a moderate force tap with the tip of the left middle finger to the client's right distal radius.

POST TREATMENT TESTING AND INQUIRY

Use the standard post treatment procedure for mobility testing and question asking detailed in the introduction to treatment methods section. Either treat this same area further, as indicated by this inquiry, or return to general assessment.

Load and tap example 3

ASSESSMENT

General assessment suggests the right lower limb. An inhibitory contact at the right greater trochanter supports this assessment. An inhibitory contact at the right lateral malleolus rules out the foot and ankle.

An inhibitory contact at the knee suggests that the primary lesion is at the knee. A manual thermal sweep of the leg shows thermal projections at the anteriolateral knee and anterior mid shin. The client is placed supine on the table. Local listening and inhibition between the two areas of thermal projection finds the anteromedial knee more primary. The local listening is at the medial aspect of the right patella.

Local listening has a slight curve, suggesting the lesion is deep to the investing fascia, but not much deeper. Layer listening suggests the

knee joint capsule. In this area, the joint capsule attaches to the outer perimeter of the hockey puck-like low cylinder of the patella. Thus, the capsule runs over the lateral and medial walls of the patella before continuing to attach to the distal femur and proximal tibia. Normally there is joint lubricant continuing from the knee joint to the glide plane between the joint capsule and the sides of the patella. Since knees both get used hard and banged, adhesions of the joint capsule to the periosteum of the sides of the patella are frequent occurrences.

MOBILITY TESTING

Observe the client walking with particular attention to knee function. With the client in side-lying positions, check the mobility range of each knee. Side-lying is preferred for this examination, as in supine, both the knee and hip must be moved to check the range of the knee. Then with the client in supine, the glide of each patella is tested, medial, lateral, superior, inferior, and at a succession of four 45-degree angles between these cardinal directions. It is found that the right patella does not easily glide medially. It is observed that the right patella sits displaced slightly lateral. An adhesion of the joint capsule to the lateral surface of the patella is hypothesized. To test this, stand at the client's right side near mid-calf, facing the client's head. With the right hand, dynamically stabilize the right patella. With the tip of the left index finger, touch the medial aspect of the right patella, sinking into the depth of the joint capsule. Attempt to drag the joint capsule over the periosteum superior and inferior. No glide is found in the inferior three-quarters of this glide plane.

TREATMENT

Using the second through fifth fingers of the right hand, stabilize the right patella. With the right thumb, sink to contact the joint capsule over the medial aspect of the right patella. Apply a superior force to the capsule establishing a shear load between the capsule and the periosteum. Starting with the left shoulder, make a whip motion to deliver a moderate force tap with the tip of the left middle finger to the anterolateral corner of the patella adjacent to the right thumb contact.

Mobility test the glide of the joint capsule over the underlying periosteum as before. Note any improvement. If glide is not ideal, retreat, so long as no hint of edema has appeared.

POST TREATMENT TESTING AND INQUIRY
Use the standard post treatment procedure for mobility testing and question asking detailed in the introduction to treatment methods section. Either treat this same area further, as indicated by this inquiry, or return to general assessment.

TECHNIQUES IN WHICH THERAPEUTIC ENGAGEMENT IS MADE BY THE THERAPIST AND UNWINDING MAY OR MAY NOT OCCUR

In most techniques where the therapeutic engagement is made by the client's tissue, unwinding will occur. The presence of unwinding as a component of the therapeutic process is more variable with techniques in which therapeutic engagement is made by the therapist. Some therapist-initiated therapeutic engagement techniques encourage and support unwinding. Other therapist-initiated therapeutic engagement techniques forbid unwinding.

This section describes a third subset of therapeutic techniques where tissue engagement is made by the therapist where unwinding may or may not occur.

In these techniques, unwinding is neither encouraged nor discouraged. Unwinding is permitted in these techniques and may be useful but is not an essential element of the technique.

Treatment method 20: first barrier stretch

Origin
Traditional osteopathic method. Discoverer not known.

Concepts
COLLAGEN AND ELASTIN IN CONNECTIVE TISSUE
The many varieties of connective tissue in our bodies including tendons, ligaments, articular cartilage, and membranes are all composed largely of elastin and collagen. As its name suggests, elastin fibers are elastic. Collagen fibers are not elastic. Each tissue has the right mix of elastic and non-elastic fibers, and the right total fiber content, to be able to do its job.

For example, tendons have a high total fiber content and more collagen than elastin. A little elasticity in tendons is useful for shock absorption, but too much elasticity would not allow them to transfer the contractile force of a muscle to a bone.

Loose areolar tissue just under the skin is almost all elastin, and has low total fiber content. The stretch in this tissue allows skin to move over the tissues deep to it.

HEALING RESPONSE IN CONNECTIVE TISSUE
When tissue is injured or inflamed, the body quickly lays down mostly collagen in the initial repair process. Later, the body reabsorbs some of the collagen and makes the remaining collagen more orderly. Still the total fiber content often stays too high, and the balance of collagen and elastin is shifted to more collagen. We experience this tissue as stiff.

In addition to increased collagen content within a tissue, collagen often grows across glide planes into adjacent tissue, so they no longer glide.

We call excess growth of collagen fibrosity. We call fibrosity within a tissue a contracture. We call fibrosity between tissues an adhesion. Both varieties of fibrosity reduce mobility but in different ways. It is possible to have contracture and adhesion of the same tissue.

TREATMENT OF FIBROSITY
To restore stretch and glide of fibrosed tissue, we artfully disrupt collagen fibers so the body will reabsorb them. Disruption of excess collagen fibers must be done gently and in modest sized steps, so the body does not perceive this as a new injury. If the treatment process creates inflammation the tissue may initially seem less stiff, but the body will respond to the inflammation by making new fibrosity, reestablishing the stiffness.

TREATMENT
METHOD 20

TREATMENT OF CONTRACTURE

The present treatment method reduces contractures. The treatment process for adhesions is similar but not identical.

Pretest

- Observe alignment in the usual way.
- Assess end range mobility in the usual way.
- Locate a specific, relatively primary element of contracture contributing to the overall stiffness of the area. Ultraslow mobility testing may be useful for this along with other assessment methods.

MULTIDIRECTIONAL MOBILITY TESTING

The same tissue may exhibit substantially less stretch in one direction than in another. For contractures, mobility test the stretch of the tissue in a series of directions like a compass rose, at least four sets of opposed directions on 45-degree variations.

FOCAL END RANGE MOBILITY TESTING

Before beginning to treat, test the stretch of the tissue by elongating it with two hands until a firm barrier, approaching but not at end range, is felt. *Always respect the normal span of the tissue. Never force anything.*

ASSESS RESTING RELATIONSHIP OF
THE TISSUE TO ITS FIRST BARRIER

For a given direction in a particular tissue at equilibrium with neighboring tissues, there are two possibilities: 1) the tension in the tissue is greater than its first barrier, or 2) the tension in the tissue is less than first barrier. In theory, a third condition could be found where the tissue is resting precisely at a first barrier, but in practice this is not found.

Finding and treating at the first barrier

1. Use two contacts, usually two hands, to slack the tension in the tissue. To accomplish this, contact the tissue at two points and slowly shorten the tissue, so it becomes more slack.

2. Very slowly release the pressure required to slack the tissue.

   a. If the first barrier is more slack than equilibrium, here is what you will observe. To slack this tissue, you had to stretch other tissues engaging them like a stretched spring. As you very slowly release the force required to load this spring, watch for a moment when the springiness of the tissue suddenly seems to push less hard into your hands. You are now at the first barrier. If you arrive back at equilibrium without observing this, then:

   b. Slowly begin to stretch the tissue beyond its resting state until there is a small but usually sharp rise in the force required to stretch the tissue. You are now at the first barrier.

3. Once at the first barrier, wait until a release sign is observed. Then proceed very slowly in the direction of stretch until a new first barrier is felt.

4. Proceed in this way through a succession of first barriers. If you started from a slack position, this succession of barriers will move through and past the equilibrium position.

5. When a more generalized release is felt, or one of the other signs of completion is felt, you are done.

6. Gently retest the near end range span of tissue in this direction to end range in the direction treated.

7. Retest the near end range span of the tissue in other directions.

8. Continue to treat the other directions as needed.

9. At the first subtle sign of swelling or edema in the tissue, *stop*. Make a note to recheck this tissue at the next treatment. It may have improved on its own or may benefit from additional treatment.

TREATMENT
METHOD 20

First barrier stretch

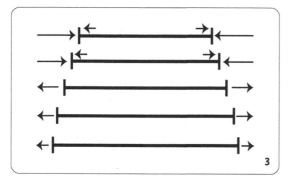

In some circumstances, a goal is to elongate the resting length of a particular tissue. The initial length and amount of stretch on this tissue will be in equilibrium with several other connected tissues.

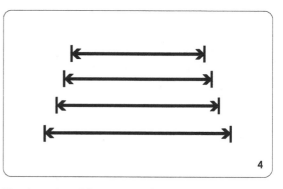

Therefore, it is important to first slack the tissue we wish to elongate, to make sure it has less than a first barrier stretch on it, then let it slowly spring back out until the first barrier is encountered.

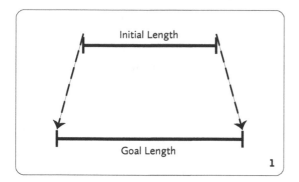

From the length where the first barrier is encountered, allow the tissue to lengthen, keeping a first barrier load on it. The felt sense of the first barrier will change as the equilibrium point with related tissues is passed.

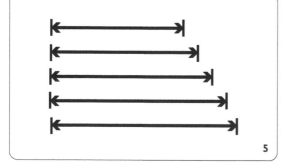

The elongation of the tissue may happen symmetrically in both directions throughout the lengthening of the tissue,

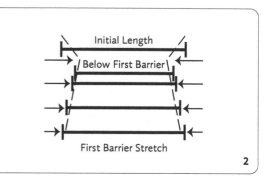

or the lengthening may be all toward one direction from a seeming fixed end,

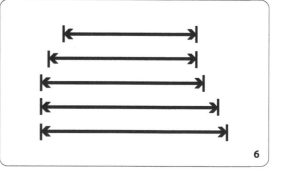

or the elongation may happen in several increments, sometimes symmetrically to both ends, sometimes in both directions but asymmetrically, and sometimes exclusively toward one end.

TREATMENT METHOD 20

Six factor model: First barrier stretch

TISSUE ENGAGEMENT

Tissue engagement is made by gently elongating the tissue to a first barrier. While unwinding phenomena commonly occur, engagement is not made by letting the client's body initiate the unwinding.

FORCE

First barrier.

SPEED

Slow. Follow the tissue's lead as it releases, never rushing it.

CONSTRAINT

Low. Release is allowed in most directions, just not shortening in the direction in which the tissue is being stretched.

DIRECTIVENESS

Moderate to high. At any given moment, the tissue is being loaded in a particular direction. There is a distinct message given to the tissue— elongate in this direction.

RELATIONSHIP TO FIRST BARRIER

Treatment of this variety is all done at a first barrier. The location of the first barrier usually changes as the tissue releases. Thus, treatment is applied at a succession of first barriers until a final release is felt, or other signs indicate it is time to stop.

First barrier stretch example 1

ASSESSMENT

General assessment leads to the right upper limb. There is a lean into the right upper chest/shoulder area which is localized to the upper limb by a witness point at the right olecranon process.

In local assessment, a gliding inhibition leads to the right wrist area. Manual thermal assessment, local listening, layer listening, and applied kinesiology questioning lead to skin on the back of the right wrist.

CLIENT INQUIRY

Ask the client:

- how they have been feeling in general, and
- of their awareness of their wrists and hands.

MOBILITY TESTING

Active

Ask the client to:

- flex and then extend each wrist, and
- make a circumduction of each wrist.

Passive global

Ask the client to lie supine on the table. Instruct the client to allow you to move their hand and arm without either resisting or assisting. One at a time test the ranges of motion of:

- each wrist
  - flexion
  - extension
  - ulnar deviation
  - radial deviation
- each elbow
  - flexion
  - extension.

Passive focal tests

- With fingers of both hands, make a two-point contact on the skin of the back of the wrist with one contact on the radial side and one on the ulnar side.
- With this contact, attempt to gently stretch the skin. Rearrange your finger

contacts to make a proximal–distal stretch of the skin.

- For comparison, try the same thing on the forearm a few inches proximal to the original contact. Try all the same tests on the other wrist.

TREATMENT

For the skin on the back of the wrist, choose the direction of least restriction:

- proximal–distal
- radial–ulnar
- diagonals 45 degrees each way between the above directions.

With fingertips of two hands, engage the skin in this direction and slowly stretch it to a first barrier. Maintain a dynamic load in this axis until release is felt. Retest all four axes of movement. Retreat as needed in the same and/or other axes. Stop when either sufficient skin elasticity is achieved, or the first hint of edema is felt.

POST TREATMENT TESTING AND INQUIRY

Use the standard post treatment procedure for mobility testing and question asking detailed in the introduction to treatment methods section. Either treat this same area further, as indicated by this inquiry, or return to general assessment.

First barrier stretch example 2

ASSESSMENT

General assessment leads to the central part of the lower neck.

Local assessment such as manual thermal assessment, local listening, layer listening, and yes–no questions pinpoints this as the interspinous ligament between the spinous processes of the sixth and seventh cervical vertebrae. The interspinous ligaments spanning between each adjacent spinous process collectively form a check strap limiting forward flexion of the spine.

CLIENT INQUIRY

Ask the client:

- how they have been feeling in general, and
- of their awareness of their neck and cervico-thoracic junction area.

MOBILITY TESTING

Global active

- Ask the standing client to make neck movements, flexion, extension, left and right side bending, and left and right rotation.

Global passive

- With the client supine on the table, ask the client to allow you to move their head in various directions without either assisting or resisting.
- Sit at the head of the table. Put your hands under and around the sides of the client's head.
- At a moderate pace, move their head in flexion, extension, left and right side bending, and left and right rotation.

Focal passive

- Place the palms of your hands under the client's occiput.
- With the tips of your two third fingers, contact the spinous process of the fourth cervical vertebra, with the finger pads on the inferior–posterior surface of it.
- Move the head and vertebrae C1–C4 as a unit to make a focal flexion of C4 on C5. Note the range and ease of movement.
- Then move your fingertips one spinal segment inferior to make a similar focal

flexion of C5 on C6. Compare this movement to the movement of the segment above.

- Proceed inferiorly one segment at a time to make focal flexions of C6 on C7, and C7 on T1.

TREATMENT

Having noted the apparent elasticity of each of the interspinous ligaments, return your fingertip contact to C6. Use your hands and fingers to move the head and all vertebrae C1–C6 as a unit into mild extension. Return out of this toward flexion until a first barrier is felt. Maintain a dynamic first barrier stretch on the C6–C7 interspinous ligament, feeling for increments of softening and lengthening.

POST TREATMENT TESTING AND INQUIRY

Use the standard post treatment procedure for mobility testing and question asking detailed in the introduction to treatment methods section. Either treat this same area further, as indicated by this inquiry, or return to general assessment.

First barrier stretch example 3
ASSESSMENT

General assessment leads to a superior part of the anterior chest wall near the midline.

Local assessment such as manual thermal assessment, local listening, layer listening, and applied kinesiology questioning pinpoints a primary restriction in the left third costal cartilage. On each side of the sternum each of the first four ribs has a separate bar of flexible cartilage articulating the rib with the sternum. Inferior to the fourth ribs, costal cartilages bridge together.

CLIENT INQUIRY

Ask the client:

- how they have been feeling in general

- of their awareness of their anterior chest, and
- of their awareness of their breath.

MOBILITY TESTING
Global active

- Ask the client to walk; observe gait, particularly how movement flows through the upper thorax.
- Ask the client to exhale fully, then inhale fully.

Focal passive

- Describe to the client what you will do and explain the reason for your contact on the anterior chest wall. Use anatomic models and illustrations.
- Ask the client to lie supine on the table. The costal cartilage of interest is on the left side.
- Compare the flexibility of the left third costal cartilage to all the other first four costal cartilages on each side. Begin with the right side. For each cartilage, exert moderate fingertip pressure posteriorly on the cartilage, observing the extent to which the cartilage will bow posteriorly.
- The left third costal cartilage is expected to be stiffer than other cartilages in this cluster; however, it may be only the most primary of several stiff cartilages. In which case, treating the primary cartilage may improve the flexibility of other cartilages.

TREATMENT

With one of your hands, contact and control the sternal end of the left third rib. With your other hand, contact and control a portion of the sternum adjacent to the left third costal cartilage. Gently and slowly distract these two bones away from each other, thereby exerting a gentle stretch on the costal cartilage, to a first barrier. More of the slight movement will be for the rib; your action on the sternum will be closer to a dynamic stabilization, though some movement is available. Maintain this first barrier stretch in a dynamic way, so that as the cartilage lengthens a little, your stretch load stays at a first barrier, even though your hands move slightly away from each other.

POST TREATMENT TESTING AND INQUIRY

Use the standard post treatment procedure for mobility testing and question asking detailed in the introduction to treatment methods section. Either treat this same area further, as indicated by this inquiry, or return to general assessment.

Treatment method 21: first barrier shear

Origin

Traditional osteopathic method. Discoverer not known.

This is like the first barrier stretch technique except the goal is to restore glide rather than stretch. It is worth noting that often where there is an adhesion between two structures there is often also a contracture in one or both of the adhered elements. It is usually easier to release the contractures after the adhesion is released. However, occasionally it is useful to soften the whole assembly before attempting to release the adhesion. Yes–no questions are useful for prioritizing these actions.

Method

1. Mobility test glide between two surfaces in several directions. Test at least eight directions varying by 45 degrees.

2. Choose the direction in which there is the least restricted glide.

3. Apply a first barrier load in this least bound direction, with the intent to *gently* shear the fibers adhering the two surfaces together.

4. Observe a succession of releases to incrementally increase glide excursion.

5. When a more generalized release or other final release is felt, stop.

6. Retest glide in other directions. Treat the next least bound direction, cycling steps 3, 4, and 5.

7. Cycle steps 1–6 until either glide is completely free or step 8 below.

8. At the first subtle sign of swelling or edema in the tissue, *stop*. Make a note to recheck this tissue at the next treatment. It may have improved on its own or may benefit from additional treatment.

First barrier shear

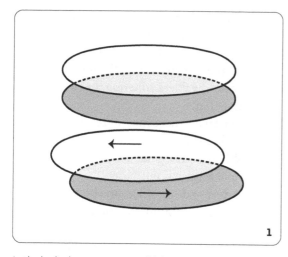

In the body there are many well lubricated glide planes.

Examples of glide planes include between organs, the dural tube through the vertebrae, and joint capsule over bone at the margins of joints.

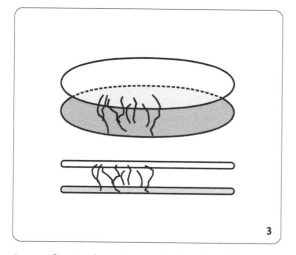

As part of healing from injury or infection, fiber often grows through the lubricant between structures which should glide on each other. We call this an adhesion.

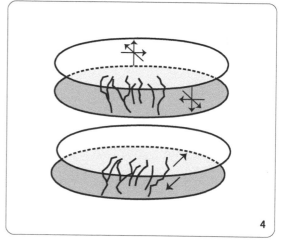

Adhesions can often be separated with gentle, slow shear forces through the adhesion. To set up a first barrier shear force treatment, begin by gently attempting to move the two structures in opposite directions in several axes. Movement will be slight due to the adhesion. Select the direction of greatest movement. Move the two structures in opposite directions in the axis of greatest available movement. As you maintain this gentle shear load, a little more movement will become available.

TREATMENT
METHOD 21

First barrier shear (*cont.*)

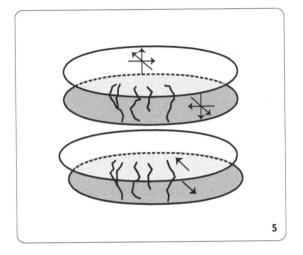

5

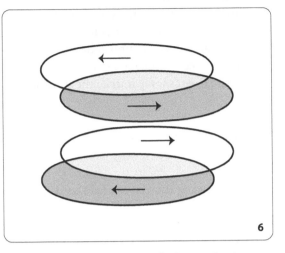

6

Retest the glide plane between the two structures to see which direction now has the greatest movement. This may be the same direction as in the previous step or not. Once again, move the two structures in opposite directions in the axis of greatest movement. Maintain this gentle shear until a little more movement is felt. Repeat mobility testing and tissue loading in this fashion until

either the two structures can glide freely on each other, in which case you are done, or stop as soon as the first hint of fluid filling, swelling, or edema is felt. Stop to avoid creating any inflammation in this area. Make a note to retest the glide of these structures on each other at the next treatment. More glide will often become available between appointments. If the glide is perfect, that treatment is done; if it is not perfect, treat it again in a future appointment. Depending on the strength of the adhesion, two or more episodes of treatment may be necessary in a succession of appointments.

Six factor model: First barrier shear

TISSUE ENGAGEMENT

Therapeutic engagement is made by the therapist, who gently applies a shear force to the tissue at a first barrier. While unwinding phenomena commonly occur, engagement is *not* made by letting the client's body initiate the unwinding.

FORCE

First barrier.

SPEED

Slow. Following the tissue's lead as it releases, never rushing it.

CONSTRAINT

Low. Release is allowed in most directions, just not shortening in the direction in which the tissue is being elongated.

DIRECTIVENESS

Moderate to high. At any given moment, the tissue is being loaded in a particular direction. There is a distinct message given to the tissue-shear adhesion fibers to restore glide.

RELATIONSHIP TO FIRST BARRIER

Treatment of this variety is all done at a first barrier. The location of the first barrier incrementally changes as the tissue releases. Thus, treatment is applied at a succession of first barriers until either a final release is felt or edema is observed. Direction of force application is also usually changed several times during the treatment.

First barrier shear example 1

ASSESSMENT

General assessment leads to the right lower limb, confirmed by inhibition at the witness point at the right greater trochanter. A negative witness point result at the lateral malleolus rules out the ankle and foot.

In local assessment, a gliding inhibition on the leg suggests a primary restriction at the knee.

Manual thermal assessment, local listening, layer listening, and applied kinesiology questioning pinpoint a joint capsule adhesion on the medial aspect of the knee joint with the joint capsule adhered to the periosteum superior to the joint line.

CLIENT INQUIRY

Ask the client:

- how they have been feeling in general, and
- of their awareness of their knees.

MOBILITY TESTING

Active

- Ask the client to walk; observe gait, particularly with respect to the knees.

Passive knee joint

- Ask the client to lie supine on the table.
- Instruct the client to allow you to move their leg without either resisting or assisting.
- One at a time, test the range of motion of each knee, checking both range and ease of movement.

Passive capsular glide

- The joint capsule of the femero-tibial joint, like the capsule for most synovial joints, attaches to bone, not right at the joint line but some distance back on the bone. Stand at the side of the table on the side of the leg you are testing. Place a hand under the distal femur to provide dynamic stabilization.
- With a finger pad of the other hand, sink in to engage anterior–lateral focal areas of the material of the lateral aspect of the knee joint capsular, and attempt to glide

it medially and laterally on the distal centimeter of the femur.

- Shift your contact a finger width posterior and again engage the capsule and attempt to glide it posterior and anterior over the periosteum. Continue this pattern to incrementally test your way posterior around the distal femur.
- In this fashion, you can define the area of joint capsule which is adhered to the periosteum too close to the joint line. If more than one area of capsular adhesion is found, use local listening and inhibition to learn which is the more primary area.

TREATMENT

- Dynamically stabilize the distal femur with one hand. With the tip of the right index finger, sink to the depth of the adhesion between the joint capsule and the periosteum.
- At a moderately slow pace, drag this portion of capsular tissue posterior to a first barrier load.
- Maintain this dynamic load. As the adhesion begins to release, the capsular tissue will move a little. As it moves, maintain a first barrier load.
- This process may fully release the adhesion. Mobility test the glide of the capsular material just treated over the periosteum. If it is not fully freed, again engage the capsular material and load it anteriorly (opposite to the previous load). Again, wait for a series of releases.

POST TREATMENT TESTING AND INQUIRY

Use the standard post treatment procedure for mobility testing and question asking detailed in the introduction to treatment methods section. Either treat this same area further, as indicated by this inquiry, or return to general assessment.

First barrier shear example 2

ASSESSMENT

General assessment leads to an area of the lower right anterior chest wall.

Local assessment methods, including manual thermal assessment, local listening, layer listening, and yes–no questioning, refine this to an adhesion in the anterior portion of the right costo-diaphragmatic recess. This is a common adhesion of the parietal peritoneum on a portion of the respiratory diaphragm to the parietal peritoneum on the chest wall. Look for flaring out of portions of the costal arch. This is a signature for costo-diaphragmatic recess adhesion.

CLIENT INQUIRY

Ask the client:

- how they have been feeling in general
- how their breath has felt lately, and
- how they feel in the area of the primary restriction.

MOBILITY TESTING

Active

- Ask the client to extend their torso:
  - straight back
  - angled left back
  - angled right back.
- Ask the client to exhale fully and then take a full deep breath.

Passive

- Ask the client to lie supine on the table. Contact a portion of the costal arch and lower rib cage lateral to the area of the primary restriction. Sink into the chest wall.
- At a moderate pace, attempt to glide that focal area of chest wall superior. Allow this tissue to rest back to neutral.

- Shift your hand to the area of the primary restriction. Again, attempt to glide this portion of the chest wall superior. Compare these two areas.
- Shift your attention to the other side of the inferior chest wall. Make the same tests on that side for comparison.

TREATMENT

Again, contact the chest wall in the primary area of costo-diaphragmatic adhesion. Sink to the depth of the chest wall. At a moderately slow pace, move that portion of chest wall superior until a first barrier is encountered. Maintain a dynamic first barrier load in a superior direction. Each time the client takes a breath, the diaphragm will attempt to pull down away from the chest wall.

Do not instruct the client to take active control of their breath or even to focus awareness on breath; if you do, the client will inadvertently add tension to the system. Incrementally, you will feel release under your hand and the portion of chest wall you are loading will move a little more superior.

POST TREATMENT TESTING AND INQUIRY

Use the standard post treatment procedure for mobility testing and question asking detailed in the introduction to treatment methods section. Either treat this same area further, as indicated by this inquiry, or return to general assessment.

First barrier shear example 3

ASSESSMENT

General assessment points toward the central part of the lower abdomen just above the pubic symphysis.

Local assessment including local listening, manual thermal assessment, layer listening, and applied kinesiology questioning leads to a primary restriction which is an adhesion between some loops of small intestine and the floor of the peritoneum.

The inferior surface of the parietal peritoneum forms the partition between the abdominal cavity and the pelvic cavity, attaching to most of the perimeter of the true pelvis. The bladder is naturally attached to this portion of the parietal peritoneum. Normally there is a well lubricated glide plane of the loops of small intestine on the superior surface of this membrane.

CLIENT INQUIRY

Ask the client:

- how they are feeling in general
- of their awareness of their lower abdomen, and
- about bladder function.

Describe the situation to the client. Use anatomy illustrations and/or models.

MOBILITY TESTING

Active

- Ask the seated client to make trunk rotations left and right.

Passive

- Ask the client to lie supine on the table. Ask the client to give you a physical landmark by touching the superior surface of the pubic symphysis. Once the client has shown you this, use the fingers of one hand to contact the lower abdomen about one finger width superior to the pubic symphysis.
- Place the fingers of your other hand just superior to and adjacent to the fingers of the first hand. Sink in at a moderate pace until moderate resistance is felt. Attempt to glide the loops of the small intestines left then right on the dynamically stabilized tissue inferior to them.

TREATMENT

Return your hands to the original midline position. Move your hands slowly opposite each other to a first barrier. Maintain this first barrier as a dynamic load. Wait for tissue release which usually comes incrementally but may release all at once. Once substantial release is felt, remobility test this glide plane. If you need to treat it again, try a shear in the opposite direction.

POST TREATMENT TESTING AND INQUIRY

Use the standard post treatment procedure for mobility testing and question asking detailed in the introduction to treatment methods section. Either treat this same area further, as indicated by this inquiry, or return to general assessment.

Treatment method 22: middle barrier technique

Origin

Traditional osteopathic method. Discoverer not known.

Pretest

Observe alignment in the person's body both locally and globally. Test the end ranges of motion in the area to be treated. It is often useful to point these out to the client.

Treatment method

SETUP PHASE

At a moderate pace, compress the tissue to be treated noting the first barrier; continue to compress to near end-feel. Then, at a moderate pace, gradually release pressure until the first barrier is reached; do not release to less than the first barrier. Then compress again to near end-feel. Finally, at a moderate pace, release pressure just to a middle barrier.

TREATMENT PHASE

Maintain pressure at a middle barrier and follow unwinding, gently encouraging each release at its end. As needed, adjust the level of pressure within the middle third of the range to find a pressure that encourages release.

End of treatment

Several releases will be felt. Eventually there may be a larger or more general release, after which the sequence of releases will stop and the tissue will feel quieter, more relaxed, and more at ease.

Post test

Retest the end range in each dimension to see what change has occurred. Observe any change in alignment compared to the pretreatment condition.

VARIATION A

Combine with alternate interrupt unwinding: allow the first leg of unwind; when the second leg of unwind starts, give just enough counter force to prevent it. When the tissue changes to a new direction of unwind, allow this; as soon as it tries to change direction again, prevent the next movement. Continue to allow and prevent alternate movements.

See alternate interrupt method, page 113.

VARIATION B

Initiate treatment with stretch rather than compression. Stretch to near end range. Return to, but not less than, first barrier. Stretch to near end range, return to a middle barrier, and allow unwind.

This may be combined with variation A.

Middle barrier technique

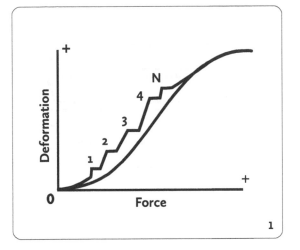

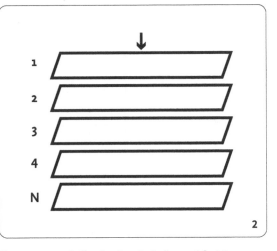

If a substance of uniform composition and texture is stretched, bent, or compressed it will exhibit a force-deformation curve similar to the smooth one in this illustration. Substances of mixed composition exhibit stepped deformation curves like the one in this frame. The steps in the curve are felt as small increases in resistance to pressure. We refer to these steps as effort barriers. We call the first step encountered as the first barrier, etc.

The sequence of effort barriers, including end-feel, is schematically visualized here as a series of surfaces. These do not represent actual surfaces or separate structures of any kind, rather they are the steps up in force showing in the diagram in frame 1.

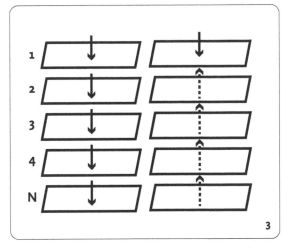

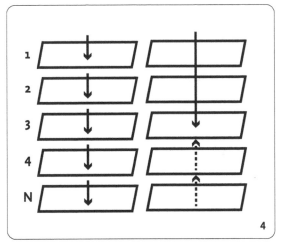

To begin this type of treatment, slowly compress, stretch, or bend the tissue, noting each effort barrier until end-feel is reached. Then slowly reduce the compressive, stretching, or bending load, again noting effort barriers in passing until the first effort barrier is reached. Do not release force to less than first barrier.

Again, slowly compress, stretch, or bend the tissue, noting each effort barrier until end-feel is reached. Begin to reduce the force applied until a middle barrier is released. This diagram shows five effort barriers, so the middle one is 3; there may be any number of barriers even or odd; choose one in the middle of the sequence.

Middle barrier technique (*cont.*)

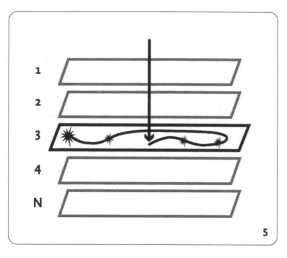

5

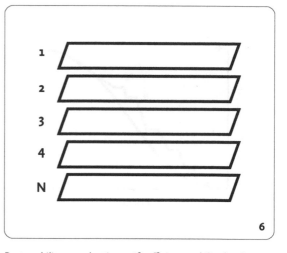

6

At this middle barrier, an unwind will begin. This may be treated as a classic unwind, alternate interrupt unwinding, or augmented unwinding. As usual, there will be several increments of release ending in a larger, more general release. Remove your hand.

Post mobility test the tissue. If sufficient mobility has been achieved you are done with this part of the treatment; return to general assessment. If mobility is not sufficient and if no hint of new inflammation is felt, treat the tissue again with either the same method or a different method. If any hint of inflammation is felt, make a note to reassess the area another day, and for now return to general assessment.

Six factor model: Middle barrier technique

TISSUE ENGAGEMENT

Tissue engagement is made by the therapist.

FORCE

Compressive force in the setup phase oscillates between first barrier and near end range.

SPEED

Low. Speed of inherent movement in the client's body is followed and matched. Due to the constraint applied in this method, fast tissue movement as a defense is very rarely seen. In these rare cases, when the speed is perceived as too high, the therapist slows the movement of the tissue.

CONSTRAINT

Low. During the treatment phase moderate compression is applied, but no movement is forbidden.

DIRECTIVENESS

None. No specific movement is sought.

RELATIONSHIP TO EFFORT BARRIERS

Setup: Using compression, move at a moderate pace from first barrier to end range, back to first barrier, again to end range, and out to a middle barrier.

Middle barrier example 1

Caution—This treatment and the associated testing must not be done on clients known to have osteoporosis or who have risk factors for osteoporosis but have not been recently tested for osteoporosis. Any other condition known to cause bone fragility is also a contraindication.

ASSESSMENT

General assessment leads to the right upper limb. Local assessment, including local listening, layer listening, manual thermal assessment, and applied kinesiology questions, leads to bone in the left humerus.

MOBILITY TESTING

Global active

- Ask the standing client to make several movements of each arm, one arm at a time:
  - elbow flexion, then extension
  - forward flexion of the arm at the shoulder
  - abduction of the arm at the shoulder
  - internal and external rotation at the shoulder
  - shoulder circumduction.

Global passive

- Standing at the client's right side, use your left hand to provide a gentle dynamic stabilization of the upper arm.
- Flex the elbow, return it to its natural hanging position, then gently attempt to hyperextend the elbow.

Repeat these tests on the other arm for comparison.

- Standing behind your seated client, place your left hand on the top of the right shoulder girdle. With your right hand, contact and control the right elbow so you can make shoulder joint movements while maintaining the elbow in a comfortably extended position:
  - forward flexion of the arm at the shoulder
  - abduction of the arm at the shoulder, then let the arm rest to the side
  - internal and external rotation at the shoulder
  - shoulder circumduction.

Repeat these tests on the other arm for comparison.

TREATMENT METHOD 22

Local passive

- Explain to the client what you propose to do, and its purpose.
- Ask the client to lie supine on the table.
- Sit behind or stand at your client's right side.
- With your two hands, grasp the two ends of the right humerus.
- Slowly attempt to bend the humerus a few degrees in a succession of directions:
  - frontal plane medial bow
  - frontal plane lateral bow
  - sagittal plane posterior bow
  - sagittal plane anterior bow
  - spiral around a longitudinal axis clockwise
  - spiral around a longitudinal axis counterclockwise.

Repeat these tests on the other humerus for comparison.

TREATMENT

With your client still supine on the table, sit or stand comfortably at the client's left side. With your two hands, grasp the proximal and distal ends of the humerus. At a moderately slow pace begin to make a longitudinal compression of the bone. Note the succession of barriers in passing. Do not pause for unwinding. When you arrive at a comfortable end-feel, begin to reduce your compression at a similarly moderate rate, noting barriers as you go. Also, in this phase, do not pause for unwinding to occur. Do not release your load to less than first barrier. When your pressure load has arrived at a first barrier, begin to compress again on the same longitudinal axis much as you did before. This time, when you arrive at end-feel, promptly begin to decompress until you arrive at a barrier in the middle third of the sequence of barriers. Fish for a barrier in the middle third where a robust unwind will proceed. Continue to treat at this force barrier near the

middle of the sequence of force barriers until unwinding stops in the usual way.

POST TREATMENT TESTING AND INQUIRY

Use the standard post treatment procedure for mobility testing and question asking detailed in the introduction to treatment methods section. Either treat this same area further, as indicated by this inquiry, or return to general assessment.

Middle barrier example 2

ASSESSMENT

General assessment points to the upper right limb, confirmed by an inhibitory contact at the right olecranon process.

Local assessment, including a gliding local listening, manual thermal assessment, layer listening, and yes–no questions, leads to an adhesion in the right subdeltoid bursa.

MOBILITY TESTING

Global active

- Ask the standing client to make several movements of each arm, one arm at a time.
  - forward flexion of the arm at the shoulder
  - abduction of the arm at the shoulder, then let the arm rest to the side
  - internal and external rotation at the shoulder
  - shoulder circumduction.

Global passive

- Standing behind your seated client, place your left hand on the top of the right shoulder girdle.
- With your left hand, contact and control the right elbow so you can make shoulder joint movements while maintaining the elbow in a comfortably extended position.

- forward flexion of the arm at the shoulder
- abduction of the arm at the shoulder, then let the arm rest to the side
- internal and external rotation at the shoulder
- shoulder circumduction.
- Repeat these tests on the other arm for comparison.

Local passive

- Explain to your client the purpose and method of the test you will do.
- With your client still standing, stand at your client's right side. Place your left hand on the medial aspect of the upper arm as superiorly in the axilla as you can comfortably go. Grasp the humerus and associated musculature.
- With your right hand, grasp the deltoid muscle. At a comfortable moderate pace, make anterior and posterior shearing movements between the tissue in your two hands to explore the integrity of the glide plane in the subdeltoid bursa.
- Perform the same test on the left arm for comparison.

TREATMENT

Ask the client to lie on the table in a supine position. Alternatively, a seated position may be used. Place your left hand as for the mobility test on the medial aspect of the upper right arm to give you control of the humerus. Place your right hand on the middle portion of the right deltoid muscle. At a moderately slow pace, begin to compact your two hands toward each other. This compresses tissue, including the adhered subdeltoid bursa. As you begin to compact, note the first force barrier in passing. Note each successive barrier, but do not stop to allow an unwinding. When you have arrived at a comfortable end range, begin to slack your pressure at a moderate rate, noting force

barriers as you back out. Stop at the first barrier; do not pass the first barrier. Promptly begin to compress the tissue again in the same fashion as before, noting force barriers as you go, but not pausing for unwinding. When you have again arrived at a comfortable end-feel, begin to reduce your compression at a moderate rate. When you have arrived at the middle of the succession of force barriers, fish for a barrier where a robust unwind will occur. Wait for the usual signs of completion of an unwind.

POST TREATMENT TESTING AND INQUIRY

Use the standard post treatment procedure for mobility testing and question asking detailed in the introduction to treatment methods section. Either treat this same area further, as indicated by this inquiry, or return to general assessment.

Middle barrier example 3

ASSESSMENT

General assessment leads to the right margin of the abdomen.

Local assessment leads to an adhesion of the lateral aspect of the visceral peritoneum of the ascending colon and the parietal peritoneum of the right lateral abdominal wall.

MOBILITY TESTING

Global active

- Ask the client to sit on a stool or bench. Ask the client to:
  - side bend right, return to center, then side bend left
  - rotate the trunk left, return to center, then rotate to the right.

Local passive

- Explain to the client the mobility test you wish to perform and its purpose.
- Ask the client to lie supine on the table. Support the client's knees on one or two

pillows to give a little slack to the abdominal wall without the client engaging muscles to hold the knees up.

- Palpate for and locate the cecum and ascending colon. Palpate for and locate the lateral border of the ascending colon and cecum. Assess the integrity of the glide plane between the lateral aspect of the ascending colon and the lateral body wall by gently attempting to glide your fingertips into this potential space. All or part of this glide plane may be adhered. If more than one portion of this glide plane is adhered, use local listening and inhibition to determine which portion of the adhesion is the more primary.

TREATMENT

With the client still supine on the table and standing or sitting comfortably at the client's right side, contact the right half of the client's abdominal wall with your two hands. Create some slack in the abdominal wall by using your hand to move tissue from the midline laterally. Sink adjacent fingertips of the two hands gently toward the potential cleft between the lateral aspect of the colon and the lateral abdominal wall. With the heels of your hands, gently compress the ascending colon and the lateral body wall toward each other. Begin to allow the tissue to spring back from this compression, watching for the first barrier and successive force barriers as you go. When you have arrived at neutral at the end of this medial–lateral compression, use your fingertips to begin to pull the ascending colon and the lateral body wall away from each other in a medial–lateral direction in a frontal plane. Continue to observe the succession of barriers. Do not pause for unwinding.

When you have arrived at a comfortable end-feel, again begin to bring the ascending colon and lateral body wall toward each other. Initially, this will be a relaxation of the stretching apart that you just made. After passing a stretch/compression neutral you will begin to compress the colon and body wall together. Do not pause to allow unwinding to occur at any barrier. Again, begin to move the right body wall and the ascending colon away from each other as you initially did. When you arrive at a comfortable end-feel, again allow the ascending colon and right body wall to begin to spring back toward each other as you progressively relax your stretch load at a moderate pace. When you have arrived at the middle of the force barrier succession, fish for a force barrier in that mid-range where a robust unwind will happen. Stay at this force barrier with a dynamic load as the tissue unwinds. Continue until the usual signs of unwind completion are felt.

POST TREATMENT TESTING AND INQUIRY

Use the standard post treatment procedure for mobility testing and question asking detailed in the introduction to treatment methods section. Either treat this same area further, as indicated by this inquiry, or return to general assessment.

Treatment method 23: flossing

Origin
Jeffrey Burch.

Concept
It is often beneficial to address issues of glide and elasticity together at the same time. The flossing method is designed to address both issues together. Request for release in particular directions make flossing more directive than many other methods.

This method was originally designed for linear structures such as nerves and blood vessels, but can be successfully applied to other structures, even blocky bones.

Method
Make two points of contact on the same structure more or less distant from each other. The contacts should be arranged so that it is possible to both gently stretch the structure between the two points of contact, and at the same time glide the structure as a whole through neighboring tissues.

Once the two points of contact are established, stretch the structure to a first barrier between the two contacts.

Once the linear stretch is established along the structure, also move both hands in the same direction to glide the structure through neighboring tissue. This results in the leading hand moving slightly faster than the following hand to maintain both stretch and glide loads at first barrier. Both aspects of load are moving targets.

The difference between the glide rate of the leading hand and the trailing hand is determined entirely by the rate of therapeutic elongation of the structure in response to the first barrier stretch established by the therapist.

When a limit of glide is reached, continue to maintain the stretch on the structure and reverse the direction of glide. Continue to glide the stretched structure back and forth several times until a more general release is perceived, and/or sufficient glide and span are achieved. While the therapist-determined direction of stretch and glide is maintained, other dimensions are allowed to unwind in the usual way. Loads applied by the therapist are all first barrier; however, this technique is neither specifically a near first barrier, nor a far first barrier technique.

This technique is highly directive; the therapist imposes his intent to concurrently lengthen the structure and to improve its glide.

Variations

1. Additional dimensions, such as torsion and side bending, can be loaded in either ease or effort. In this variation, the technique is mixed in the sense that the direction of stretch is determined by the therapist without respect to near first barrier or far first barriers, while other dimensions are loaded with respect to ease or effort first barriers.

2. Long levers may be used. For example, if you are working on a blood vessel in a limb, also move the segments of the limb being treated into combinations of ease and effort to facilitate release. For example, contact the left brachial artery and left radial artery. Set up flossing along the arterial line between the two, then fish for position with the shoulder joint, elbow, and wrist to facilitate release.

3. The client can also be directed to move slowly in ways that encourage release, particularly aspects of glide.

4. Surprisingly, flossing may be initiated with compaction rather than stretch. This variation is depicted on page 248.

Six factor model: Flossing

TISSUE ENGAGEMENT

Engagement is made by the therapist.

FORCE

Low—first barriers only.

SPEED

Slow. In the direction of glide, the movement is determined by the body's ability to release in response to a first barrier load, which will be slow. In other dimensions, inherent movements in the client's body are followed and matched, also slow.

CONSTRAINT

Mixed. In the direction of stretch and glide, the therapist determines the movement. In all other dimensions, the movement is not constrained.

DIRECTIVENESS

Mixed. In the direction of stretch and glide, dimension is strongly directive. No direction is given to movement in any other direction.

RELATIONSHIP TO EFFORT BARRIERS

In two aspects of one dimension, stretch and glide, first barrier force is consistently applied. In all other dimensions, free movement is allowed and then encouraged to a first barrier at changes of direction.

Flossing

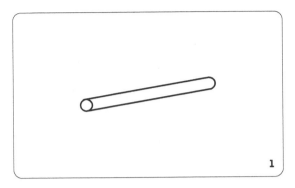

1

The flossing treatment technique was created to restore the elasticity and glide of nerves and blood vessels. Use of this treatment method has been extended to many other tissues. For nerves, long lever handles provide a measure of safety.

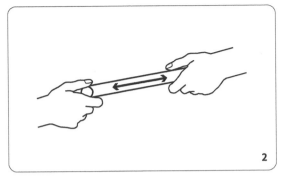

2

Using contacts at two ends of a structure, exert and maintain a first barrier stretch load.

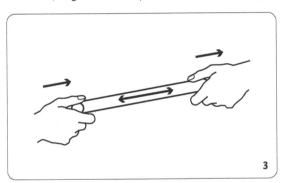

3

While continuously maintaining a first barrier stretch load, slowly glide the structure in one direction. Glide at a pace at which the tissue can easily change. This is often a first barrier load.

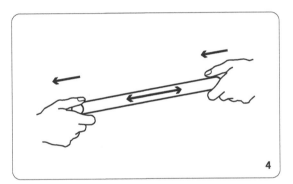

4

When a limit of glide is reached in the first direction, reverse the direction of glide, all the while maintaining the stretch load.

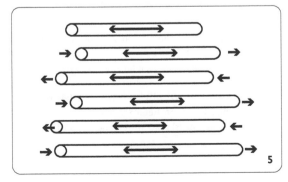

5

While continuously maintaining a stretch, load alternate directions of glide. The tissue will become progressively longer and its movement through adjacent tissue will also improve.

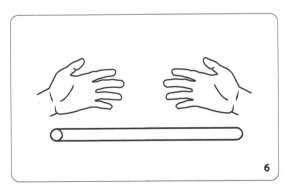

6

When a larger scale more general release is felt, stop the treatment, remove your hands, and post-mobility test.

Compaction initiated flossing

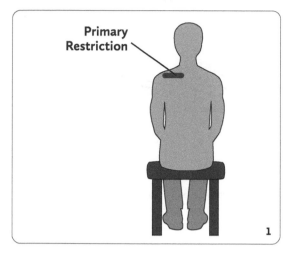

Locate a primary restriction. Mobility test the tissue.

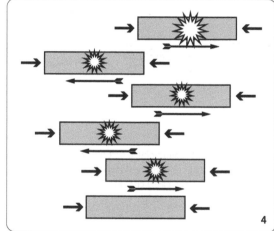

Compact the lesion along its long axis to a middle barrier.

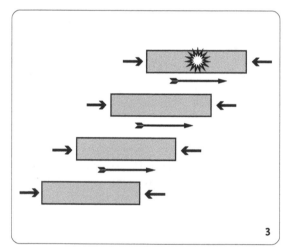

While maintaining the compaction, glide the structure in a particular direction to a comfortable anatomic limit. During this glide unwinding may or may not occur, permit unwinding if it does occur while maintaining the compaction and glide. Unwinding is less likely than with stretch-initiated flossing. A release will likely but not necessarily be felt at the end of the glide.

Continuing to maintain compaction, glide the structure in the opposite direction to a comfortable anatomic limit. Continue to glide the structure back and forth between anatomic limits. The excursion is likely to increase a little with each pass. When a larger release is felt, the treatment episode is done. Return to assessment. Perform the same mobility test(s) used in step one as a post test.

Flossing example 1

ASSESSMENT

General assessment leads to the posterior aspect of the thorax.

In local assessment, manual thermal assessment, local listening, layer listening, and applied kinesiology pinpoint a stripe of investing fascia running vertically over the right erector spinae muscles from about T3 to T9 and varying from 0.5 to 1.5 cm in width.

CLIENT INQUIRY

Ask the client:

- how they have been feeling in general, and
- of their awareness of their upper back.

MOBILITY TESTING

Global active

Ask the seated client to:

- Roll down through their spine, starting with letting their head fall forward and then progressively rolling down from the top; then reverse this stacking the spine
- Rotate the trunk left, return to center, rotate to the right, then return to center.

Global passive

- With the client still seated, sit behind the client. Use your two hands to contact the lateral parts of the thorax a little inferior to the axillae.
- From this position, make a spiral motion of the client's trunk first lifting and vertically elongating the right side as you turn the client to the left.
- Return the client to center, then lift and vertically elongate the left side of the trunk while rotating the client to the right.

Focal passive

- Have the client either seated or prone with the head in a face cradle so there is no rotation of the neck. Use your two hands to make two contacts on the skin over the right paraspinal muscles, somewhat lateral to the area of primacy.
- Sink to the level of the investing fascia. With your two hands, make a linear vertical stretch of the tissue to test to a comfortable end feel the elasticity of the investing fascia.
- Shift your hands medially to the area of perceived primacy; again stretch vertically superior–inferior to test elasticity of tissue.
- Shift your hands more medial and similarly test the elasticity of a third parallel stripe of investing fascia.

TREATMENT

Return your hands to the two ends of the primary lesion area of investing fascia overlying the right spinal erector muscles. Sink through the skin into the superficial fascia. Move your two contacts slightly toward each other creating slack in the skin and superficial fascia. Maintaining the slack in the skin and superficial fascia, sink further into the investing fascia. Stretch the investing fascia vertically to a first barrier. Maintain this first barrier stretch as you slowly move both hands in a superior direction to an anatomic limit. As you move both hands in a superior direction, maintain the first barrier stretch on the investing fascia by leading slightly with the superior hand and maintaining a slight drag with the inferior hand. After you have arrived at an anatomic limit, reverse directions, now leading inferiorly with the inferior hand. Continue inferiorly to an anatomic limit. Again, reverse directions. Work back and forth alternately superiorly and inferiorly until a general sense of release is felt.

POST TREATMENT TESTING AND INQUIRY
Use the standard post treatment procedure for mobility testing and question asking detailed in the introduction to treatment methods section. Either treat this same area further, as indicated by this inquiry, or return to general assessment.

Flossing example 2
ASSESSMENT
General assessment leads to the right side of the face.

In local assessment, manual thermal assessment, local listening, layer listening, and applied kinesiology pinpoint this as extracranial branches of the right facial nerve serving the cheek. The external branches of the facial nerve (cranial nerve VII) emerge from the neurocranium through the stylomastoid foramen in the temporal bone. The branches indicated here spread out anteriorly in the cheek.

CLIENT INQUIRY
Ask the client:

- how they have been feeling in general, and
- of their awareness of their head, face, jaw joints, and neck.

MOBILITY TESTING
Active focal

Ask the client to move their mandible in a succession of directions:

- open mouth wide
- thrust jaw forward
- move jaw left
- move jaw right.

Passive focal

- Ask the client to lie supine on the table.

Sit comfortably at the head end of the table.
- Place your left hand broadly on the left side of the head to support it. Place the fingers of your right hand broadly on the right cheek. With your right hand, gently stretch tissue on the right cheek anterior.
- Reverse these directions to test the left cheek. While stiffness in other structures could limit this stretch it is specific for facial branches of the seventh cranial nerve.

TREATMENT
This treatment will utilize a method known as source and target treatment. In this method, the bone(s) that a nerve emerges from is used to control one end of a nerve, and the tissue the nerve innervates is used to control the other end of the nerve. This is a double long lever treatment which is a safer way of working on a nerve than contacting the nerve directly.

Shift your right hand so the fingers and portions of the palm are under the occiput and the thumb lies anterior-laterally on the mastoid process of the temporal bone. Reach across with the fingers of your left hand to contact the right cheek. Sink into a moderate depth. Initially slack the tissue on the right cheek posteriorly. From there, use the fingers of your left hand to slowly move tissue of the right cheek anteriorly to a first barrier. At this first barrier engagement, you will also feel a tendency of the right mastoid process to move anterior-laterally. Initially provide just enough back pressure to dynamically prevent this movement of the mastoid process. Once this first barrier stretch of these branches of the facial nerve is established, use the thumb of your right hand to slowly move the mastoid process further posterior-medial. Maintaining the stretch load to the cheek at a first barrier level, allow the fingers of your left hand to move posteriorly following the pull on the facial nerve generated by your movement of the mastoid process. When you reach end-feel, promptly reverse directions using your left hand to slowly drag tissue of the right cheek anterior, as you slack your right thumb pressure on the mastoid process at a rate which maintains the first barrier stretch between your two hands. When end-feel is encountered at an anatomic limit in this direction, again reverse directions. Continue to work back and forth in this fashion between your mastoid contact and your cheek contact until a generalized release is felt.

POST TREATMENT TESTING AND INQUIRY

Use the standard post treatment procedure for mobility testing and question asking detailed in the introduction to treatment methods section. Either treat this same area further, as indicated by this inquiry, or return to general assessment.

Flossing example 3

Caution—Do not perform vascular manipulation if there is any known vascular fragility or the slightest suspicion of it. This includes but is not limited to: vascular type Ehlers Danlos syndrome, any clotting disorder, either phlebitis or insufficient clotting, aneurism current or past, or current use of blood thinners.

Question thoroughly. Err on the side of caution.

ASSESSMENT

General assessment leads to the right upper limb. This assessment is supported by a witness point at the right olecranon process.

In local assessment, manual thermal assessment, local listening, layer listening, and applied kinesiology pinpoint this as the right radial artery.

CLIENT INQUIRY

Ask the client:

- how they have been feeling in general, and

- of their awareness of their right arm and hand.

MOBILITY TESTING

Global active

Ask the client to make a fist, then extend the fingers, and check the following:

- Wrist mobility
  - flexion
  - extension
  - radial deviation
  - ulnar deviation
  - circumduction.
- Elbow mobility
  - flexion
  - extension.

Global passive

- With your hands, move the client's hand and forearm in all the above directions noting range, and ease within range.

Focal passive

- Perform an Allen's test for perfusion of the hand discriminating the contribution of the radial artery and the ulnar artery.
- Client makes a clenched fist and holds it for 30 seconds.
- With the fist still clenched, use your thumbs to put pressure on both the radial and ulnar arteries on this hand at the wrist, just enough to occlude blood flow.
- Client opens and relaxes the hand, which should appear blanched.
- Release pressure on the ulnar artery only. Note how well and quickly the hand re-perfuses.
- Repeat the above steps but release the ulnar radial artery only. Again, note how well and quickly the hand re-perfuses.

- Perform the same test on the other hand for comparison.
- Sink in to contact the right radial artery at the wrist. Gently drag it first distally and then proximally. Release the artery.
- Sink in to contact the right ulnar artery at the wrist. Gently drag it first distally and then proximally. Release the artery.
- With the fingers of one hand, locate the pulse of a distal portion of the right brachial artery on the medial side of the upper arm in the cleft between the biceps and triceps muscles. With a finger of the other hand contact the radial artery. Gently move these two contacts away from each other to assess the elasticity of the artery. Repeat this test for the ulnar artery.

TREATMENT

Using the contacts on the right brachial and ulnar arteries used in the last mobility test, gently move the fingers of the two hands away from each other, the brachial end proximal, and the radial end distal. Load this arterial continuity to a first barrier. Leading with the brachial end, glide the gently stretched artery proximal to a soft, comfortable end-feel. The force applied in gliding the artery should also be at a first barrier load. Reverse directions, leading with the radial end to drag the artery distal while maintaining the first barrier stretch on it. When a soft comfortable end-feel is encountered, again reverse directions. Continue to gently drag the artery alternately proximally and distally while maintaining a dynamic first barrier stretch on it, until a generalized release is felt.

POST TREATMENT TESTING AND INQUIRY

Use the standard post treatment procedure for mobility testing and question asking detailed in the introduction to treatment methods section. Either treat this same area further, as indicated by this inquiry, or return to general assessment.

Treatment method 24: circle flossing

Origin
Jeffrey Burch.

Concept
Flossing treatment technique was originally developed for long linear structures. Sometimes these structures bend around corners, so flossing technique takes on a rope on pulley shape. Flossing was originally initiated with a gentle tissue stretch. Later it was discovered that flossing could be initiated with a gentle compaction. Combining and extending these ideas provides a way to treat structures located deep in the body where linear flossing is not possible.

This method is particularly useful for small joints deeper in the body such as spinal facet joints. It may be used for other structures which are not fully accessible.

Pretreatment assessment

- Assess mobility both active and passive.
- Assess alignment.

Treatment
The outer surface of facet joints are approachable with compressive long levers. Portions of the joint farther from the surface of the body cannot be so directly contacted.

Consider a joint as a circle perpendicular to the surface of the body. The portion of the circumference of this circle nearest the surface of the body will present as a line which can be described as having left and right, or superior and inferior, ends. Approach this projected line segment with the tips of two fingers, one finger at each end. Compress moderately with both fingers toward the ends of the projected line. From this initial moderate two-point compression, increase the pressure on only one of the fingers while slowly decreasing the pressure on the other point. This will result in a pressure wave around the deeper portions of the circumference of the joint. Maintain a sense of contact between the two fingertips through this circumference. As you reach a limit of compression with one finger, change directions so you are now slowly reducing the compression with that finger at the same time you correspondingly increase pressure with the other finger, all the while maintaining the sense of circumferential pressure wave between the two fingers. Continue in this direction until an anatomic limit is reached. Then again reverse directions. Continue to alternate the pressure between the two fingers. Tissue will be felt to soften as you progress through several alternations of pressure wave.

Stop when any of the following occur.

- A broader, more generalized sense of tissue relief is felt.
- Fluid filling of the area occurs, possibly accompanied by warming. This is a sign of inflammation.
- Substantial release is felt to have occurred.

Post treatment testing and inquiry
Use the standard post treatment procedure for mobility testing and question asking detailed in the introduction to treatment methods section. Either treat this same area further, as indicated by this inquiry, or return to general assessment.

Six factor model: Circle flossing
TISSUE ENGAGEMENT
Made by the therapist.

FORCE
Moderately low. The amount of force used is the minimum to establish a felt sense of connection around the deep side of the structure being treated.

SPEED

Slow. Speed is adjusted along with force to maintain a connection around the deep side of a structure at a pace which allows tissue to change. Too slow will lose control for staying in the therapeutic range. Too fast will engage defenses.

CONSTRAINT

None to low. Specific movements are not expressly forbidden, but movement other than the required movement is unlikely due to the level of directiveness.

DIRECTIVENESS

High. While a dialog is maintained with the tissue to stay in a therapeutic range of forces, direction is constantly given for how the tissue is to move.

RELATIONSHIP TO EFFORT BARRIERS

None. First, second, or subsequent barriers are not assessed. Force used is gauged by therapeutic response. The force used is moderately low but not calibrated with respect to force barrier steps.

Circle flossing

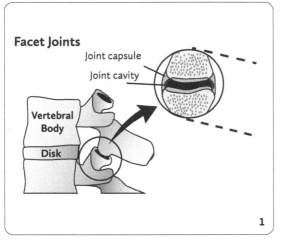

Circle flossing is useful for any structure such as a facet joint where it would be anatomically challenging to set up linear flossing on the deep side of the structure.

Here we see the facet joint in its relationship deep to the skin. It would be physically difficult to organize a flossing treatment for the joint capsule around its full perimeter.

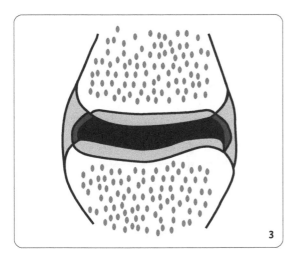

Here we are looking down on the facet joint through the skin as if the skin and muscle were transparent.

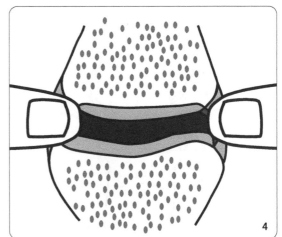

With two finger pads, contact the skin over the margins of the facet joint. With both fingers, sink in to engage the capsule of the facet joint.

Circle flossing (*cont.*)

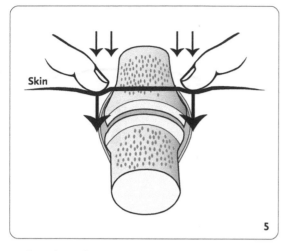

5

Apply moderate fingertip pressure through the skin down toward each side of the joint capsule. The pressure is initially equal on the two sides.

6

Slowly reduce the pressure on one side of the joint while maintaining the same pressure on the other side of the joint. This will produce a circular pressure wave through the deep side of the joint capsule.

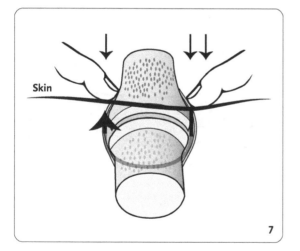

7

Continuing to maintain a constant pressure connection between the two finger contacts down around the deep side of the joint, slowly reverse the pressures applied by the two fingers. Start by slowly pressing in with the finger that was less deep before; as you feel the pressure response in the other finger, allow that fingertip to slowly rise up, maintaining the pressure wave connection between the two fingers.

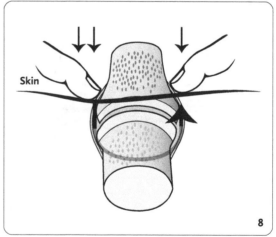

8

Continue to toggle the pressure slowly back and forth between the two fingers until a generalized softening is felt. Then lift both fingers off. Then mobility test the joint again to see how much mobility improvement has been made.

Circle flossing example 1

ASSESSMENT

General assessment points to the left lower limb. This general assessment is supported by an inhibitory contact at the left greater trochanter and refined to the foot or ankle by an inhibitory contact at the left lateral malleolus.

Local assessment including manual thermal assessment, local listening and inhibition, layer listening, and applied kinesiology questioning refines this to the medial articulation of the talo-calcaneal joint complex. The broad articulation area between the inferior surface of the talus and the superior surface of the calcaneus usually has three separate synovial joints with a hollow area between them. The most medial of these three synovial joints is between the sustentaculum-tali projection of the calcaneus and a corresponding medial projection of the talus.

CLIENT INQUIRY

Ask the client:

- how they are feeling in general, and
- in their feet.

MOBILITY ASSESSMENT

Global active

- Ask the client to walk barefoot. Observe gait, particularly with respect to the feet and ankles.

Local active

- Ask the client to lie supine on the table with feet just off the end of the table. In this position ask the client to:
  - dorsiflex and plantarflex each foot
  - circumduct each foot.

Local passive

- Explain to the client the method and purpose of your test.

- With the client supine on the table, heels just off the end of the table, use one of your hands to dynamically stabilize the talus bone with one hand. With the other hand, control the calcaneus bone. Move the calcaneus in a succession of directions on the talus:
  - anterior glide
  - posterior glide
  - medial glide
  - lateral glide
  - circumduction in a transverse plane
  - tilt the inferior part of the calcaneus medial, opening the lateral part of the joints
  - tilt the inferior part of the calcaneus lateral, opening the lateral part of the joint.
- Make a similar set of local active and passive tests on the other hindfoot for comparison.

TREATMENT

Ask the client to lie left side down on the table. Offer pillows for the client's head, in front of their torso, and one under the right leg, which is flexed at knee and hip, so the right foot lies anterior to the left foot. Stand behind the client facing their left foot. Locate the left sustentaculum-tali bony projection of the calcaneus, and the joint at its superior surface. Place the tip of one index finger at the posterior edge of the sustentaculum-tali joint, and the tip of your other index finger at the anterior edge of the sustentaculum-tali joint. With both fingers slowly press into the soft tissue at the anterior and posterior margins of this joint to a comfortable end-feel. Then slowly begin to reduce the pressure with your right index finger. As you reduce this pressure, you will find the tip of your left index finger sinking in deeper. Following this natural tendency, maintain a sense of connection between your two fingers around the deep side of the joint. At a point where pressure with the retreating right fingertip approaches losing contact with this pressure wave around the deep side of the joint, reverse your pressure loading, slowly sinking the right fingertip in deeper and allowing the left index finger to retreat from its deeper loading while maintaining the sense of connection between the two fingertips around the deep side of the sustentaculum-tali joint. Continue to toggle the pressure between these two fingers back and forth until a more general sense of release is felt.

POST TREATMENT TESTING AND INQUIRY

Use the standard post treatment procedure for mobility testing and question asking detailed in the introduction to treatment methods section. Either treat this same area further, as indicated by this inquiry, or return to general assessment.

Circle flossing example 2

ASSESSMENT

General assessment points to the right upper limb. This general assessment is supported by an inhibitory contact at the right olecranon process.

Local assessment including manual thermal assessment, local listening and inhibition, layer listening, and applied kinesiology questioning refines this to the right acromioclavicular joint.

CLIENT INQUIRY

Ask the client:

- how they are feeling in general, and
- in their shoulders.

MOBILITY ASSESSMENT

Global active

- Ask the client to walk barefoot. Observe gait, particularly with respect to arm swing.

Global passive

- Stand behind the client with your body shifted a little to the right rather than centered behind the client. Place your left hand on the top of the client's right shoulder girdle, creating a dynamic stabilization of the shoulder girdle. With your right hand, hold the client's right elbow so you can passively circumduct the right gleno-humeral joint while gently maintaining the elbow in comfortable extension.

- Move your left hand to the top of the client's left shoulder girdle as close to the base of the neck as possible. Place the tip of your left thumb against the left lateral aspect of the first thoracic spinous process. Use these contacts to dynamically stabilize the upper trunk. Place the palm of your right hand over the right upper deltoid muscle area with your fingers on the glenoid region of the scapula. With your right hand, successively protract, retract, and elevate the scapula over the trunk, allowing the shoulder girdle to rest to neutral between each movement.

Local active

- Ask the client to sequentially circumduct each shoulder.
- Ask the client to sequentially protract, retract, and elevate each shoulder.

Local passive

- Explain to the client the method and purpose of your test.
- Ask the client to lie supine on the table. Stand at the head end of the table.
- With your left hand, make a dynamic stabilization of the distal end of the right clavicle.
- With fingers of your right hand, control the right acromion process, and the rest of your hand more distal on the

shoulder. With this right-handed control of the scapula, move the scapula on the clavicle successively sheared anterior, posterior, superior, and inferior, then successively protracted and retracted.

- Make a similar set of local passive movement tests on the left shoulder for comparison.

TREATMENT

With the client still supine on the table, place the tip of your left index finger on the anterior edge of the right acromioclavicular joint, and the tip of your right index finger on the posterior edge of the same acromioclavicular joint.

With both fingers, slowly press into the soft tissue at the anterior and posterior margins of this joint to a comfortable end-feel. Then slowly begin to reduce the pressure with your right index finger. As you reduce this pressure, you will find the tip of your left index finger sinking in deeper. Following this natural tendency, maintain a sense of connection between your two fingers around the deep side of the joint. At a point where pressure with the retreating right fingertip approaches losing contact with this pressure wave around the deep side of the joint, reverse your pressure loading. Slowly sink the right fingertip in deeper and allow the left index finger to retreat from its deeper loading while maintaining the sense of connection between the two fingertips around the deep side of the acromioclavicular joint. Continue to toggle the pressure between these two fingers back and forth until a more general sense of release is felt.

POST TREATMENT TESTING AND INQUIRY

Use the standard post treatment procedure for mobility testing and question asking detailed in the introduction to treatment methods section. Either treat this same area further, as indicated by this inquiry, or return to general assessment.

Circle flossing example 3

ASSESSMENT

General assessment points to the right lower limb. This general assessment is supported by an inhibitory contact at the left greater trochanter. A negative result for inhibition at the right lateral malleolus rules out the foot or ankle.

Local assessment, including manual thermal assessment, local listening and inhibition, layer listening, and applied kinesiology questioning, refines this to the bursa between the iliopsoas tendon and the femur immediately superior to the insertion of the iliopsoas tendon at the lesser trochanter.

CLIENT INQUIRY

Ask the client:

- how they are feeling in general, and
- in their hips and legs.

MOBILITY ASSESSMENT

Global active

- Ask the client to walk barefoot. Observe gait, particularly with respect to the hips.

Local active

- Ask the client to make a gentle lunge movement with each leg. Compare relative extension of the two hips.

Global passive

- Ask the client to lie supine on the table. Stand at the client's right side.
- With your right hand, support the right leg a little distally to the knee joint to rotate and abduct the right leg while dynamically stabilizing the right hemi pelvis with your left hand on the anterior ilium concurrently, internally.
- Note range and ease of movement. Return

the leg to its resting position. Test the same movement for the other hip.

Local passive

- Explain to the client the method and purpose of your test. Place fingertips of your right hand on the anterior–medial thigh at the level of the inferior edge of the greater trochanter. Glide your left hand under the client's upper thigh to place fingertips directly posterior to the tips of your right hand. Let the palms of both hands be in contact with the thigh. Working between your fingertips and your palms, attempt to glide the tissue immediately adjacent to this superior–medial portion of the femur successively anteriorly and posteriorly with respect to the femur. This tests glide in the bursa.
- Test the same area on the left thigh in the same way for comparison.

TREATMENT
In the other circle flossing examples in this section, the flossing was around half to two-thirds of the circumference of a joint. This one is at most around the curve of one-third of the circumference of the femur, yet the principles and method are the same.

Return to stand or sit at the client's right side. Place your hands as you did for the bursa glide test with the fingertips of one hand anterior to the medial aspect of the shaft of the femur just inferior to the greater trochanter, and the other hand immediately posterior to it.

With both fingers, slowly press into the soft tissue approaching the medial portion of the femur from anterior and posterior, thus approaching the bursa and adjacent surfaces of the femur. With the fingertips of both hands, press in toward the bursa to a comfortable end-feel. Then slowly begin to reduce the pressure with your left index finger. As you reduce this pressure, you will find the tip of your right index finger sinking in deeper. Follow this natural tendency, maintaining a sense of connection between your two fingers around the medial surface of the proximal femoral shaft. At a point where pressure with the retreating left fingertip approaches losing contact with this pressure wave around the deep side of the joint, reverse your pressure loading, slowly sinking the left fingertip in deeper and allowing the right index finger to retreat from its deeper loading while maintaining the sense of connection between the two fingertips around the medial side of the femur. Continue to toggle the pressure between these two fingers back and forth until a more general sense of release is felt.

POST TREATMENT TESTING AND INQUIRY
Use the standard post treatment procedure for mobility testing and question asking detailed in the introduction to treatment methods section. Either treat this same area further, as indicated by this inquiry, or return to general assessment.

LEVERAGE PRINCIPLES THAT MAY BE USED WITH MANY TECHNIQUES

This section discusses ways in which leverage is applied for treatment. There are several possibilities and combinations.

- Treatment may be made directly in contact with a structure.
- Treatment can also be accomplished from a distance using other tissues for leverage.
- It is possible to have one hand directly in contact with a structure and the other hand applying treatment from a distance.
- Another possibility is leverage from each of two distant areas, one in each of the therapist's hands.
- The client can also be asked to position some of their body parts to change the leverage situation internally.

Treatment levers: long and short and mixed for functional methods

Origin
Early osteopathic technique. Likely discovered by A. T. Still MD.

Definition
Treatment can be made either directly on a structure or by use of leverage from a distant body part. We call treatment directly on a structure short lever treatment, and treatment from a distant part long lever treatment.

Treatments may be mixed long and short with one contact directly on the structure being treated and the other hand at some distance away.

In Europe, the term "short lever" is synonymous with "functional direct technique," and "long lever" is synonymous with "functional indirect technique." The lever length names are the more descriptive, and knowing about them helps make sense out of the direct/indirect terminology. In North America, the terms "direct" and "indirect" have taken on meanings which are not only entirely different from the European use of the words, but also highly inconsistent among North American therapists, to the point of being contradictory: see A proposal for clear terminology in the introduction to this part.

EXAMPLES
Tensor fascia lata muscle

- Treatment directly contacting the muscle is short lever treatment.
- Treatment with one hand stabilizing the pelvis and the other hand moving the leg from the knee and calf is long lever treatment.
- Treatment with one hand on the muscle and the other manipulating the leg from the calf is mixed long and short lever treatment.

Pubovesical ligament

- Treatment by fingertip pressure directly on the ligament is short lever treatment.
- Treatment by grasping the pubic bone with one hand and the bladder with the other is long lever treatment.
- Treatment with a finger directly on the ligament and the other hand on the bladder is mixed long and short lever treatment.

Application in conjunction with other methods
Long and short levers are not standalone methods. Whether the leverage is long, short, or mixed, treatment choices may be any other methods.

Anatomical choice limitation and relativity

Some structures such as the dural tube or the spleen cannot be contacted directly and therefore may only be treated with long lever methods.

Perspective

Few structures other than skin can be contacted directly. Most treatment is therefore long lever. For all tissues other than skin, the question becomes "How long is the lever?" rather than "Is the lever short or long?"

Reverse long lever treatment

While working with any structure in any form of leverage, long, short, or mixed, a line of tension may be noted toward any more or less distant structure or region. Noting this line of tension toward any more or less distant structure is called *referred listening*. An additional line of treatment may then be established from the structure being treated toward the distant structure.

Multiple long levers and chains of lesions

Returning to the example of the tensor fascia muscle, this muscle is innervated by the superior gluteal nerve that arises from L4, L5, and S1. There may be physical tension in one or more of these nerve roots that creates apparent physical tension in the muscle. To assess this, have the client lie supine. Reach under, and with relaxed fingertips contact L4, L5, and S1. With the other hand, contact the tensor fascia lata muscle. Gently traction the muscle anterior–inferior and observe any relative motion of L4, L5, and S1. If, for example, L5 rotates when the muscle is tractioned, this suggests the nerve root extending from it toward the muscles has physical tension in it. Try physically rotating the vertebra further in this direction and then retest the stretch of the TFL muscle; if the muscle now seems less tense, this adds evidence to the possibility of tension in the nerve. Then move the vertebra in the opposite direction and again test the stretch of the TFL muscle. If the TFL now appears more tense than before, this adds yet further evidence for tension in the TFL muscle.

Treatment can now be organized using the vertebra as a long lever handle. This can be combined with the other hand directly on the TFL muscle to give one long and one short lever. Alternatively, one hand can be on the vertebra and the other hand supporting and controlling the lower leg giving two long levers. Choices of near first barrier, far first barrier, or mixed first barriers can be made in either of these configurations.

Client-assisted long levers

A referred listening may be noted when the therapist's hands are fully occupied. In this situation, the client can be asked to very slowly move body parts to achieve long lever treatment.

Example: If a facet joint restriction is noted in the neck, treatment can be organized by contacting the transverse process of the lower segment and the spinous process of the upper segment. Since the ligaments of the facet joint are not directly contacted, this is a double long lever treatment. Client-assisted long levers can then be added in several ways, including:

1. Client has both knees up. Both knees are moved extremely slowly left or right. At some point, a line of tension will be observed into the joint being treated.
2. Client slowly rolls an arm internally or externally until a line of tension is noted into the area being treated.
3. Client moves the mandible left, right, anterior, posterior, and/or opening/closing the mouth until lines of tension are noted.
4. Client slowly shifts the eyes to gaze left, right, superior, and inferior until lines of tension are noted.
5. Any number of client-assisted long levers may be added.

Normal process

The usual methods of pretest, treatment method choice, recognition of end of treatment, and post testing are used.

Laughlin method
Origin

This method was first taught by A. T. Still's grandson, George Laughlin DO, who learned it from William Garner Sutherland DO, who learned it from osteopathic creator A. T. Still MD. Since Laughlin first taught this method more widely, it bears his name.

Concept

This is not a separate technique, but rather a complex long lever approach that may be employed as an extension of many different techniques. The Laughlin method is easier to use with treatment methods that apply more directiveness or constraint and least easy to use with pure unwinding.

Laughlin technique applies long lever treatment concurrently along a series of connected somatic dysfunctions discovered by extended listening processes.

In this method, the therapist first sets up a treatment at a particular area, then uses his contacts with that area to set up long lever treatment of a related area, which is then used to organize a treatment on a third area and so forth.

The somatic dysfunctional chain to be treated by this complex long lever process can be discovered in any of several ways:

- Find a primary somatic dysfunction, then engage the tissue in that area to discover an extended listening. Shift contact to the new area and find yet another extended listening. Repeat this process incrementally, discovering a somatic dysfunctional chain. Once the chain of dysfunctions is discovered, work from one or both ends of the chain to set up a complex treatment on all elements of the chain.

- As a variant of the above, note a symptomatic area from conversation with the client, then find a primary somatic dysfunction not at the location of the symptom. Work with a sequence of extended listening until a chain of connection is found between the symptomatic area and the primary somatic dysfunction.

- Find a primary somatic dysfunction. As you set up a treatment for this area, watch for an extended listening. When the extended listening is observed, work from the therapeutic setup on the primary to set up a treatment on the extended. Maintaining contact on the primary, continue this process incrementally along the somatic dysfunctional chain. It may or may not be useful to have the client gently position themselves in particular ways which you as the therapist direct, to help engage the segments of the chain.

The treatment method applied at each link in the somatic dysfunctional chain may be the same, and this is easier to keep track of; however, different treatment methods may be used at several somatic dysfunctions along the chain.

The usual pre and post assessment of mobility and alignment must be applied.

Since this is not a specific technique but rather an organizing perspective, the six factors describing functional methods is not directly describable; however, for any specific Laughlin setup using one or more specific techniques, the use of the six factors can be described.

Laughlin method

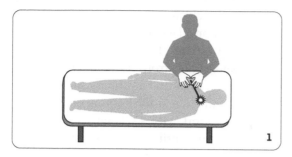

Begin with extended listening to notice any pull that may be present from the primary restriction you are treating to another area.

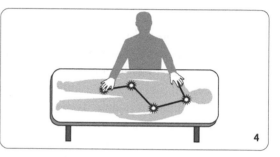

As you establish a long lever treatment on the second area, you may notice a third area. The three areas found so far will be connected by a segmented line.

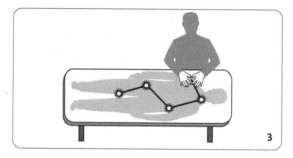

Any number of additional areas may be felt, connected by further line segments. Continue to set up long lever treatments on each.

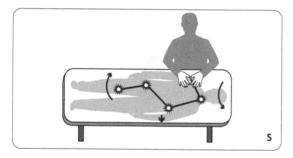

Alternatively, one hand may be moved to the other end of the segmented line, or to any other convenient point along the line.

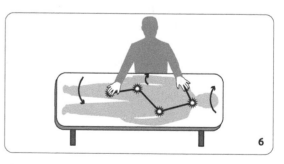

Another possibility is to treat from the primary area, setting up treatments on each area found along the line, and also ask the client to move slowly in specific ways to find positions that facilitate treatment.

These treatment elements may be combined, using both hands on two areas and client positioning. Consider also bolstering areas of the body to find positions that facilitate treatment.

The Laughlin treatment method is an expansion of the extended listening method to include several points and the lines between them in treatment. In some situations, this makes for a stronger or more thorough treatment. In other instances, a simple treatment produces the best result.

PART 4

Five In-Depth Treatment Protocols

One of the joys of this work is the splendid diversity of bodily structures to find and to treat. The companion pleasure is the fascinating kaleidoscopic journey of finding the succession of best places to work.

The number of possible structures, or parts of structures, to treat in the body is very large. The number of potential assessment pathways to arrive at any one of these is also large. There are many potential ways to treat any one lesion, either with shorter or longer leverage. Altogether, the number of possible permutations approaches uncountable.

What follows are five examples of how assessment and treatment might play out in a particular situation. These should be taken as suggestive of the broad range of possibilities. In the decades of your practice, you may never see exactly any one of these.

These five examples are written in a range of depth, providing simpler and more complex viewpoints, and emphasizing different aspects of the process.

Treatment example 1

Question or activity	Answer or result
Is it safe and beneficial to treat?	Yes
Can I find the primary restriction with general listening?	Yes
Can I find the primary restriction with general lift?	No
Can I find the primary restriction with general tap?	Yes
General listening	Twist on top of head, and head does not move on neck
General tap	Echo from just superior to the anterior margin of the left ear
Local tap frontal bone	Echo from left squamous suture
Local tap left mastoid process	Echo at left squamous suture
Manual thermal scan	Heat signature anterior half of left squamous suture
Local listening near area of heat signature	Shape consistent with anterior half of left squamous suture. The pull has a mild curve consistent with the depth of the suture.
Questions about tissue type	
Skin	No
Superficial fascia	No
Investing fascia	No
Vasculature	No
Nerve	No
Bone	No
Cranial suture	Yes

cont.

Questions about tissue type	
Portion of left squamous suture	Yes
Anterior half of left squamous suture	A weak yes (the weakness of the yes may be due to the approximate nature of the "half" designation)
Approximate anterior half of left squamous suture	Yes
Mobility tests	
distensibility of finger-width segments of the right squamous suture	Normal mobility full length
distensibility of finger-width segments of the left squamous suture	Posterior half normal, anterior half stiff
Treatment method choice	
Does the best treatment method for the anterior half of the left squamous suture utilize unwinding in any fashion?	No
Hoover technique	No
Reconstructed A. T. Still technique	No
Recoil technique	No
First barrier stretch technique	Yes
Apply first barrier stretch treatment to a succession of finger-width increments along the anterior half of the left squamous suture	
Post treatment mobility test	Mobility test of left squamous suture in finger widths is now normal and matches the mobility of the right squamous suture
Is the left squamous suture sufficiently treated?	Yes
This treatment segment is complete.	

Return to general assessment methods to begin to locate the next primary.

DISCUSSION

This example is the application of the protocol to a single primary dysfunction. In a full treatment, a succession of structures would be treated. Each of the succession of structures to be treated would be discovered first by general assessment methods, and then further specified with local assessment methods.

Treatment example 2

Client's primary complaint: left knee will not fully extend.

EXAMINATION

In both standing and in gait the left knee appears to not quite fully extend. The right knee appears to have normal extension in active movement. Passively, neither knee appears to hyperextend, and the left knee will not fully extend, with an eight-degree lack. Bilateral ankle and hip mobility appear normal, both actively and passively. Standing alignment is good with a mildly exaggerated thoracic kyphosis giving a mildly head forward posture, and mild bilateral scapular protraction.

Right knee examination

- No edema evident
- Palpated temperature is normal and matches the other knee
- Color normal and matches the other knee
- Normal flexion and extension range and ease of passive movement
- Medial and lateral collateral ligaments have normal span
- Patellar grind test normal
- Drawer test normal
- McMurray test normal

Left knee

- No edema evident

- Palpated temperature is normal and matches the other knee
- Skin color is normal and matches the other knee
- Normal passive full flexion with mildly increased effort at end range
- Extension stops about ten degrees short of full extension
- More than usual effort is required to achieve the last five to eight degrees of available extension
- Collateral ligaments have normal span
- Patellar grind test normal
- Drawer test normal
- McMurray test normal

A succession of primary restrictions are found and treated in the first treatment session. None of the primaries found are at or near the symptomatic knee. During this first treatment the thoracic kyphosis becomes somewhat less. The client notes easier breathing. Effortful breathing had not been a complaint and the client enjoys the improvement.

In the second treatment session, a succession of primary restrictions are found. Neck range of motion improves. The client had not complained of limited neck mobility, but the client is grateful for more ease and range of neck movement. One of the primary restrictions found is in the left patella. Releasing this patellar intraosseous strain somewhat improves ease of movement through the range in the knee, but does not increase the end range movement of the knee.

In the third treatment session, after the initial interview, the first three primary restrictions found are stiffness in the left subtalar joint complex, right sacroiliac joint capsule stiffness, and stiffness in the cartilage of the left costal arch. At that point, discussion with the client leads to a decision to target the area of complaint more specifically at this time.

Question or activity	Answer or result
Is it safe and beneficial to specifically target assessment and treatment of left knee extension at this time?	Yes
Will the use of the ultraslow mobility testing assessment method for the extension of the left knee provide useful information for improving the extension range of motion of the left knee?	Yes
Is there a means of investigating the extension of the left knee more effectively than ultraslow mobility testing at this time?	No
Will it be safe and beneficial to treat based on the findings of ultraslow mobility testing at the left knee?	Weak yes
Will it be safe to treat based on findings of ultraslow mobility testing at the left knee?	Yes
Will it be beneficial to treat based on findings of ultraslow mobility testing at the left knee?	Weak yes

The client is placed in a side-lying position with the left leg up. Both hips are in slightly flexed neutral position. Pillows are provided to provide comfort and stability. The left knee is passively fully extended and fully flexed without moving the hip. Both the end ranges of mobility and the ease of movement of the knee joint are noted.

Without displacing the hip, the left knee is fully flexed, then extension is initiated extremely slowly. The first hint of resistance is felt after about five degrees of movement and is located deep in the left mid-calf. Layer listening followed by mobility testing shows this to be related to fibrosity in the intermuscular septum between the gastrocnemius and soleus muscles. This is treated with a compressive reconstructed A. T. Still technique. Extension of the knee is again tested, and range of motion is found to be slightly improved.

In the same position, ultraslow mobility testing is again initiated for the left knee. The perceived first pull is now noted at or near the left patella. Investigation with local listening, manual thermal assessment, and layer listening shows this to be intraosseous strain in the patella. This is treated with Hoover's centralizing technique. Full extension is again tested. Range is not increased but ease of movement in the last five degrees of movement is markedly improved.

With the client in the same side-lying position ultraslow mobility testing is again applied. The first resistance is in a focal area in the posterior-medial knee just superior to the joint line. Local listening, manual thermal assessment, layer listening, and mobility testing show a focal capsular adhesion of the knee joint capsule to the periosteum of the distal femur in this area. This adhesion is released by a first barrier shear technique. Passive extension is again tested, and range of motion is found to be significantly but not quite fully improved.

The client is asked to stand, walk a few steps, then come to standing again. Both in movement and standing the knee now extends notably more than before but not quite fully.

Question	
Is it safe and beneficial to proceed with local assessment of the left knee guided by ultraslow mobility testing and treatment of the results of this testing?	No

The normal assessment protocol is resumed. Thirty-five minutes of the treatment session have been used. Fifteen minutes remain. A succession of four more primary restrictions is found, including:

- an adhesion of the second leg of the sigmoid colon to the parietal peritoneum in the left iliac fossa
- right olecranon bursa adhered
- right #2 metatarsophalangeal joint capsule fibrosed
- stiff skin overlying the left lateral malleolus.

Gait is observed at the end of the treatment session. Both legs appear more fluid. The left knee now has about one-third of the extension limitation that it did at the beginning of this treatment session.

DISCUSSION

It would have been possible to use ultraslow mobility testing and other methods earlier in the series of treatments to target the symptomatic area. However, in chronic situations, symptoms are, at best, weak guides as to where one should treat to resolve the symptoms. Often symptoms will resolve best by treating a series of primary restrictions, few if any of which may be at or near the symptomatic site. That said, there is the relationship with the client to consider. Seeming to attend more directly to the symptomatic area helps the client feel heard and attended to. In some but not all cases, working local to the symptom may also lead to some reduction of symptoms earlier in the series of treatments, though, in the end, treating locally may not be the most efficient path to full symptom reduction.

In this example, two and one third sessions were completed following the usual assessment protocol. This has untangled the big picture enough that the person's body responds to a question agreeing it is safe and beneficial to attempt some more local work. However, after three local moves, the body says to move back to the larger ecology. It is possible that in a future session additional local work will be useful.

Treatment example 3
Client: Baby, two months old, brought by both parents.

Chief complaints

- Head always sits tilted to the right
- Frequent distressed crying, difficult to comfort

Question or activity	Answer or result
Is it safe and beneficial to treat?	Yes
Can the primary restriction be found with horizontal general listening?	Weak yes
Can the primary restriction be found with general tap?	Weak yes
Is it safe to use general tap?	Weak yes
Is the reduced safety of general tap due to open fontanels?	Yes
Can local tap be safely and effectively used?	Yes
Can the primary restriction be found with lift (stretch) listening?	Weak yes
To make lift (stretch listening) more effective at finding the primary restriction, is it valuable to do it from hands and feet as well as from the head?	Weak yes
Is assessment of the PRM useful as a step to finding primary dysfunction?	Yes
At this time, is use of the PRM as an assessment more useful than any of the general assessment methods?	Yes
Monitor PRM from occiput and greater wings of sphenoid.	Flexion motion preference and positionally a right-side bending rotation (R-SBR).
Maintaining occiput and greater wings of sphenoid contact, gently slack the neck inferiorly.	R-SBR corrects, but not the flexion PRM preference, suggesting that the R-SBR is created and maintained by a pull up through the neck, but the flexion fixation is not.
Comparing cranial R-SBR and flexion, is one more primary than the other?	Yes
Is R-SBR more primary than flexion?	No
Is it beneficial to treat the cranial flexion restriction with induction?	Yes
Is there any treatment method for the cranial flexion restriction that is more beneficial than induction?	No
Treat cranial flexion with induction.	Result is the flexion preference is corrected and the R-SBR is more accentuated.
Is the cranial flexion restriction sufficiently treated?	Yes
Again, gently compact neck while monitoring the occiput and sphenoid.	R-SBR is diminished but not eliminated.
As slowly, allow neck to lengthen.	A pull is felt down the right side of neck anterolateral.
Is the pull establishing the cranial right side bend vascular?	No
Is this pull in a nerve?	Yes
Is this pull the right vagus nerve?	Yes
Is the right vagus nerve the most primary restriction now?	No
Can the current primary be found with lift (stretch) listening?	Weak yes
Can the current primary be found with a succession of local taps?	No
Can the current primary be found by lift (stretch listening from a limb)?	Yes
From an upper limb?	No
From right lower limb?	Yes
From left lower limb?	No

cont.

Question or activity	Answer or result
Test traction from right ankle.	Line of tension to the right lower abdominal quadrant.
Gently compact right lower limb superiorly from heel, then very slowly let it spring out.	A linear pull to the lower right abdomen quadrant, almost vertical near McBurney's point.
Is the primary dysfunction a contracture?	No
Is the primary dysfunction an adhesion?	Yes
Is the primary dysfunction an adhesion involving the colon?	Yes
Is the primary restriction between a portion of the ascending colon and loops of the small intestine?	Yes
Manual thermal scan	A radiated heat signature in a vertical line consistent with the above description of an adhesion between the ascending colon and loops of the small intestine.
Mobility test glide planes between the ascending colon and loops of the small intestine.	A focal area of adhesion just superior to the ileocecal valve.
Treatment method decision:	
Does the best treatment method utilize unwinding?	Yes
Does the best treatment method utilize tissue engagement by client?	Yes
Is the best treatment method for this adhesion pure unwinding?	No
Is the best treatment method for this adhesion augmented unwinding?	Yes
Post mobility test the glide plane between the colon and the small intestine.	Normal glide
Post mobility test traction of the right leg.	Normal and equal to the left leg
Reassess PRM at occiput and sphenoid	
Is the ascending colon–small intestine adhesion sufficiently treated?	Yes
Is it safe and beneficial to treat?	Yes
Gently compress neck.	Right SBR does not change with this maneuver.
Is the remaining R-SBR anchored in the head?	Yes (This confirms the result of the previous test.)
Is this head restriction anchoring a R-SBR now primary?	No
Local taps?	No
General listening?	Weak yes
General listening from head?	No
Listening from a lower limb?	No
Listening from the left upper limb?	No
Listening from the right upper limb?	Yes
Is it best to general listen from the metacarpal heads?	Yes
Fold baby's right hand into loose fist. Apply gentle pressure on metacarpal heads toward the shoulder.	Resistance to scapular elevation is felt deeply.
Can the primary restriction be described as a single tissue type?	Yes
Is the primary restriction in bone?	No
Is the primary restriction in an intermuscular septum?	No

Is the primary restriction in a nerve?	No
Is the primary restriction in vasculature?	No
Is the primary restriction in a bursa?	Yes
Is the primary restriction in the right subscapular bursa?	Yes
Mobility test the glide of both scapulae.	The glide of the right scapula has less excursion and requires more effort than the left.
Choice of treatment method:	
Does the best treatment method for the right subscapular bursae utilize unwinding?	No
Is the best treatment method Hoover's centralizing technique?	No
Reconstructed A. T. Still technique?	No
First barrier shear?	Yes
Treat the right subscapular bursae with first barrier shear. Mobility test the glide of the right scapula.	Scapular glide 70% improved
Is the right subscapular bursae sufficiently treated?	Yes
Is it safe and beneficial to treat?	No
Is it safe to treat?	Weak yes
Is it beneficial to treat?	No
Would an SSOT-4 maneuver improve receptivity to treatment?	No
How long before it will be safe and beneficial to treat?	
Seconds	No
Minutes	No
Hours	No
Days	Yes
3 days	No
4 days	No
5 days	Yes
Make a new appointment for 5 or more days in the future.	

DISCUSSION

Initially it was challenging to find a method to discover the primary. Question asking suggested that none of the general assessment methods would be adequately useful. Further question asking suggested that the use of monitoring the craniosacral rhythm and cranial bone position would show a primary restriction. This method showed two kinds of cranial aberrations: a flexion preference, and a right-side bending rotation (R-SBR). Question asking showed that the flexion preference was the more primary than the R-SBR. The flexion preference was treated with induction, achieving good correction of the flexion preference. At this point, it would have been tempting to treat the R-SBR; however, the fact that the flexion preference was primary to the R-SBR does not mean that the R-SBR is the next most primary dysfunction. In addition, treating anything shuffles the deck so that if the R-SBR had been the next most primary dysfunction, after treating the flexion preference, the R-SBR may no longer be next most primary. Question asking showed that the R-SBR is not now primary. Further question asking showed that general assessment methods which were previously weakly useful are now more useful. Use of a general assessment method showed an abdominal adhesion as the current primary.

When the scapular glide was treated, a 70 percent correction was achieved, and then question asking stated this was sufficient. It is often best practice to treat to less than full release. The body will continue to change for weeks after treatment, generally improving. It often works out best to allow this normal bodily process rather than taking the tissue to full correction during the treatment session.

The treatment was brief. It is often so with babies. The right amount of treatment is important. It is easy to overtreat.

At the next appointment, ten days later, the baby's mother reported that the right head tilt was about one-third corrected, the frequency of distressed crying was reduced by about half, and it was easier to calm the baby.

Treatment example 4

Question or activity	Answer or result
Is it safe and beneficial to treat?	No
Is it safe to treat?	Yes
Is it beneficial to treat?	No
If I were to perform a standing sacro-occipital type 4 maneuver (SOT-4), would it then be beneficial to treat?	Yes
Assess pelvis and sacrum position.	Moderate degree of right anterior ilium. The sacrum is right facing on a right diagonal axis (the positions of the ilia and sacrum are incongruent).
Perform standing variant of SOT-4 technique.	
Reassess pelvis and sacrum position.	Slight right anterior ilium but with sacrum now in a slight left on left position. (The position of the sacrum is now congruent with position of the ilium.)
Question: Is it safe and beneficial to treat?	Yes
Can I find the primary restriction with general listening?	Yes
Can I find the primary restriction with lift listening?	Yes
Can I find the primary restriction with general tap?	No
Perform general listening.	Lean left forward, seemingly at the left ankle.
Perform general lift.	Lean left forward toward the left lower limb.
With one hand on the top of the head, touch the point at left greater trochanter, thus asking if primary restriction is in left lower leg.	No lean. Therefore, the primary dysfunction is in the left lower limb.
Touch the witness point at left lateral malleolus with inhibitory intent. This asks if the primary dysfunction is in the left ankle and/or foot.	No lean. Therefore, the primary dysfunction is in the left foot and/or ankle.
Can the primary dysfunction be described as a single tissue type?	No
Does the primary dysfunction involve two tissue types?	Yes
Does the primary dysfunction involve only two tissue types?	Yes
Is the primary dysfunction in:	
Skin?	No
Superficial fascia?	No

Investing fascia?	No
Vasculature?	No
Nerve?	No
Bone?	No
Tendon?	No
Bursa?	No
Joint capsule?	Yes
Periosteum?	Yes
Is the primary dysfunction an adhesion of joint capsule to periosteum?	Yes
Is more than one foot joint to be treated now?	No
Lie client down supine, with the client's feet just off the end of the table.	
Manual thermal assessment	Three hot spots in left foot/ankle:
	Anterior talocrural joint
	First tarso-metatarsal joint
	Talonavicular joint
Local listening with inhibition shows this primacy order:	1. Talonavicular joint
	2. First TMT joint
	3. Anterior talocrural joint
Assess right foot joint mobility:	
Talonavicular joint	50% range of motion
First tarso-metatarsal joint	Normal
Talocrural joint	Normal
Assess left foot joint mobility:	
Talonavicular joint	Moderately effortful through full range
First tarso-metatarsal joint	Moderately effortful through full range
Talocrural joint	Moderately effortful through full range
Treatment method choice:	
Does the best treatment method utilize unwinding?	No
Is the best treatment method A. T. Still reconstructed?	Yes
Is the best treatment method compaction-initiated A. T. Still?	No
Is the best treatment method stretch-initiated A. T. Still?	Yes
Treat the right talonavicular joint with stretch-actuated reconstructed A. T. Still technique.	
Reassess mobility of right foot and ankle joints: talonavicular joint.	85% range of motion
First TMT joint	Normal
Talocrural joint	Normal
Reassess mobility of joints in left foot.	
Talocrural joint	Normal
Talonavicular joint	Normal
First TMT joint	Moderately stiff (unchanged)

cont.

Question or activity	Answer or result
Is the right talocrural joint sufficiently treated?	Yes
Stand client up for next assessment episode.	

Question or activity	Answer or result
Gently compact right lower limb superiorly from heel, then very slowly let it spring out.	A linear pull to the lower right abdomen quadrant, almost vertical near McBurney's point.
Is the primary dysfunction a contracture?	No

DISCUSSION

The general listening and general lift assessment methods give results that are consistent, though as typical, the general lift provides less specific information for a primary dysfunction more inferior in the person.

In mobility testing, the right talonavicular joint showed distinctly the least mobility of the joints tested; it might be tempting to treat it based on the mobility test. However, assessment had shown that the primary restriction is at the *left* talonavicular joint. When the left talonavicular joint was treated, the mobility of both talonavicular joints improved. This is typical. Everything in the body is connected by multiple pathways. Often the greatest improvement is obtained by working at primary restrictions geographically distant from the area of client complaint, or greatest tested dysfunction.

Treatment example 5

Question or activity	Answer or result
Is it safe and beneficial to treat?	Yes
Can I find the primary dysfunction with general listening?	Yes
Can I find the primary dysfunction with general tap?	Weak yes
Can I find the primary restriction with lift listening?	Yes
Is the most informative place to do lift listening from the occiput and mandible?	Yes
General listening	Right subcostal area
Inhibitory contact (fishing in the area)	Quite focal near tip of ninth rib
Lift listening	Right subcostal
General tap	Diffuse area in lower right thorax
Manual thermal sweep	2 cm diameter area right subcostal below tip of ninth rib
Is the primary restriction in a costal cartilage?	No
Is the primary restriction any part of the biliary system?	Yes
Is it beneficial to check the functionality of all sphincters?	Yes
Sphincters	
Superior esophageal	Normal
Gastro esophageal	Normal
Pylorus	Normal

Sphincter of Oddi	Semi-functional
Duodenojejunal junction	Offline
Ileocecal valve	Semi-functional
Valves of Houston	Normal
Inhibit between sphincters to assess relative primacy.	Primacy sequence
	1. Oddi
	2. Duodenojejunal
	3. Ileocecal valve
Inhibit from limbic system of the brain.	The limbic system is not primary to any of the sphincters.
Questions to the client:	
How has your digestion been lately?	Not bad, a little bloated
Have you had any pain under your right front ribs?	Occasional mild discomfort
Press gently under left costal arch ninth rib level, then similar on the right. Ask the client to compare sensation.	Client says slight discomfort to pressure on the right.
Gently palpate gallbladder.	Normally full contour
	Not hot
	No pain or discomfort to gentle palpation
Is it beneficial to perform the whole biliary system treatment protocol?	No
Mobility test hepatoduodenal ligament.	Stiff
Is it safe and beneficial to treat the hepatoduodenal ligament?	Yes
Does the best treatment method for the hepatoduodenal ligament utilize unwinding?	No
Is the best treatment method for the hepatoduodenal ligament:	
First barrier stretch?	No
Flossing?	Yes
Treat the hepatoduodenal ligament with flossing.	
Retest stretch of the hepatoduodenal ligament.	50% reduction in stiffness
Is the hepatoduodenal ligament sufficiently treated?	Yes
Is it beneficial to now treat any other element of biliary system?	Yes
Is it now beneficial to treat:	
the common bile duct?	No
the sling of peritoneum under the gall bladder (GB)?	Yes
In addition to sling of peritoneum under the GB are there more elements of the biliary system to treat now?	No
Does the best treatment method for the peritoneum under the GB utilize unwinding?	Yes
Does the best treatment method for the peritoneum under the GB utilize therapist-initiated tissue engagement?	No
Is the best treatment method for the peritoneum under the GB:	
pure unwinding?	No
augmented unwinding?	No
alternate interrupt?	Yes
Assess the elasticity of the sling of peritoneum under GB.	Moderately stiff

cont.

Question or activity	Answer or result
Treat the sling of peritoneum under GB using the alternate interrupt unwinding technique.	
Reassess span of peritoneal sling under gall bladder.	25% less stiff
Is the sling of peritoneum under GB sufficiently treated?	No
Is it best to use the alternate interrupt method again?	No
Does the best treatment method utilize unwinding?	No
Is it best to use accordion technique?	No
Is it best to use Hoover's centralizing technique?	Yes
Treat with Hoover's centralizing technique.	
Is the sling of peritoneum under the GB sufficiently treated?	Yes
Reassess the stretch of sling under peritoneum.	80% improved
Reassess all sphincters.	All sphincters normal except for the IC valve which remains semi-functional.
Is it beneficial to treat the ileocecal valve at this time?	No
Return to general assessment to find the next primary.	

DISCUSSION

In this example, the general assessment methods pointed to the biliary system. Then, the sphincter of Oddi, a component of the biliary system, tested as semi-functional. Two other sphincters also tested as less than fully functional, the duodenojejunal junction, and the ileocecal valve.

Comparing the three dysfunctional sphincters using inhibition showed the sphincter of Oddi as the most primary of the three sphincters, which appeared consistent with the general assessment methods having pointed to the biliary system. Based on this, it might have been tempting to treat the sphincter of Oddi; however, question asking showed that other elements of the biliary system were more primary than the sphincter of Oddi, specifically the hepatoduodenal ligament, and the sling of peritoneum underlying the gall bladder. Those two elements were successively treated, which resulted in full correction of the functionality of the sphincter of Oddi and the duodenojejunal junction.

The ileocecal valve remained unchanged, and it could have been tempting to treat that sphincter; however, question asking showed that the primary dysfunction now lay elsewhere, leading to a decision to again utilize general assessment methods to locate the current primary dysfunction.

PART 5

Appendices

APPENDIX 1: RECOMMENDED READING

Barral, J. P. (2005) *Manual Thermal Evaluation.* Seattle, WA: Eastland Press.

Barral, J. P. (2007) *Manual Therapy for the Peripheral Nerves.* Edinburgh; New York: Churchill Livingstone/Elsevier.

Barral, J. P. (2007) *Visceral Manipulation II.* Seattle, WA: Eastland Press.

Barral, J. P. (1991) *The Thorax.* Seattle, WA: Eastland Press.

Barral, J. P. and Mercier, P. (2005) *Visceral Manipulation.* Seattle, WA: Eastland Press.

Barral, J. P., Anderson, S. and Bensky, D. (1993) *Urogenital Manipulation.* Seattle, WA: Eastland Press.

Cailliet, R. (1982) *Hand Pain and Impairment.* 3rd ed. Philadelphia, PA: F.A. Davis.

Cailliet, R. (1983) *Foot and Ankle Pain.* 2nd ed. Philadelphia, PA: F.A. Davis.

Cailliet, R. (1988) *Soft Tissue Pain and Disability.* 2nd ed. Philadelphia, PA: F.A. Davis.

Cailliet, R. (1991) *Neck and Arm Pain.* 3rd ed. Philadelphia, PA: F.A. Davis.

Cailliet, R. (1992) *Head and Face Pain Syndromes.* 1st ed. Philadelphia, PA: F.A. Davis.

Cailliet, R. (1992) *Knee Pain and Disability.* 3rd ed. Philadelphia, PA: F.A. Davis.

Cailliet, R. (1993) *Pain: Mechanisms and Management.* Philadelphia, PA: F.A. Davis.

Cailliet, R. (1995) *Low Back Pain Syndrome.* 5th ed. Philadelphia, PA: F.A. Davis.

Cain, S. (2015) *Becoming Sherlock: The Power of Observation and Deduction.* Seattle, WA: CreateSpace Independent Publishing Platform.

Croibier, A. (2012) *From Manual Evaluation to General Diagnosis: Assessing Patient Information Before Hands-on Treatment.* Berkeley, CA: North Atlantic.

DeJarnette, M. B. (2007) *Compendium of Sacro Occipital Technique: Peer reviewed Literature 2000–2005.* Sacro Occipital Technique Organization-USA.

Gelb, M. J. (2000) *How to Think Like Leonardo da Vinci: Seven Steps to Genius Every Day.* New York, NY: Dell.

Goodheart, G. J. in Robert Frost Ph.D. (2012) *Applied Kinesiology, Revised Edition: A Training Manual and Reference Book of Basic Principles and Practice.* Berkeley, CA: North Atlantic.

Goodman, C. C. and Snyder, T. E. K. (2000) *Differential Diagnosis in Physical Therapy.* 3rd ed. Philadelphia, PA: Saunders.

Groopman, J. (2007) *How Doctors Think.* New York, NY: Houghton Mifflin Co.

Hoover, H. V. (1937) Osteopathic Concept of Allergy. *The Journal of the American Osteopathic Association 37*(126).

Hoover, H. V. (1945) Use of Respiratory Movement as Aid in Correcting of Osteopathic Spinal Lesions. *The Journal of the American Osteopathic Association 45*(109).

Hoover, H. V. (1953) Diagnosis and treatment of lesion patterns and complicated lesions. *The Journal of the American Osteopathic Association 52*(11), 553 -5.

Hoover, H. V. (1958) *Functional Technique, Yearbook*. Academy of Applied Osteopathy.

Hoover, H. V. (1969) *Selected Osteopathic Papers, Yearbook*. Academy of Applied Osteopathy.

Hoppenfeld, S. and Hutton, R. (1976) *Physical Examination of the Spine and Extremities*. New York, NY: Appleton-Century-Crofts.

Konin, J. G. (2006) *Special Tests for Orthopedic Examination*. 3rd ed. Thorofare, NY: SLACK.

Laughlin, G. M. (2011) *Notes on The Practice of Osteopathy: From the Lectures of Dr. George M. Laughlin, Dr. George a Still, and Dr. Frank L. Bigsby*. Charleston, SC: Nabu Press.

Lederman, E. (1997) *Fundamentals of Manual Therapy: Physiology, Neurology, and Psychology*. New York, NY: Churchill Livingstone.

Lesondak, D. (2022) *Fascia—What it is and Why it Matters.* 2nd ed. Edinburgh: Handspring Publishing Limited.

Levangie, P. K. and Norkin, C. C. (2005) *Joint Structure and Function: A Comprehensive Analysis*. 4th ed. Philadelphia, PA: F.A. Davis.

Lewis, J. (2012) *A. T. Still: From the Dry Bone to The Living Man*. Dry Bone Press.

Liem, T., Tozzi, P., and Chila, A. (Eds). (2017) *Fascia in the Osteopathic Field*. Edinburgh: Handspring Publishing Limited.

Lowe, W. W. (1997) *Functional Assessment in Massage Therapy: A Guide to Orthopedic Assessment of Pain and Injury Conditions for the Massage Practitioner*. 3rd ed. Bend, OR: Orthopedic Massage Education and Research Institute.

Magee, D. J. (2008) *Orthopedic Physical Assessment*. 5th ed. St. Louis, MO: Saunders Elsevier.

Schneiderman, H. and Peixoto, A. J. (1997) *Bedside Diagnosis: An Annotated Bibliography of Literature on Physical Examination and Interviewing*. 3rd ed. Philadelphia, PA: American College of Physicians.

Still, A. T. (2016) *The Philosophy and Mechanical Principles of Osteopathy*. London: Facsimile Publisher.

Still, A. T. (2018) *Autobiography of Andrew T. Still: With a History of the Discovery and Development of the Science of Osteopathy, Together with an Account of the School of Osteopathy, Osteopathic Medicine and Manipulation Techniques*. Lulu.com.

Still, A. T. (2018) *Philosophy of Osteopathy*. Lulu.com.

Still, A. T. (2022) *Osteopathy Research and Practice*. Legare Street Press.

Sutherland, A. (1962) *With Thinking Fingers*. The Cranial Academy.

Sutherland, W. G. (1800) *Contributions of Thought*. Sutherland Cranial Teaching Foundation.

Sutherland, W. G. (1948) *The Cranial Bowl*. Free Press Company.

Sutherland, W. G. (1990) *Teachings in the Science of Osteopathy*. Rudra Press

Sutherland, W. G. (2003). *Teachings in the Science of Osteopathy*, Sutherland Cranial Teaching Foundation.

Tz, E. H. and Cyriax, J. H. (1975) *Manipulation Past and Present: With an Extensive Bibliography*. London: Heinemann Medical.

Van Buskirk, R. L. (2006) *The Still Technique Manual*. 2nd ed. Indianapolis, IN: American Academy of Osteopathy.

Best Treatment Type
Decision Tree

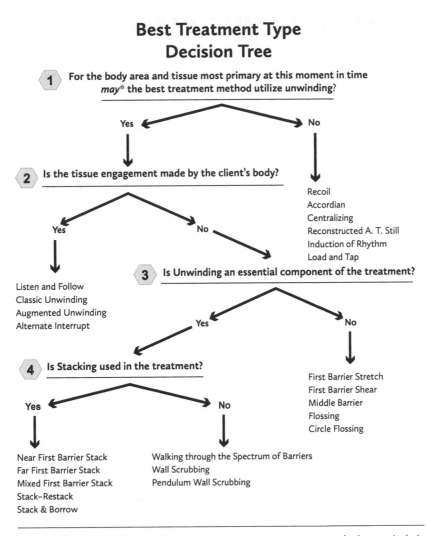

1 For the body area and tissue most primary at this moment in time
may* the best treatment method utilize unwinding?

Yes — No

2 Is the tissue engagement made by the client's body?

No →
Recoil
Accordian
Centralizing
Reconstructed A. T. Still
Induction of Rhythm
Load and Tap

Yes — No

3 Is Unwinding an essential component of the treatment?

Listen and Follow
Classic Unwinding
Augmented Unwinding
Alternate Interrupt

Yes — No

4 Is Stacking used in the treatment?

No →
First Barrier Stretch
First Barrier Shear
Middle Barrier
Flossing
Circle Flossing

Yes — No

Near First Barrier Stack
Far First Barrier Stack
Mixed First Barrier Stack
Stack–Restack
Stack & Borrow

Walking through the Spectrum of Barriers
Wall Scrubbing
Pendulum Wall Scrubbing

---

*The word *may* in the first question is important, as some treatment methods must include unwinding; in other methods unwinding *may* or *may not* occur during the treatment. In yet other treatment methods unwinding cannot occur or may be forbidden.

Best treatment type decision tree

APPENDIX 2: HOW THIS BOOK CAME TO BE: A BIOGRAPHICAL APPENDIX

I was always interested in the body, how it is put together and how it functions. One evening when I was five years old my mother, father, and I were sitting in the living room by the fireplace. As was their habit, each of my parents was reading a book. I was brushing my mother's hair. As I worked, gently combing out the tangles, I became fascinated with the minutiae of the structure of her head. At a certain moment I wished I had her skull out of her head so I could study it. I was immediately struck by the morbidness of my thought. Ashamed and frightened by the activity in my mind I quickly completed my task and moved on to something else. Hindsight being 20/20, I now recognize this as a budding anatomist.

My interest in anatomy continued. I spent regular time at my grandfather's farm and participated in butchering animals, where I came to be regarded as a nuisance, getting lost in the details of anatomy rather than getting on with the task at hand.

I dissected roadkill. I cleaned and dressed the wounds of my cat, and later neighbors' cats and dogs. My parents noticed my interest and by age nine I had anatomical models. In fifth grade, a pet turtle died in the classroom of my all-time favorite teacher Geraldine Dawson. Another student and I performed an autopsy, finding an inflamed gall bladder.

The summer before my first year of high school I took a year of high school biology compressed into a summer session. The next year I took chemistry, then in succeeding years advanced placement (AP) biology and AP physics.

Along the way, I had begun to hunt pheasants, quail, rabbits, and deer. This offered more butchering opportunities, where my reputation for dragging out the process as I got sidetracked into dissection continued.

I considered medicine as a career but found the thinking model not to my liking. I wandered in college through some universities and a larger number of majors before settling into a biology major with an emphasis on genetics. I took classes in many areas simply because I was interested in them. I graduated with a lot more credits than necessary for a bachelor's degree.

During my college years I visited friends at another campus. A friend suggested I attend the lecture that evening on Rolfing®. I had never heard of Rolfing before, but the Rolfing talk was the only thing happening that evening, so I went. The speaker was Don Hanlon Johnson, a recently certified Rolfer who would later found the California Institute of Integral Studies. His previous career as a Jesuit may have contributed to his good public speaking ability. He talked about the work of Ida P. Rolf PhD: structural integration, which claimed to alter the alignment of the human body so it could begin to make use of the field of gravity as an energy source rather than fighting it. I found this idea both intriguing and one of the odder things I had ever heard of. I tucked it away in the back of my mind.

A couple of years later I had a bicycle crash in which the front forks on my French racing bicycle collapsed, locking up the front wheel and pitching me over the handlebars onto the pavement. The immediately obvious injury was deep bruises and abrasions on my left knee. Three days later my back went into spasm. I went to the student health service where I was prescribed a muscle relaxant. The Flexeril relaxed the muscles in my back and relaxed my mind. Trying to take in a biochemistry lecture while on Flexeril was useless. Then my injured knee swelled up like a watermelon. I spent four days in a hospital on IV antibiotics, followed by a week on oral antibiotics. The infection in my knee was cured. My back still hurt a lot.

I remembered Johnson's talk on Rolfing and decided to give it a try. At the time there were about a hundred Rolfers in the world. The nearest one was 500 miles away. The term at school was over. I traveled to where a few Rolfers were, found one, and began receiving Rolfing. Three treatments later, my back pain was gone and in some ways my body worked better than ever.

I went back to school, picking up the next term. A year later I graduated with my degree in biology. I found myself back at my old summer job working for the US Forest service, which wasn't nearly as much fun as it had been in earlier years. I began thinking through what to do next in life. I considered several options, including graduate school. Remembering my good experience with Rolfing, I considered it as a career path. As a Rolfer I would be able to help people, I could work for myself, and there would be no end of opportunity to learn, all things that appealed to me. I applied to study at the Rolf Institute of Structural Integration.

At the time I graduated from the Rolf Institute in August 1977 there were 174 Rolfers in the world, mostly in the US. Through a mailing list for the Association for Humanistic Psychology I found groups of people in Europe that wanted Rolfing. I spent the next year with a very busy itinerant practice working in several European cities and one trip to Tehran in the last days of the Shah.

During this year I met European trained osteopaths. Returning to Boston in the middle of that year for a continuing education class, I met a US osteopath. Starting to read the works of the founder of osteopathy, Andrew Taylor Still, and other osteopaths, I recognized that everything in Dr. Rolf's philosophy of therapeutics was a part of osteopathy. I learned that Dr. Rolf had studied extensively with osteopaths on the way to developing her work, including prominent osteopaths Kenneth Little DO and Amy Cochrane DO.

In time, I began to study with European trained osteopaths, notably Jean-Pierre Barral DO and his associates, and Alain Gehin DE.[1]

I first heard the term "functional methods" from A. J. de Koenig DO (Netherlands) at a Barral visceral manipulation class in Toronto. De Koenig described functional methods as an umbrella term including the few treatment methods taught in the Barral curriculum and pointed out more of these methods. In describing functional methods, de Koenig spoke of Herbert Hoover DO of Tacoma, Washington and his landmark 1954 presentation to the American Osteopathic Association (AOA) and follow up publication in the yearbook of the AOA.

I got a copy of Hoover's article and read it. In the article, Hoover chided his colleagues for having lost sight of mobility as an equal partner to alignment. He proposed a very gentle treatment method which would improve mobility. Hoover used the term "functional" in this context to mean mobility. Hoover's treatment method improved mobility equally, complementing improved position of spinal segments.

As I continued to follow this thread, I was to learn that Hoover's landmark presentation and publication led to many brilliant workers in the decades since developing a wide spectrum of gentle technique all aimed at improving mobility. This development continues to this day. Collectively, these techniques are known as functional methods. The diversity of functional techniques is astonishing. All of them are effective. Many of these functional methods are presented in this book.

I began to wonder why, if all the functional methods are effective, did people continue to invent more and more of them? Why was Dr. Hoover's original method not enough? Was this just free-floating creativity which would not be quenched? No. While it turns out that each of the methods will be effective most of the time, there are some situations in which each of them will not be effective. And for each situation, there are some functional methods which are more efficient and

---

1   Etiopathy, a variant of osteopathy developed in France in the 1960s, is currently taught in schools at four locations in France.

effective than others. Great! Does that mean we can organize a chart directing the use of method A for situation type 1, method B for situation types 2 and 5, etc.? Alas, no. There are some exclusions where certain methods are not considered safe on specific inherently fragile tissues. There are other situations where performing a particular treatment method would be difficult or impossible to do. But overall, most methods may be used on most tissues. In time, I would learn methods to discern the best treatment method for the uniqueness of each situation. This book presents methods to determine which method or methods may be most fruitful for a given situation.

I learned that as the number of functional methods to improve mobility increased, the number of accompanying assessment methods kept pace. Before treating, it is essential to know what one is working on and why. Assessment is key. In my basic Rolfing training the number of assessment methods taught was small. In later years, more assessment methods have been added to the Rolfing curriculum.

Both at the Rolf Institute and later in a class with Jean-Pierre Barral DO we were told to ask constantly as we face our client, "Where can I work in this person's body that will make the most positive change for the whole person?"

Everything in our bodies is interconnected. The interconnections are of many kinds, through the connective tissue matrix, through the nervous system, hormonally, and more. We select a place to work on the body, but the effects are never just local. Immediate change is always visible at a distance. Then change continues to unfold for weeks. Any intervention we make will continue to ripple out through the body for weeks.

All our bodies change all the time. We are not today as we were yesterday, and certainly not as we were a year ago. In this dynamic situation, we cannot change something and say, "There, that is done, that is fixed, end of story." In this situation of constant change, what we as therapists can do is change the direction of development. We must choose our interventions with care for they shall echo long.

No one assessment method will tell us everything about a person; each method has its limitations. In addition, each assessment method can give true readings or errors. Therefore, we must use and compare the results of multiple assessment methods to learn where we should work in the body and what we should do there. This book presents more than a dozen assessment methods and how to use them in concert to arrive at this best estimate.

As I continued to study these assessment and treatment methods in their grand diversity, I looked both for the common ground, and for dimensions of variability. Discerning some of these dimensions led me to develop several new assessment and treatment methods.

This book is the story of how all the assessment and treatment methods can be brought together into a coherent whole guiding therapeutic effectiveness and efficiency.

APPENDIX 3: MECHANICAL FORCE TYPES

Mechanical forces are classified by engineers into six types. As therapists, knowing and understanding these force variations helps us organize treatments. In manual therapy these forces are used both in assessment and in treatment. Situations with mixed force types are common. Below are the six types of force described.

1. **Tensile force**
    Stretching something either in one direction from a fixed point or in two opposite directions.
    Mechanical examples
    a. a stretched rubber band
    b. a rope supporting a swing
    c. when a nut is tightened on a bolt there is a tensional force in the long axis of the bolt.
    Therapy examples
    a. stretching a muscle
    b. a gentle stretch load on a fascia initiating an unwind
    c. positioning and moving a limb by a client to gently stretch a nerve or blood vessel.

2. **Compressive force**
    Squeezing or compacting an object either against a fixed structure or from two opposite sides.
    Mechanical examples
    a. a post supporting a roof
    b. a carpet under a foot
    c. pressing a doorbell button.
    Therapy examples
    a. pressing into a muscle to test its springiness before and then after a treatment
    b. gentle superior pressure on a part of the soft tissue of a leg to encourage lymph flow
    c. loading tissue in the preparatory phase of a recoil treatment.

3. **Bending force**
    A force tending to change the angle between two parts of an object either locally or over a longer run.
    In some force classification systems bending is not considered a separate force since across the thickness of an object being bent one side will be under compression while the other side is under tension. While bending can be considered a mixed force it has enough unique characteristics to warrant a separate name and description.
    Mechanical examples
    a. gravitational load on a bridge span between two supports causing the bridge to sag, however slightly
    b. load on a diving board increasing as a diver walks to its end
    c. force on a piece of paper as you bring its two ends toward each other with your hands.
    Therapy examples
    a. passively side bending the neck for mobility testing
    b. one dimension of load on a tissue as part of creating a three-dimension force stack as part of any of several different treatment methods
    c. first immediate effect of an HVLA thrust on a bone before the bone moves.

4. **Torsional force**
    Twisting an object. This is related to

bending but creates a spiral deformation rather than a bend in one plane.

Mechanical examples

a. force applied to a tuning peg when tuning a guitar

b. force applied to a cleaning rag to wring it out

c. force on strands of fiber when they are twisted together to make yarn or rope.

Therapy examples

a. force applied to a joint when its long axis rotation is passively mobility tested

b. long axis rotary movement observed in the knee during flexion or extension when the knee's screw home mechanism is tested

c. load applied along the long axis of the petrous ridge of a temporal bone by applying gentle posterior–medial pressure on the mastoid process to create shear loads in the joints of the petrous ridge to the occiput and to the sphenoid.

5. **Shear force**

A lateral force focused along a particular plane.

Mechanical examples

a. Tightly screwing a lid onto a glass jar creates a shear force at the base of each spiral ridge of glass engaged by the lid. Note, this also creates torsion; see below.

b. Place a pencil extending over the edge of a desk, hold down the portion of the pencil on the desk with one hand, then use the other hand to exert a downward force on the portion of the pencil just off the edge of the desk. Note this is different from bending the pencil down from farther away from the edge of the desk.

c. Hold a toothpick between the thumb and forefinger of one hand. Then also grasp the same toothpick with the thumb and forefinger of the other hand, with the thumb and fingers of one hand touching the thumb and finger of the other hand. Now make straight opposite movements of the two hands, one away from you and the other toward you. Notice how this is different from bending the toothpick.

Therapy examples

a. Hold two adjacent muscle bellies such as the long and short heads of the biceps brachii, one in each of your two hands. Gently move the two muscle bellies in opposite directions to assess how well they glide on each other.

b. With a client supine on the table and seated at the client's head, use opposite finger pressure on cervical spinous processes to assess lateral glide between vertebrae.

c. With two hands, exert gentle counter pressure, a first barrier load, between two adjacent portions of intestine which are adhered to each other. Dynamically maintain this pressure as the glide plane is gradually restored.

6. **Torsional shear force**

Torsional shear is combined shear and torsion and is recognized in engineering as the most destructive mechanical force. When designing machinery, situations where torsional shear forces would be found in the device are carefully avoided unless the goal of the device is to take something apart along a particular line or plane.

Mechanical examples

a. A paper cutter. The torsion happens around the pivot of the cutting arm. Shear happens along an advancing series of points between the edge of the paper support table and the shearing arm.

b. Scissors cutting cloth. Similar to a paper cutter, the torsion occurs around the pivot of the scissors and the shear happens along an advancing series of points across the cloth between the two blades of the scissors. Pure shear by itself is ineffective for cutting most cloth. Torsion is of similarly low value for separating cloth. Shear and torsion together cut cloth easily.

c. As a bolt is tightened, there is torsion within all parts of the bolt and shear forces within the threads of the bolt which may separate the threads from the shaft of the bolt if the bolt is tightened too tight.

Therapy considerations

a. Torsional shear is included here for completeness of the list of mechanical force types. However, it is seldom used in manual therapy. Due to the highly destructive nature of torsional shear, it is usually avoided as a too-strong intervention. Simple shear or simple torsion are almost always sufficient.

APPENDIX 4: SPACE BETWEEN THE STARS

One day as I was working on a client, the client and I disappeared and there was only a beautiful star-filled summer night sky. I waited in the luminous emptiness. Being in this state felt delicious for me. After a few minutes, the scene shifted back to conventional reality. Fine changes had occurred for the client.

In the months and years after that, this same thing would very occasionally occur, always followed by good changes for the client.

I tinkered to try to find a way to induce this state, by manipulating the stars in various ways. After eight years of failure, I had an insight that it was not about the stars. It was more useful to work with the space between the stars. If I focused on the luminous emptiness, I could begin to induce this state.

Continuing to experiment with how to interact with the space between the stars, I found it useful to slowly zoom in, so the stars got farther apart until there was just the luminous emptiness. Pace was important. Too fast would not work. The image of a piece of down floating down through the air was the most useful pace for sinking in.

In the sky, stars are not uniformly distributed; some parts of the sky have many stars, some parts of the sky have fewer stars. I experimented with where to sink in. Most fruitful was to sink into where there were the most stars, and to sink into the space between those stars until there were no stars. The changes produced could be quite various, moving the person the next steps toward integration.

This could be done with contact anywhere on the body. Location seemed not to be important. Often, I did this with a classic cranial hold with thumb pads on the greater wings of sphenoid and finger pads 4 and 5 on the occiput, giving the appearance of doing cranial work.

When I would induce this space between the stars there would be a good effect in the person's body; however, it was never as good as when it happened spontaneously. I learned to ask the person's system if working with the space between the stars was the most beneficial thing I could do for the client at that moment. I seldom get a yes. Over time, I came to see that this state is usually best worked with when it arises spontaneously.

About the Author

Jeffrey Burch received a BA in biology from the University of Oregon in 1975, after which he trained at The Dr. Ida Rolf Institute® in Boulder, Colorado, receiving his Certification as a Rolfer in 1977.

He received his Rolfing Advanced Certification in 1990, after which he again began studying at the University of Oregon, where he received a second BA in Psychology in 1993 and a Master of Science in Counseling in 1995. His Master's thesis "Alexithymia and Dissociation" explores topics related to psychosomatic conditions.

Jeffrey has been a member of the Rolf Institute board of directors. He served for many years on the Rolf Institute ethics committee. He founded the International Association of Structural Integrators (IASI) Yearbook journal. He is a member of the Rolf Institute research committee.

In 1998, Jeffrey began intensively studying Craniosacral Therapy through the Upledger Institute, Cranial Manipulation with French Etiopath Alain Gehin, and Visceral Manipulation with Jean-Pierre Barral and his associates. Jeffrey completed the apprenticeship to teach

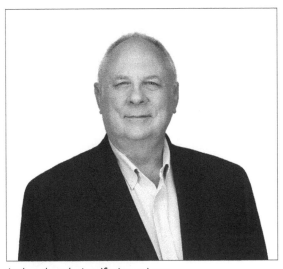

Author photo by Jennifer James-Long

visceral manipulation. Teaching internationally, he offers foundational and advanced courses in assessment methods and treatment methods.

Starting in 2010 he began to develop groundbreaking new methods to assess and release adhesions and contractures in joint capsules, bursas, and tendon sheaths. He now teaches these methods.